1992
YEAR BOOK OF
SURGERY®

The 1992 Year Book® Series

Year Book of Anesthesia and Pain Management: Drs. Miller, Abram, Kirby, Ostheimer, Roizen, and Stoelting

Year Book of Cardiology®: Drs. Schlant, Collins, Engle, Frye, Kaplan, and O'Rourke

Year Book of Critical Care Medicine®: Drs. Rogers and Parrillo

Year Book of Dentistry®: Drs. Meskin, Currier, Kennedy, Leinfelder, Matukas, and Rovin

Year Book of Dermatologic Surgery: Drs. Swanson, Salasche, and Glogau

Year Book of Dermatology®: Drs. Sober and Fitzpatrick

Year Book of Diagnostic Radiology®: Drs. Federle, Clark, Gross, Madewell, Maynard, Sackett, and Young

Year Book of Digestive Diseases®: Drs. Greenberger and Moody

Year Book of Drug Therapy®: Drs. Lasagna and Weintraub

Year Book of Emergency Medicine®: Drs. Wagner, Burdick, Davidson, Roberts, and Spivey

Year Book of Endocrinology®: Drs. Bagdade, Braverman, Horton, Kannan, Landsberg, Molitch, Morley, Odell, Rogol, Ryan, and Sherwin

Year Book of Family Practice®: Drs. Berg, Bowman, Davidson, Dietrich, and Scherger

Year Book of Geriatrics and Gerontology®: Drs. Beck, Abrass, Burton, Cummings, Makinodan, and Small

Year Book of Hand Surgery®: Drs. Amadio and Hentz

Year Book of Health Care Management: Drs. Heyssel, Brock, King, and Steinberg, Ms. Avakian, and Messrs. Berman, Kues, and Rosenberg

Year Book of Hematology®: Drs. Spivak, Bell, Ness, Quesenberry, and Wiernik

Year Book of Infectious Diseases®: Drs. Wolff, Barza, Keusch, Klempner, and Snydman

Year Book of Infertility: Drs. Mishell, Paulsen, and Lobo

Year Book of Medicine®: Drs. Rogers, Bone, Cline, Braunwald, Greenberger, Utiger, Epstein, and Malawista

Year Book of Neonatal and Perinatal Medicine: Drs. Klaus and Fanaroff

Year Book of Nephrology®: Drs. Coe, Favus, Henderson, Kashgarian, Luke, Myers, and Strom

Year Book of Neurology and Neurosurgery®: Drs. Currier and Crowell

Year Book of Neuroradiology: Drs. Osborn, Harnsberger, Halbach, and Grossman

Year Book of Nuclear Medicine®: Drs. Hoffer, Gore, Gottschalk, Sostman, Zaret, and Zubal

Year Book of Obstetrics and Gynecology®: Drs. Mishell, Kirschbaum, and Morrow

Year Book of Occupational and Environmental Medicine: Drs. Emmett, Brooks, Harris and Schenker

Year Book of Oncology: Drs. Young, Longo, Ozols, Simone, Steele, and Weichselbaum

Year Book of Ophthalmology®: Drs. Laibson, Adams, Augsburger, Benson, Cohen, Eagle, Flanagan, Nelson, Reinecke, Sergott, and Wilson

Year Book of Orthopedics®: Drs. Sledge, Poss, Cofield, Frymoyer, Griffin, Hansen, Johnson, Simmons, and Springfield

Year Book of Otolaryngology–Head and Neck Surgery®: Drs. Bailey and Paparella

Year Book of Pathology and Clinical Pathology®: Drs. Gardner, Bennett, Cousar, Garvin, and Worsham

Year Book of Pediatrics®: Dr. Stockman

Year Book of Plastic, Reconstructive, and Aesthetic Surgery: Drs. Miller, Cohen, McKinney, Robson, Ruberg, and Whitaker

Year Book of Podiatric Medicine and Surgery®: Dr. Kominsky

Year Book of Psychiatry and Applied Mental Health®: Drs. Talbott, Frances, Freedman, Meltzer, Perry, Schowalter, and Yudofsky

Year Book of Pulmonary Disease®: Drs. Bone and Petty

Year Book of Speech, Language, and Hearing: Drs. Bernthal, Hall, and Tomblin

Year Book of Sports Medicine®: Drs. Shephard, Eichner, Sutton, and Torg, Col. Anderson, and Mr. George

Year Book of Surgery®: Drs. Schwartz, Jonasson, Robson, Shires, Spencer, and Thompson

Year Book of Transplantation: Drs. Ascher, Hansen, and Strom

Year Book of Ultrasound: Drs. Merritt, Mittelstaedt, Carroll, and Nyberg

Year Book of Urology®: Drs. Gillenwater and Howards

Year Book of Vascular Surgery®: Dr. Bergan

Roundsmanship '92–'93: A Student's Survival Guide to Clinical Medicine Using Current Literature: Drs. Dan, Feigin, Quilligan, Schrock, Stein, and Talbott

1992

The Year Book of SURGERY®

Editor

Seymour I. Schwartz, M.D.
Professor and Chair, Department of Surgery, University of Rochester, School of Medicine and Dentistry, Rochester, New York

Associate Editors

Olga Jonasson, M.D.
Robert M. Zollinger Professor and Chair, Department of Surgery, The Ohio State University, Columbus

Martin C. Robson, M.D.
Chief of Division of Plastic Surgery, University of Texas Medical Branch, Galveston

G. Tom Shires, M.D.
Professor and Chairman, Department of Surgery, Texas Tech University, Lubbock, Texas

Frank C. Spencer, M.D.
George David Stewart Professor of Surgery; Chairman, Department of Surgery, New York University; Director, Department of Surgery, New York University Medical Center and Bellevue Hospital

James C. Thompson, M.D.
John Woods Harris Professor and Chairman, Department of Surgery; Chief of Surgery, University Hospitals, The University of Texas Medical Branch, Galveston

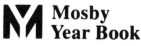 **Mosby Year Book**

St. Louis   Baltimore   Boston   Chicago   London   Philadelphia   Sydney   Toronto

Editor-in-Chief, Year Book Publishing: Kenneth H. Killion
Sponsoring Editor: Nancy Puckett
Manager, Literature Services: Edith M. Podrazik
Senior Information Specialist: Terri Santo
Senior Medical Writer: David A. Cramer, M.D.
Assistant Director, Manuscript Services: Frances M. Perveiler
Associate Managing Editor, Year Book Editing Services: Elizabeth Fitch
Senior Production/Desktop Publishing Manager: Max F. Perez
Proofroom Manager: Barbara M. Kelly

Editorial Office:
Mosby-Year Book, Inc.
200 North LaSalle St.
Chicago, IL 60601

International Standard Serial Number: 0090-3671
International Standard Book Number: 0-8151-7791-7

Table of Contents

Journals Represented

Mosby–Year Book subscribes to and surveys nearly 900 U.S. and foreign medical and allied health journals. From these journals, the Editors select the articles to be abstracted. Journals represented in this YEAR BOOK are listed below.

Acta Chirurgica Scandinavica
American Journal of Epidemiology
American Journal of Infection Control
American Journal of Medicine
American Journal of Pathology
American Journal of Surgery
American Journal of the Medical Sciences
American Surgeon
Anesthesia and Analgesia
Angiology
Annals of Internal Medicine
Annals of Plastic Surgery
Annals of Surgery
Annals of Thoracic Surgery
Annals of Vascular Surgery
Archives of Otolaryngology—Head and Neck Surgery
Archives of Surgery
British Journal of Cancer
British Journal of Plastic Surgery
British Journal of Surgery
British Medical Journal
Burns
Cancer
Cancer Research
Circulation
Circulatory Shock
Clinical Radiology
Complications in Surgery
Critical Care Medicine
Digestive Diseases and Sciences
Diseases of the Colon and Rectum
European Journal of Cancer
European Journal of Clinical Investigation
European Journal of Vascular Surgery
Gastroenterology
Head and Neck
Hepatology
Immunology
Intensive Care Medicine
International Journal of Cancer
International Journal of Pediatric Otorhinolaryngology
Journal of Applied Physiology
Journal of Burn Care and Rehabilitation
Journal of Cardiac Surgery
Journal of Cardiovascular Surgery
Journal of Clinical Endocrinology and Metabolism
Journal of Clinical Immunology
Journal of Clinical Investigation
Journal of Emergency Medicine
Journal of Family Practice

Journal of Immunology
Journal of Laboratory and Clinical Medicine
Journal of Parenteral and Enteral Nutrition
Journal of Pediatric Surgery
Journal of Surgical Research
Journal of Thoracic and Cardiovascular Surgery
Journal of Trauma
Journal of Vascular Surgery
Journal of the American Academy of Dermatology
Journal of the American College of Cardiology
Journal of the American Medical Association
Journal of the National Cancer Institute
Journal of the Royal College of Surgeons of Edinburgh
Lancet
Medicine
Nature
New England Journal of Medicine
Orbit
Otolaryngology–Head and Neck Surgery
Plastic and Reconstructive Surgery
Proceedings of the National Academy of Sciences
Quarterly Journal of Medicine
S.A.M.J./S.A.M.T.–South African Medical Journal
Scandinavian Journal of Gastroenterology
Science
Southern Medical Journal
Surgery
Surgery, Gynecology and Obstetrics
Transplantation
World Journal of Surgery

STANDARD ABBREVIATIONS

The following terms are abbreviated in this edition: acquired immunodeficiency syndrome (AIDS), the central nervous system (CNS), cerebrospinal fluid (CSF), computed tomography (CT), electrocardiography (ECG), human immunodeficiency virus (HIV), and magnetic resonance (MR) imaging (MRI).

Publisher's Preface

This volume is the 22nd and final volume of YEAR BOOK OF SURGERY led by Seymour I. Schwartz, M.D., as editor-in-chief. When Dr. Schwartz assumed that role with the 1971 volume, he joined a line of succession that started in 1901 with John B. Murphy and continued with Albert J. Ochsner, Evarts A. Graham, and Michael E. De Bakey.

To represent the diversity and complexity of surgery, Dr. Schwartz recruited an extraordinary team of associate editors—John S. Najarian, Erle E. Peacock, Jr., G. Tom Shires, William Silen, and Frank C. Spencer. Drs. Shires and Spencer have worked with Dr. Schwartz on all 22 of these volumes; Dr. Silen was succeeded by James C. Thompson in 1985, Dr. Najarian by Olga Jonasson in 1986, and Dr. Peacock by Martin C. Robson in 1991.

A glance back at the 1971 volume reveals the consistency of purpose of Dr. Schwartz's tenure. In his Preface to that volume, Dr. Schwartz wrote, "In this age of 'information explosion,' it becomes increasingly pertinent to attempt to focus on the novel, the analytic, and the provocative contributions to surgical literature." This could well describe the contents of the 1992 volume also.

In addition, the Publisher's Note to that volume concluded, "We are certain that the reader will find [the editors'] choice of material interesting and their comments incisive." These are words we can stand by today, 21 years later. We are deeply grateful to Dr. Schwartz and his colleagues for the strength of their commitment and the consistency of their performance.

It has been a great privilege to work with Dr. Schwartz and the talented surgeons on his editorial team. In addition, we are grateful to Ms. Wendy Husser, Dr. Schwartz's long-time associate in Rochester, who coordinated many of the editorial details for most of these 22 volumes.

The sixth editor-in-chief of the YEAR BOOK OF SURGERY, Edward M. Copeland, III, of the University of Florida, has already begun work on the 1993 volume, along with a diverse team of talented associates. We believe our readers will be stimulated by their new perspective.

As publishers, we feel challenged to seek ways of presenting complex information in a clear and readable manner. To this end, the 1992 YEAR BOOK OF SURGERY now provides structured abstracts in which the various components of a study can easily be identified through headings. These headings are not the same in all abstracts but, rather, are those that most accurately designate the content of each particular journal article. We are confident that our readers will find the information contained in our abstracts to be more accessible than ever before. We welcome your comments.

Annual Overview

General Considerations

There is a growing spectrum of surgical diseases in patients infected with HIV. An operation should not be denied patients who have these troublesome symptoms if they can be alleviated by operation.

Seymour I. Schwartz, M.D.

Shock

During the past year there has been a remarkable increase in the amount of research effort being devoted to the pathophysiology and management of both hemorrhagic and septic shock. The greatest increase in effort during the past year has clearly been focused primarily on the increasingly expanded role of mediators as a major source of mortality and morbidity in both hemorrhagic and septic shock. Initial resuscitation from shock is still a major concern, and there are continuing efforts to improve resuscitation even more. A significant number of papers have been written during the past year investigating the resurgent interest in hypertonic fluids, both saline and saline with dextran. Experimental studies continue to show a significant number of serious problems with the use of hypertonic saline. One study from the home of the resurgent interest in hypertonic saline demonstrates that with rapid administration of even small volumes of hypertonic saline, significant hypotension can and will occur. This is accompanied by a remarkable decrease in systemic vascular resistance. This kind of study adds weight to evidence indicating that even a small bolus of hypertonic saline alone produces remarkable vasodilatation systemically and a decrease in systemic vascular resistance. Another recent study has shown that hypertonic saline alone may contribute to significant clotting abnormalities. Although the studies show that hypertonic saline would be necessary in larger volumes than are currently being used, it is also apparent that on even a transient basis, small amounts of hypertonic saline might contribute to clotting abnormalities. Specifically, the activated partial thromboplastin time and prothrombin time were significantly prolonged with hypertonic saline alone. In addition, platelet aggregation was impaired. These even transient alterations in clotting ability might well be compounded by other alterations in injured patients such as hypothermia, acidosis, hypoperfusion, tissue trauma, or consumptive coagulopathy. All of these effects of trauma, coupled with an infusion of dextran solution that is known to reduce clotting ability, may well be compounded by hypertonic saline. Additional experimental studies have shown clearly that there is significant hypernatremia and hyperosmolarity associated with reduced survival after administration of hypertonic saline. In addition, other studies have shown that the effects of hypertonic saline in uncontrolled hemorrhagic shock in animals are more pronounced when large vessel or uncontrolled hemorrhage is produced. This was quantitated in the past year and, clearly, the larger the vessel size that is injured, the more likely the hypertonic saline is to exacerbate the hemorrhage as well as increase the mortality rate. Further, a multi-institutional trial was conducted to test the efficacy and safety of prehospital fluid resuscitation with a small volume of 7.5% sodium chloride and 6% dextran 70. Although there was no difference in the use of hypertonic saline dextran compared with balanced saline solution, the volume of balanced saline solution was far less than is generally used in patient fluid resuscitation and, in fact, was no greater than the hypertonic saline dextran solution. Further, these patients were all resuscitated in an urban center with rapid transit time, and previous authors have shown that the difference in overall survival in this setting is probably not influenced by fluid therapy in any event. Consequently, it would appear that no real conclusions should be drawn from such a clinical trial.

Other resuscitative fluids have been investigated, and there is continuing evidence that the oxygen-delivering capacity of stroma-free hemoglobin manipulated in a number of ways will deliver oxygen adequately. All of the experimental studies appear to support the use of this substance, but these studies have been done in lower animals, and the queston of endotoxin-free solution remains.

Good summary articles have been written this year describing once again the remarkable influence of tumor necrosis factor (TNF) in response to injury. It is still clear that TNF is a proximal mediator turned on by either hemorrhagic shock or sepsis, and that this proximal mediator then activates a number of downstream cytokines that produce the effects seen in what had previously been thought attributable to bacterial endotoxin. It also became more apparent during the past year that the downstream activity of these cytokines basically results in cell damage by the release of oxygen free radicals and hydroxyl radicals at the cell membrane level. It is clear that antibody to TNF given before injury prevents virtually all of these downstream effects. However, because patients are not seen early enough for this antibody to be effective, many studies have concentrated on the antioxidant agents that would either counteract or prevent the release of oxygen free radicals. These include several vitamins, as well as ibuprofen. These antioxidants may also have their effect by stabilizing neutrophils in addition to preventing oxygen free radical damage by acting as an oxygen radical scavenger. Ibuprofen, α-tocopherol, ascorbic acid, and a few other agents are being tried as oxygen free radical scavengers, but surely more and better scavengers will appear soon.

Trauma

Better management of specific injuries continues to evolve. Furthermore, there are now more accurate measurements to monitor the effects of improved trauma care. One such study appearing recently compared the effects of management between patients with severe injuries treated in trauma centers with those treated in nontrauma centers. This interesting study, which contrasted strictly comparable injuries in the two settings, found that there was, in fact, a remarkable difference in the mortality and morbidity rates—patients treated in the trauma center had much lower rates of mortality and morbidity than similar injured patients treated in a nontrauma center. This kind of outcome data should be useful in improving trauma center efforts around the nation. Other papers continue to describe even better scoring systems for patients with multiple injuries, a new one this year being the Functional Independence Measure. This system covers five general categories: self-care, sphincter control, mobility, locomotion, and communication skills. Long-term follow-up (over a year) of these patients indicated that this is a good predictive scoring system.

The relationship between cytokines and tissue injury has been examined more carefully. It appears that cytokine release in the plasma after graded surgical trauma indicates that TNF and interleukin (IL)-6 levels appeared promptly after significant tissue trauma, whereas IL-2 and IL-1 levels showed no increase in activity after trauma. This kind of study tends to substantiate that most of the mediator activity for TNF is generated locally and is a paracrine effect, and that a continuing endocrine effect occurs with the spill of TNF into plasma. Clinical trials of antioxidant vitamin therapy have also been tried in patients with blunt injuries to see once again what the antioxidant effect might be; this was specifically measured based on the mobility of polymorphonuclear leukocytes in patients who sustained serious blunt trauma. There was evidence of effectiveness in this category as well.

During the past year, the clearly documented and reproducible bacterial translocation to mesenteric lymph nodes in response to injury and infection in the laboratory was examined in two studies in patients who had sustained trauma. Bacterial translocation was not found to occur in patients undergoing trauma by the techniques used. However, serious questions are raised by these studies, because the patients had all received antibiotics before the operative procedure; also, most of them did not have systemic infection, so that one would not have expected prolonged bacterial translocation. This entire fascinating subject, i.e., translocating bacteria to initiate the cytokine response and produce multiple organ failure, still is undergoing intense scrutiny and will for quite a while.

New additions to previously existing technologies appeared this past year, including the apparent utility of measuring amylase and alkaline phosphatase in peritoneal lavage fluid. It appears that in a significant number of patients with an injured hollow viscus and without bleeding, these enzymes are elevated in the lavage fluid. One other technical advance would be continuous arterial venous hemofiltration with dialysis as an alternative to hemodialysis in the mass casualty situation. This is an easy system to use technically, but it requires an arterial and a venous catheter.

New studies during the year also indicated that a single agent given as the presumptive antibiotic in patients with penetrating abdominal trauma is as effective as multiple antibiotics alone. This past year even β lactam as a single agent appears to be equally advantageous when compared with multiple antibiotics.

The use of some form of mesh, whether vicryl or polypropylene, continues to enjoy increased popularity for the management of crush injuries to such organs as the liver and spleen and apparently achieves significant success. More aggressive vascular control for renal trauma when major vessels are injured and large hematomas are present continues to receive renewed interest and support. Retroperitoneal hematomas are being better managed, and the mortality rate is being reduced by more aggressive management, particularly of central retroperitoneal hematomas as well as lateral ones. The experience with lower abdominal retroperitoneal hematomas is still better with nonoperative intervention. The value of peripheral arteriography in extremity vessel injuries has been reaffirmed repeatedly during the past year. Computed tomography continues to receive support in several clinical articles in evaluation of penetrating injuries to the back and flank. With the combination of clinical and CT evaluation, potentially serious penetrating back and flank injuries can be assessed with a high degree of accuracy.

Fluid Electrolytes and Nutrition

Additional clinical studies during the past year evaluating crystalloids vs. colloids as fluid resuscitation in randomized controlled trials have indicated no advantage of colloids over crystalloid. Because the cost of colloids is extremely high, even if one is a colloid champion, certainly the cost alone would favor crystalloid therapy, which is demonstrated nicely in clinical trials. The addition of sodium bicarbonate to treat lactic acidosis is belittled in a number of clinical studies, indicating that volume repletion to remove the low-flow state cause of lactic acidosis is far preferable. An interesting new technique for more rapid restoration from hypothermia is the use of the new rapid fluid warmer without cardiopulmonary bypass. There is little doubt that normothermia can be reached much more quickly with arterial venous rapid warming of the patient's own blood.

An interesting study during this past year confirmed the capillary leak that occurs with sepsis as compared to hemorrhagic shock. This was true during the initial resuscitation and certainly after adequate resuscitative fluid therapy.

A huge cooperative study conducted this past year attempted to assess the benefits of 2 weeks of total parenteral nutrition preoperatively in surgical patients. This study showed convincingly that only very severely malnourished patients had fewer noninfectious complications than controls when total parenteral nutrition was applied perioperatively. Several papers also appeared this year attempting to document clinically that the use of early enteric feeding is far preferable to total parenteral nutrition.

This seems to be true from several standpoints, but particularly in reducing activation of mediators following injury.

Wound Healing

As has been the case in recent years, knowledge in the wound healing field is exploding. The ability to clone large quantities of recombinant growth factors has made research regarding their use in wound healing quite feasible. Animal models are being described to look at specific processes of the wound healing scheme. This past year, specific papers appeared demonstrating the comparative utility of various growth factors for extracellular matrix deposition, contraction, and epithelialization. By choosing models specific to each wound healing process, the function of growth factors can be specifically determined. This allows a more specific choice for wound pharmacology in the clinical situation.

One of the first human trials for a recombinant peptide growth factor in chronic ulcerated wounds was reported. In a crossover study of ulcerated wounds of various etiologies, epidermal growth factor was suggested to be efficacious in healing these indolent wounds.

As wound pharmacology becomes more prevalent, other host factors that may affect wound healing must be clarified. One group attempted to show the effect of smoking on subcutaneous oxygen levels and found that smoking a single cigarette may significantly lower subcutaneous oxygen levels. It was suggested that α-adrenergic blocking agents might overcome the effects of smoking and promote healing in patients who refused to cease smoking. The suggestion that oxygen is beneficial to wound healing has been intensified with reports of the use of therapeutic hyperbaric oxygen. However, it appears from animal studies that hyperbaric oxygen is necessary only to establish an angiogenic gradient in hypoxic, poorly perfused wounds, e.g., radiated wounds. Breathing 100% oxygen at 1 ATA should provide the necessary gradient to stimulate angiogenesis in most wounds.

As methods are found to modulate normal wound healing, objective measures for determining the results of that modulation are necessary. Determining wound collagen content is one such measure. However, this has been a fairly complex biochemical technique in the past. A new, simplified radioimmunoassay technique was described to measure on-line levels of type I collagen. Type III collagen can be measured by such a simple technique, and the new methodology for measuring type I collagen should be quite useful.

As more and more knowledge is made available regarding wound healing, it is clear that many of the processes are the same as those in tumor stroma generation. Cell adhesion, migration, and proliferation are important events in both processes. As one manipulates the processes of wound healing, it will be necessary to determine the possible effect on neoplastic tumors.

Infection

The infection of most concern for surgeons during the past year has been that caused by the HIV. Two papers were chosen from the many excellent papers on this subject. The first shows that because a positive HIV state can occur in patients with no known risk factors, universal precautions are recommended in all surgical cases. The second paper demonstrates that these precautions are not universally followed. More alarmingly, even after educational programs regarding universal precautions were instituted, compliance by surgical team members was unsatisfactory.

Just as universal precautions are necessary, infection surveillance programs are also becoming necessary. To institute continuing quality improvement, nosocomial infection rates and wound infection rates must be monitored prospectively. It was shown that surgeons' opinions regarding their wound infection rates are not necessarily accurate. Because data are kept in a prospective manner, patient categories must be continuously subselected to allow for homogeneous subgroups. Patient risk factors were shown to be an important adjunct to the usual categories ranging from clean to dirty.

As data are prospectively maintained for outcomes, more sophisticated input to decision making on infections are being provided. For instance, in the management of intra-abdominal abscesses, the Apache II score was shown to be useful, as were delayed-type hypersensitivity tests. Using this more detailed sophistication appears to be helpful both in determining the type of intervention as well as being predictive of outcome.

The more frequent use of newer technologies has also been demonstrated to be effective in improving diagnoses in complex wounds. Magnetic resonance imaging spectroscopy was shown to improve the diagnosis of hidden abscesses in diabetic foot infections, and ^{111}In-labeled oxyquinolone leukocyte scans were shown to increase the accuracy of diagnosing osteomyelitis in the same lesion.

With these improvements in diagnostic technique, improvements were also shown with antibiotic treatment. In areas of massive contamination, it was demonstrated experimentally that a combination of systemic and topical antimicrobials was more efficacious than either alone. However, in levels of moderate contamination, systemic and topical antimicrobials were found to be equally efficacious and not synergistic when used together.

Burns

Advances were made in all aspects of burn care during the past year. Resuscitation techniques continue to be refined. It appears that, as more and more is learned about the various inflammatory mediators released as a result of thermal trauma, neutralizing the mediators or preventing their formation should result in therapeutic advances. The use of antioxidants has been investigated recently, and in this past year the beneficial effect of an iron chelator, deferoxamine, was demonstrated in animals. These experiments not only increase the knowledge of the pathophysiology of fluid shifts following burning, they may well prove to be useful clinically for more physiologic resuscitation in the near future. Although protein-free resuscitation fluids have been in vogue for the past few years, new data have become available suggesting that colloid oncotic pressure gradients can be better maintained by the use of protein in the early resuscitative period.

Macrophage activation, which is becoming so important in wound healing, may be detrimental in inhalation injury. It was demonstrated that activated wound macrophages are present in inhalation injury, and that these may lead to the increased fibrosis seen in conditions such as adult respiratory distress syndrome.

Nutritional support is rapidly becoming recognized as one of the keys to survival after major burns. The timing of nutrition as well as its component parts are being evaluated. This past year showed the clinical superiority of a new nutritional formula that has been carefully worked out for a series of animal experiments. If multiple burn center teams can achieve the same results as reported by the authors, this will be a major advance in early treatment of the seriously burned patient.

Other aspects of burn care were carefully addressed this year. Pain management was shown to be improved by the use of patient-controlled analgesia. Although this technique has been used in many other fields, it has not been popular for burn patients. In this past year a paper appeared suggesting that it is useful not only in adults but also in children.

Burn rehabilitation was addressed in an excellent review of the follow-up care provided to children in Russia by a combined United States/ Russian burn team. These children were followed carefully during their rehabilitative phase, and techniques not commonly applied in our country appear to yield striking results. The use of hyaluronidase electrophoresis alternated with hydrocortisone without compression dressings appears to result in less scarring than is commonly the case in burn units in the United States. Certainly, prospective trials of this new therapy seem justified. Long-term problems after burn injuries have included the ability of burn-injured women to maintain a normal pregnancy and delivery. A longitudinal study from the Shriners Burns Institute showed that very few problems connected with pregnancy occurred after women sustained circumferential trunk burns. Rather, normal pregnancies with uncomplicated vaginal deliveries appear to be the rule.

Transplantation Immunology

A number of studies during this past year have focused on immunosuppression—the mechanisms of drug actions, effectiveness of new drugs, and the powerful immunosuppression potential of the prostaglandins. More exciting, however, have been the advances in understanding of T cell activation and inactivation, specifically, studies related to immunologic tolerance. Recommended to the readers are a number of excellent overviews of this topic, such as those of von Boehmer and Kisielow in the *Scientific American* (October 1991), Streilein (*Transplantation* 52:1–10 1991); and Kroemer and Martinez-A (*Lancet* 338:1246–1249, 1991). As Kroemer and Martinez-A point out, several complementary mechanisms for self-tolerance exist side by side: clonal deletion, inactivation, and suppression. The mechanism of clonal deletion may well be at play in the elegant experiments of Posselt, Naji, Roark, Markmann, and Barker. These investigators inoculated pancreatic islet cells into the thymus, and then were able to successfully transplant genetically identical islets into the portal vein of diabetic rats with cure of diabetes, even when the diabetes was the result of an autoimmune islet destruction. Remuzzi, Rossini, Imberti, and Perico went a step further by inoculating glomeruli into the thymus and following with a vascularized kidney transplant—also successful without further immunosuppression. Introduction of tissue-specific antigens into the thymus may have resulted in deletion of clones of potentially destructive cytotoxic T lymphocytes and avoidance of rejection. The importance of tissue-specific antigens was emphasized by Miller's group from the University of Miami, who demonstrated substantial differences between liver and kidney in this regard.

The continuing saga of the immunosuppressive effects of blood transfusion may be narrowing to mechanisms of immunologic blockade and suppressor cells, as suggested in the several papers discussed in this section on the effect of blood transfusions on transplant outcome. It is clear that positive suppression is induced, whether by absence (deletion?), inactivation (anergy?), or blockade (anti-idiotypic antibodies). Experimentally, blood transfusion can be made to cause tolerance under certain circumstances, and in clinical series increased graft survival and a reduced rate of rejection are documented even in the face of effective immunosuppression. Each of the papers selected suggests a different mechanism, but all invoke some degree of incompatibility between blood donor and recipient. Blockade of binding sites of endothelial cells by anti-idiotypic antibodies may also be present, as suggested by the work of Hardy and his co-workers at Columbia University.

The endothelial cell as the boundary between graft and host has received considerable attention. Introduction of a gene into the endothelial cells to prevent activation of complement was strikingly successful in the test tube, even in a discordant xenograft model, and may have great promise given the advances now possible with genetic engineering and transgenic animals. Adhesion molecules, platelet-activating factors, and complement activation are all subjects of intense investigation.

More information has become available about the long-term beneficial effect of matching kidney donor and recipient for HLA antigens. A distinct positive cost-benefit ratio can be demonstrated, and organ sharing on the basis of matching seems inevitable. The imperfections of HLA typing have been highlighted by molecular techniques, but the serologic typing results of providing kidneys with no mismatches for the recipient are apparent. Whether by matching or induction of tolerance, reduction of immunosuppression by pharmacologic means is important; the incidence of B cell lymphomas related to Epstein-Barr virus infections appears to be increasing and is related to heavy immunosuppression. The rate of occurrence of this disease is highest in extrarenal organ transplant recipients, especially when large doses of OKT3 have been used. Bludgeoning the immune response with more and more powerful drugs seems to be having dread consequences; the development of therapeutic anti-B-cell antibodies for use in this disease is promising, but avoiding its induction would be ideal.

In summary, the advances in transplantation immunology this past year have been in the fundamental understanding of several of the mechanisms of immunity. Through these avenues, specific immunosuppression or tolerance may soon be achieved.

Tumor Immunology

The recent advances in molecular biology as applied to tumor biology have been remarkable. The role of oncogenes at various stages of the cell cycle are better understood, and it is now recognized that oncogenes are normal components of the genome, acting abnormally after transforming mutation or other events. Recently, genes that suppress cell growth or transformation have also been identified. Of these suppressor genes, whose absence or mutation has been associated with cancer development, the p53 gene has been of interest in the development of a number of types of malignancy. Using the very powerful molecular technique of the polymerase chain reaction (PCR), Kovach et al. performed simple touch preparations from fresh specimens of breast cancer and, from only a few cells, were able to detect point mutations of the p53 gene. The p53 mutations have also been detected in colon cancer and polyps, and in other malignancies such as lung tumors and osteosarcomas. The Li-Fraumeni familial cancer syndrome is marked by mutations in p53. Cossman and Schlegel (*J Natl Cancer Inst* 83:980–981, 1991) suggest that identification of p53 mutations in cells may be an important tool in the diagnosis of cancers when technologic advances make this practical. Application of these techniques, for instance, to needle biopsy specimens from difficult tumors such as pancreatic or endocrine masses, may be useful. Of basic importance, of course, is the further understanding of how these suppressor genes function in inhibition of the development of cancers—tumorigenesis mechanisms are closer to being understood.

Additional areas of interest are the mechanisms by which tumor cells metastasize. The detection of cancer cells in the bone marrow of colon cancer patients, even though bone metastases develop infrequently in this disease, leads to speculation of the mechanisms by which metastatic tumor cells protect themselves, perhaps by failing to express the major histocompatibility complex antigens necessary for T cell cytotoxicity. The PCR technology has also enabled investigators to detect as few as a single malignant melanoma cell in 2 mL of blood. The step that follows circulation of these tumor cells is adhesion to the endothelium of various organs and tissue, permitting invasion of the microvasculature. The interesting observation that certain cancer cells adhere to certain endothelial beds (e.g., colon cancer cells to the liver endothelium displaying the adhesion molecule ELAM-1) may shed light on the prediliction of tumors for organ metastases. Elaboration of cytokines by tumor-infiltrating lymphocytes (TIL cells) in response to activation by tumor-associated antigens, an inflammatory reaction, may be responsible for a number of these adhesion events by upregulating the expression of the adhesion molecules on the endothelium.

Invasion of the endothelium must be followed by establishment of a blood supply in order to develop a metastatic growth. Angiogenesis has been analyzed in breast cancer and its presence in invasive specimens has been correlated with metatastases. Folkman's group from the Boston Children's Hospital and Harvard Medical School has greatly furthered our understanding of angiogenesis and now has focused on means by which angiogenesis may be inhibited. An observation made on a contaminated cell culture dish has led to the development of a class of fungus-derived "angioinhibins," which have demonstrated considerable effectiveness in decreasing metastasis formation in an experimental tumor model and of preventing growth of cells that have invaded.

In summary, application of powerful molecular tools has carried forward our understanding of tumorigenesis and the differences between normal and malignant cells. Use of these tools in diagnosis and therapy will be areas of major development in the near future.

Skin

In the past few years synthetic skin substitutes have continued to be improved. These are necessary for replacement of natural skin secondary to burn and other injuries, as well as neoplasms. This year, an improvement was the inclusion of a slow release antibiotic. If these products prove useful, then one can begin to add other medications to them that would be useful in wound healing and possibly tumor treatment.

Skin neoplasms were the subject of many useful papers this past year. The treatment of malignant melanoma was advanced with the publication of a paper describing aggressive treatment of the recurrence of melanoma. This resulted in prolongation of life as well as marked palliation. For nonmelanotic lesions, cryosurgery was shown to be curative as well as useful in adjunctive or palliative treatment. In a large series the cure rate for basal cell carcinoma was shown to be the same as for other modalities, e.g., excision or radiation. Micrographic surgery is also useful in the management of nonmelanotic cancer (e.g., basal cell carcinoma) in the periocular area. Again, in well-chosen lesions this approach was demonstrated to be equal to excision.

With regard to benign lesions, an interesting paper appeared demonstrating the utility of the CO_2 laser for neurofibromas. This lesion often exists in hundreds of sites within the body, and the laser was shown to be simple, efficient, and time-saving, compared to excision, in management.

Definitive articles describing the vascular bases for fasciocutaneous and septocutaneous flaps have appeared. These flaps have totally revolutionized 1-stage reconstruction of skin defects. Advancement of knowledge of flap physiology, as well as continued refinement in the technology of constructing a skin replacement, should allow replacement of skin for all conditions in the near future.

Breast

A clinicopathologic study of patients with cystosarcoma phyllodes demonstrated that certain clinical variables (e.g., age, symptom duration, and size) are not valuable as prognostic tools. Local recurrence was more common in patients treated with breast-conserving operations, but there was no difference in distant metastases or survival. Needle localization biopsy should not be regarded as a totally benign procedure. Wound infections and cardiovascular complications associated with general anesthesia should be heeded. A review of patients with primary breast cancer who were younger than 35 years demonstrated 5-year and 10-year survival rates for those with stage I or stage II disease and negative axillary nodes comparable to those rates in older age groups. Patients with stage II disease and positive nodes, however, appear to have decreased survival compared to older patients. Paget's disease of the nipple is best treated by simple mastectomy. In situ carcinoma was found in 96% of the specimens, and the conclusion is that cone excision does not represent appropriate treatment. Results associated with inflammatory carcinoma of the breast remain poor. The regimens that include chemotherapy and radiation therapy followed by cytoreductive therapy and subsequent systemic therapy resulted in an 18% 5-year survival rate. The various techniques of breast reconstruction that have evolved in the past decade were reviewed.

Head and Neck

An animal model for head and neck cancer, described in this past year, may represent one of the greatest advances in recent years. Using a nude mouse to explant human laryngeal carcinoma may allow the study of tumor biology and therapeutic interactions.

The pathobiology of neoplasms may be better understood with the discovery of growth factor receptor on neoplastic cells. The potential for such a marker has only been tapped, but may show great promise in the next few years.

Reconstruction after the treatment of head and neck tumors received a lot of press during the past year. Long-term series appeared demonstrating the utility of tissue transfer by microvascular and microneural anastomosis. Functional outcome after reconstruction is becoming the benchmark by which procedures are evaluated. Voice preservation and restoration are receiving attention, and excellent results have been demonstrated for laryngeal salvage when possible and neoglottis construction when salvage is impossible.

Fibrosarcomas of the head and neck are not common enough for a single surgeon to have a large, reportable experience. An excellent institutional experience from UCLA will add useful knowledge to the management of these lesions.

Pain control has been addressed by several papers. The one chosen for inclusion documents the usefulness of patient-controlled analgesia after head and neck surgery. As described earlier in this edition for use by burn patients, this modality of pain control appears to hold real promise for the head and neck surgical patient.

The Thorax

Two different reports document again that emergency room thoracotomy is almost always futile in patients with cardiac arrest caused by blunt trauma, as well as in those who have no vital signs on arrival in the emergency room. In one series *not one* of 29 patients with blunt trauma survived. In the other series, no patient requiring cardiopulmonary resuscitation during transport survived.

The report from France of experiences with 96 pulmonary embolectomies over a period of 20 years is significant. The operative mortality of 37% must represent the critical status of the patients beforehand, for 25% had been resuscitated from cardiac arrest. It was curious (and unexplained) that massive pulmonary hemorrhage caused 8 of the 36 deaths. Recurrent pulmonary embolism was extremely rare, reflecting the effectiveness of vena caval interruption combined with anticoagulant therapy.

The nice report by Hazelrigg et al. randomized muscle sparing versus posterolateral thoracotomy. A simplistic analysis of this question would be that "smaller must be better," but the data found no meaningful difference in postoperative pulmonary function, shoulder range of motion, mortality, or hospital stay.

Whether thoracoplasty should be abandoned in favor of muscle flaps, as has virtually been done at both the Mayo Clinic and the Emory Clinic, is uncertain. The short report by Horrigan and Snow describes excellent results in 13 patients with complex problems. An obvious approach is to combine both procedures—a tailored muscle flap with a limited thoracoplasty. Although the long-term skeletal abnormalities after thoracoplasty can be significant, the primary goal with such critically ill patients is to cure the problem with as little morbidity as possible.

The role of extrapleural pneumonectomy for pleural mesothelioma seems dubious after reading the report of the Lung Cancer Study Group. Equally good results, a 2-year survival of 33%, were obtained with more limited operations.

A national survey of carcinoma of the lung that included 15,000 cases in about 10 years found no dramatic changes in therapy. Mediastinoscopy is clearly far more beneficial if restricted to patients with demonstrably enlarged mediastinal nodes on a CAT scan.

Two reports described extensive resection for bronchogenic carcinoma. Invasion of the chest wall is clearly not automatically incurable, because patients with negative nodes in the series reported by Mark Allen's group had a 5-year survival near 30%.

Mathisen and Grillo in Boston described 37 carinal resections in a period of 18 years for extensive bronchogenic carcinoma. Overall mortality was 28%, but the 5-year survival was about 20%.

For limited small cell lung cancer, the combination of chemotherapy and operation seems well established, with a 5-year survival of 51% for patients with stage I disease. With surgery alone, survival was stated to be only about 5%.

A refreshing paper was presented by Rodriguez et al., emphasizing the use of early tracheostomy as opposed to prolonged intubation. He emphasized that the widely quoted recommendations from the 1989 Consensus Conference were based partly on outmoded data. An additional development now present is the availability of fiberoptic bronchoscopy, which greatly facilitates the removal of tenacious secretions. The editor strongly recommends a tracheostomy almost routinely if intubation is required for more than 3 or 4 days. With the combination of early tracheostomy and effective tracheobronchial aspiration of secretions with the fiberoptic scope, the incidence of subsequent pneumonia is very small.

The short report by Benjamin and Curley from Sydney, Australia, documents valuable data on infant tracheostomy, finding that tracheostomy can be safely performed and subsequently removed in infants if proper attention is given to the airway, looking for granulations or other localized problems, before decannulation. These data continue to refute the long-standing myth about the insurmountable difficulties in decannulation if a tracheostomy is performed in an infant.

Congenital Heart Disease

The excellent report by Murphy et al. from the Mayo Clinic analyzed late results in 123 patients with atrial septal defect older than 25 years of age at the time of operation. The clinical implications of the study are striking. Delaying operation until after 25 years of age resulted in a significant increase in late mortality, 16% vs. 9% in those aged 25–40 years, and 60% vs. 41% in those older than 40 years. Age exerted an independent significant influence on mortality for unknown reasons.

Equally alarming is the fact that late deaths were caused by stroke in 19% of patients, all of whom were in atrial fibrillation.

Hence, as the operative risk of closure of an atrial septal defect is near zero, there would seem to be very little reason for delaying operation in asymptomatic adults once the presence of a large defect has been confirmed.

The safety of current operations for ventricular septal defect are well defined in the short report by McGrath. In 115 consecutive patients, a ventriculotomy was not required; there were no instances of heart block, and only 1 operative death.

The report by Merrill et al. describes experiences with 103 patients with atrioventricular canal treated in a 10-year period after palliative pulmonary artery banding was stopped after 1977. Overall results were quite good, although operative mortality was about 15%.

The report by Di Donato et al. indicates that neonatal repair of tetralogy of Fallot is feasible; 27 neonates had a corrective procedure. Whether or not the complex total correction, rather than a simple shunt, should be performed is not clear from the data. There were 5 deaths, 3 of which were said to be caused by "avoidable technical problems." But if lethal "technical problems" occur for a group as experienced as the surgical group at the Boston Children's, the risk seems significant. Only data from multiple institutions will provide the answer. In the meantime, the critical question remains as to which procedure is safer for the patient.

The data in the report from London by Gerosa et al. about long-term results with pulmonary autograft replacement of the aortic valve in children is quite impressive. The initial operations were performed more than 15 years ago. The autograft has shown a susceptibility to endocarditis, but there have been no instances of valve degeneration or any episodes of thromboembolism, a remarkable observation.

The strange development of aortic regurgitation after a left ventricular myomectomy in 3% to 4% of patients is described in the report by Brown et al. from the National Institutes of Health. Another series with similar observations was described in this Overview 2 years ago. The initial recognition of regurgitation months or years after operation virtually precludes an operative injury. The basic mechanism remains unclear.

There is uncertainty about the best operation for coarctation in infants—subclavian flap vs. resection. The report by Brouwer and co-workers from The Netherlands, strongly supports resection. The study by Arenas et al. describing absorbable polydioxanone suture is significant in this regard, because absorbable sutures should enhance late growth of the anastomosis.

Similar uncertainties exist about when a "hypoplastic" transverse arch in neonates requires surgical correction. What is truly hypoplastic is uncertain, because the congenital anomalies present divert blood flow from this area of the aorta. The report from France describes resection of the transverse arch when a 50% reduction in diameter is present, whereas the report by Siewers et al., who clearly documented late growth of the arch, recommends resection only if there is severe hypoplasia, i.e., a reduction in diameter to about 0.25. Quite striking in the latter report is the finding that, among a group of 18 patients studied on late follow-up, not a single one had a arm-leg pressure gradient.

Valvular Heart Disease

The short report by Gonzalez-Lavin and colleagues documents the unacceptably high rate of deterioration of pericardial valves within 10 years after operation, with an exponential increase in frequency of deterioration starting about 7 years postoperatively. This is, unfortunately, similar to results with fascia lata valves and homograft dura mater valves, both of which produced good results for at least 5 years. Hence, evaluation of biological prostheses seems to require at least 10 years of postoperative observation before their durability can be clearly determined.

The short report by Jatene's group in São Paolo about preserving the aortic valve with chronic aortic dissection is encouraging. Using the techniques of homgraft reconstruction, the aortic valve was preserved in about half of the 44 patients undergoing operation.

The short report by Roberts et al. well indicates the importance of a precise surgical technique when the Morrow operation (myocardial resection) is performed for hypertrophic subaortic stenosis. At the National Institutes of Health, among a group of 23 patients undergoing a repeat operation, there were 12 who initially were operated on elsewhere, more than 50% of whom were treated by repeat myomectomy. The availability of intraoperative echocardiography should greatly facilitate the effectiveness of performing an adequate operation. The basic anatomical guidelines were well described in the classic article by Morrow years ago, but they must be carefully followed with a dry sterile operative field and excellent exposure. To the editor's knowledge, in the past 15 years, none of the patients undergoing outflow tract resection at NYU where the principles of the Morrow operation are very familiar have required repeat operation.

There is growing enthusiasm for mitral valve reconstruction rather than replacement. Carpentier describes good results in a small, unusual group of 12 patients in whom a large amount of calcium was débrided from the annulus of the mural leaflet before reconstruction was undertaken. David et al., in Canada, described the use of Gortex sutures to create artificial chordae in 43 patients, as mentioned in this review last year. Further, 2 different reports describe reconstruction of tricuspid leaflets affected by endocarditis, operating in the presence of active endocarditis in some patients. Similar reports were described in this Overview in 1991. Hence, reports from several institutions show that localized tricuspid endocarditis can be treated effectively by tricuspid valve reconstruction rather than by total excision or replacement.

Coronary Heart Disease

A 10-year follow-up by the Coronary Artery Surgical group of the 780 patients originally randomized to bypass or medical therapy was published. Survivors were similar in both groups, but a key point, often overlooked, is that angina developed in 40% of the group initially randomized to medical therapy, who were then treated with bypass. This 40%

crossover rate within 10 years constitutes a major challenge to the effectiveness of "medical therapy." If dietary measures could slow or stop the atherosclerotic process, such a high crossover rate should not occur.

Enthusiasm for the use of bilateral mammary grafts in patients undergoing reoperation was reported by Galbut and co-workers. A significant point is that 20% of the patients had an intra-aortic balloon inserted beforehand. Morbidity was clearly increased, but overall mortality was not.

The search for arterial conduits continues, with reports describing both the gastroepiploic and the inferior epigastric. The key question, of course, is the patency observed on angiography 1 or more years after operation. In the enthusiastic search for new arterial conduits, it is most important to remember that the final decision may depend on angiograms obtained 5–10 years after operation. Vein grafts appear very good for at least 5 years after operation, but a disappointingly high number of them become atherosclerotic in the next 5 years.

The problem of emergency bypass after failed angioplasty remains a significant one, as addressed in the report by Bottner et al. who used a different type of cardioplegia. An unknown question is how much of the myocardial injury following failed angioplasty is reversible with urgent bypass, because total regional ischemia in a warm, beating heart can produce irreversible injury within 30–45 minutes.

The report by Hinkamp et al. about combining coronary bypass with excision of an abdominal aneurysm is thought provoking. The familiar question is not whether it *can* be done, but *should* it be done? An alternative approach would be to perform the coronary bypass and proceed with excision of the abdominal aneurysm within a few days, certainly during the same hospitalization.

Finally, the short article on meralgia paresthetica is a valuable one, describing an uncommon but perplexing complication.

Miscellaneous Cardiac Conditions

STERNOTOMY INCISION

The interesting report by Nishida et al. describes what may be the lowest frequency of infections ever reported after sternotomy, .16% among 3,118 patients. Minimal use of electrocautery was considered by the authors to be the key factor. Using the cautery with a low frequency for pinpoint hemostasis, rather than more extensive cauterization with a high frequency current, should minimize any decrease in blood supply. Minimal use of bone wax, although difficult to document, is another important consideration.

The superb paper by Pairolero et al. should be studied with interest. It describes experiences with 100 patients treated with bone flaps for infected sternotomy wounds. Their data are not representative of the usual type of patient, because these patients were treated 7.5 weeks after the onset of sternal drainage—far later than ideal. Their classification of sternal infections into 3 groups well emphasizes the value of selectivity in therapy. Prompt recognition, which is possible by needle aspiration of the sternotomy incision, permits early treatment before extensive sternal osteomyelitis develops. After a few weeks, both osteomyelitis and a rigid mediastinum virtually mandate sternal resection and muscle flap interposition to correct the problem.

The elegant paper by Eastridge and colleagues may be an important clue to the puzzling problem of delayed chest wall pain from sternal wire sutures. His data support the hypothesis that simply *breaking the chromium oxide coat* on a steel wire may produce a tiny voltaic cell in the wire that subsequently leads to deposition of iron ions and a painful inflammatory response. It is hoped that this theory can be confirmed by others.

MYOCARDIAL PRESERVATION

Six different papers analyzed different aspects of retrograde cardioplegia, either warm or cold. None is definitive. The paper by Haan et al. demonstrates experimentally a much better distribution of cardioplegic solution by the retrograde method after an acute infarction. Better distribution of the cardioplegic solution is probably the main benefit of the retrograde method. Four other papers are from members of the Toronto group that evolved the concept of continuous cardioplegia. The recent surge of interest about warm vs. cold cardioplegia is the most recent innovation. The value of warm cardioplegia is primarily theoretical, with the obvious disadvantage that myocardial tolerance for interrupting the cardioplegia is much less with a warm heart. Whatever the explanation, however, it is well known that with conventional antegrade cardioplegia, emergency operations for acute myocardial ischemia (e.g., cardiogenic shock, ruptured ventricular septum, or ruptured papillary muscle) are associated with high mortality, which seems to be less with continuous retrograde techniques, either cold or warm. We hope that these data can be confirmed by other groups. It simply may be that any continuous method is safer when the myocardial substrate is badly depleted from acute ischemia.

The short report by Sun et al. describes an experimental study demonstrating that a selective degree of coronary sinus occlusion, producing a coronary sinus pressure of 25–35 mm, can be combined with antegrade injection, theoretically attaining the advantages and having the simplicity of both methods.

MORBIDITY OF CARDIOPULMONARY BYPASS

The most serious complication of coronary bypass is neurologic injury. The report by van der Linden et al. is both interesting and frustrating. The authors describe detection of air emboli with the transcranial Doppler technique in all 10 patients when the heart began to beat, but they say very little about the presence or absence of neurologic defects. The natural question arises as to whether the Doppler abnormalities detected were caused by air emboli or some other particle, or whether the emboli were too small to be of clinical significance. If the transcranial Doppler technique truly detects significant air emboli, the question could be answered quickly with studies from several large centers.

A report from Boston describes a 27% frequency of pancreatic injury after open-heart surgery, an alarmingly high figure. The observation that this correlated with the amount of calcium given, beginning with a calcium dose that exceeded 800 mg/m², seems quite significant.

ARRHYTHMIAS AND PERICARDIUM

Two papers document the impressive effectiveness of radiofrequency ablation of accessory pathways for the Wolff-Parkinson-White syndrome. The report by Bolling et al. describes a 90% success rate. That by Jackman's group describes a 99% success rate among 166 patients. There was a 9% recurrence, all treated successfully with a second radiofrequency ablation.

The report from Johns Hopkins describes the effectiveness of pericardiectomy for recurrent pericardial effusion. This was the primary indication for pericardiectomy in about 50 percent of 60 patients operated upon. Perhaps this approach should be employed more frequently, rather than resorting to prolonged non-operative therapy with an effusion that continues for weeks or months.

AORTA AND GREAT VESSELS

The report by George et al. describes experiences with 118 patients with cervicothoracic arterial injuries. The ominous outlook for patients with carotid injuries that produce hemiplegia or coma is clear. Among 20 patients, only 5 improved; 8 remained unchanged and 7 died.

The safety of the composite graft operation for replacement of the aortic root is well documented in 2 different reports. Gott and co-workers reported experiences with treatment of aneurysms in the Marfan syndrome in 100 consecutive patients. There were no hospital deaths among 92 patients undergoing elective repair, well supporting the recommendation for elective operation in these patients when the diameter of the aortic root reaches 6 cm.

Kouchoukos et al. report a similar low mortality rate among a series of 168 patients. Operative mortality was 5% but 4 of the 9 deaths occurred among patients having operations for acute dissection.

In aortic dissection, the report from Duke by Glower and colleagues confirms the reliability of aortic valve suspension, rather than replacement, for patients with a normal valve beforehand. The high late mortality, however, ranging from 29% to 46%, clearly emphasizes the need for continuing long-term follow-up.

The detailed paper by Coselli et al. from Stanley Crawford's group in Houston describes 40 patients with the dread problem of postoperative infection after prosthetic replacement of the ascending aorta or transverse aortic arch. Nineteen of the 40 patients were referred from other institutions. Long-term survival was about 70%. Several concepts were developed, including the use of omentum, not removing the entire prosthesis, and lifelong antibiotic therapy. Conclusive data are seldom possible in such complicated problems, but the fact that a significant percentage of patients survived without removal of the prosthesis is intriguing.

After traumatic rupture of the aorta, uncertainty remains about the use of a shunt with heparin, as well as what type of a shunt to employ. Virtually all reports, however, show that simple occlusion of the aorta for longer than 30 minutes leads to an increasing frequency of paraplegia, probably from ischemic infarction of the spinal cord. The paper by Zeiger et al. from the Maine Medical Center found a zero frequency of paraplegia in 14 patients repaired with a shunt but a 35% frequency in those repaired without a shunt. Their review of 16 published reports found an average frequency of paraplegia of 2.9% in patients operated on with a pump and 7.9% in those with a shunt, but 20% in 108 patients operated on without a shunt. Mortality, however, was significantly higher with heparinization, which has been the principal deterrent to the use of a shunt.

The short report from Capetown is thus of particular interest, describing the use of the Bio-Medicus pump without heparinization in a series of 5 patients. Earlier, 8 patients had been treated with simple cross-clamping, with 3 deaths and 2 instances of paraplegia resulting. The Bio-Medicus pump group had no fatalities and no paraplegia.

As has been suggested by others, the use of the Bio-Medicus pump with minimal or no heparinization may be the best approach to this difficult problem. When a shunt is used, however, the critical consideration, emphasized in several publications from the editor's institution, is that the flow rate through it must be sufficiently large to produce a distal aortic pressure of 50–60 mm to significantly decrease the frequency of paraplegia. Not shunting sufficient blood is probably the reason that data for the past decade have failed to demonstrate a major benefit with shunting as opposed to no shunting.

The report by Mangano and co-workers is of particular interest. One hundred high-risk patients had continuous monitoring for 1 week after major noncardiac surgery. Reversible ischemic episodes were identified in 27%, but the majority (84%) were silent. All 5 serious cardiac complications that occurred, either myocardial infarction or death, were preceded by an episode of ischemia in the previous 24 hours. Although the studies did not find the ideal way to prevent these ischemic episodes, the occurrence of ischemia in 1 patient in every 4 after major noncardiac surgery indicates both the frequency and gravity of the problem.

The Arteries, the Veins, and the Lymphatics

Assessment of the natural history of patients with abdominal aneurysms demonstrates that the aneurysms expand at highly individual rates. The initial diameter of the lesion is the only recognized predictor of rupture. The suggestion is that aneurysms smaller than 5 cm be followed by sequential ultrasonography. Operation for a ruptured abdominal aortic aneurysm continues to be associated with significant mortality—more than 8 times that for the same operation carried out electively. These data constitute a plea for increasing the proportion of patients operated on electively.

A plea is also made for prompt surgical repair of aortic dissections to obviate the need for peripheral revascularization. Long-term follow-up demonstrates that approximately one third of these patients die of the development and rupture of another aneurysm. A review of the literature was made concerning patients with spontaneous abdominal arteriovenous fistulas. Usually, digital compression of the vein at the fistula site allows suturing of the fistula from within the aneurysm sac. Routine aortoiliac grafting completes the operation.

A randomized trial of intra-arterial intravenous recombinant tissue plasminogen activator (rt-PA) and intra-arterial streptokinase in peripheral arterial thrombolysis demonstrates that intra-arterial rt-PA is a safer, more effective fibrinolytic regimen than conventional streptokinase treatment.

Percutaneous intra-arterial thrombolysis in the treatment of thrombosis of lower extremity arterial reconstruction can restore patency to grafts, but adjunctive surgical thrombectomy is required to remove persistent thrombi from the graft, and graft reocclusion can be expected if technical defects in the reconstruction are not revised. There are distinct limitations to the widespread use of low-dose intra-arterial thrombolysis.

Femorofemoral bypass to treat unilateral iliac artery occlusion of stenosis can be carried out with a 1-year patency rate of 91% and a 5-year patency rate of 82%. The major cause of graft failure is inadequate runoff and outflow disease progression. Patients with popliteal artery aneurysms should be treated because of the liver-threatening potential. These patients also have an increased risk of new aneurysm formation both in the popliteal artery and other locations. Femoral-distal bypass with the in situ greater saphenous vein is associated with an overall primary revised patency of 78% and a limb salvage rate of 88%. In contrast to reversed vein grafts, long infrapopliteal in situ grafts have long-term secondary patency. Infrapopliteal graft patency can be improved using a distal adjunctive arteriovenous fistula.

Symptomatic visceral ischemia has been managed by transaortic endarterectomy or bypass techniques. More than 95% of patients were very symptomatic at 1 year, and 86% were symptomatic at 5 years. Percutaneous transluminal angioplasty can be used as the initial treatment for atherosclerotic renal artery stenosis, and the procedure can be repeated if restenosis occurs. Microvascular free flaps are playing an increasing role in salvaging below-knee amputation stumps and providing the patient with improved mobility.

Although patients with advanced cancers and thromboembolic disease have a high complication rate when treated with anticoagulation or with the Greenfield filter placement, the latter appears more definitive. Leiomyosarcoma of the inferior vena cava remains a rare malignant tumor associated with a poor prognosis. Patients who receive a combination of operation, radiotherapy, and chemotherapy remain disease free for longer periods of time.

Esophagus

Laparoscopic cardiomyotomy represents an intriguing approach for achalasia. It has a distinct advantage in that it reduces trauma to the hiatus. Primary repair, with or without suture line plication, remains the backbone of therapy for spontaneous rupture of the esophagus. Plication of the esophageal suture line with gastric fundus can be used when pleura or other tissue flaps are not available. The 5-year survival of patients with Barrett's adenocarcinoma is double that of patients with non–Barrett's adenocarcinoma of the esophagus. This may be related to surveillance. Endoscopic monitoring may be improved if the biopsy specimens are obtained from within the distal 3 cm of the esophagus and esophagogastric junction. A multicenter, controlled trial evaluating postoperative irradiation after curative resection of squamous cell carcinoma of the mid and lower esophagus demonstrates that survival is improved regardless of lymph node status.

Stomach and Duodenum

It has been suggested that leukotriene receptor blockade reduces bile acid-induced superficial mucosal injury. This may constitute a method of therapy for bile gastritis. Proximal gastric vagotomy is an effective and safe method of managing a bleeding duodenal ulcer. The authors reported a recurrence rate of about 12%. Another study indicated that a substantial number of patients become symptomatic after highly selective vagotomy, and an even larger number have asymptomatic recurrences. Most patients with recurrent ulcer, however, do well with H_2 receptor blocker therapy. A multifactorial analysis provided evidence that definitive surgery for peptic ulcer yields a better, long-term quality of life than does simple closure. Unless a clinical condition exists at operation that is so precarious that prolongation of the procedure is contraindicated, definitive surgery represents the treatment of choice.

Completion gastrectomy is a reasonable approach for patients with chronic gastroparesis after an operation for gastric outlet obstruction. Nutritional requirements are readily met by Roux-en-Y esophagojenunostomy. Octreotide acetate prevents the vasomotor and gastrointestinal symptoms of severe postgastrectomy syndrome. The long-term treatment is successful and causes no major side effects. Control of the dumping syndrome can also be achieved by treatment with somatostatin analogue.

Infection with *Helicobacter pylori* is strongly associated with an increased risk of gastric carcinoma. The bacteria may cause chronic antral gastritis, which is known to represent a precancerous lesion. There is no relationship between perioperative blood transfusion and length of survival after curative resection for gastric cancer. This is contrary to previous studies that suggested that a relationship exists for colon cancer and for resection of other malignancies.

The risk of gastric cancer after partial gastrectomy remains controversial in the United States. A meta-analysis defines differences in relative risk between subgroups of postgastrectomy patients. The postoperative interval is a major risk factor, as is the type of ulcer for which initial surgery was performed. "Early" gastric cancer is redefined as carcinoma in which invasion is confined to the mucosa or submucosa without evidence of lymph node metastases. Extensive radical surgery, including dissection of lymph nodes, is advised to improve the survival rates for these patients. Splenectomy does not correlate with the length of survival in patients undergoing total gastrectomy for gastric carcinoma. Abdominal stapled suturing of esophagojejunostomy is expeditious and is as reliable as manual suturing.

Small Intestine

Both urogastrone and intestinal resection stimulate epithelialization in full-thickness bowel wall defects patched with adjacent serosal surface. Intraoperative enteroscopy plays an important role adjunctive to laparotomy for gastrointestinal bleeding localized preoperatively to the small bowel. The editor has been impressed with the ability to visualize angiodysplastic lesions by transmural illumination in a darkened room. Most patients with Crohn's disease, if observed long enough, will have recurrent disease after resection. Because radical resection does not protect against this recurrence, conservative removal of the bowel is indicated. It is safe, in these patients, to suture the inflamed bowel. Crohn's disease is 20 times more frequent in first-degree relatives of patients who have had the disease than it is in nonrelatives. The prevalence of ulcerative colitis in first-degree relatives of patients with Crohn's disease is 6 times greater than it is in nonrelatives.

Modern nutritional support provides excellent survival and a good quality of life for patients with the short bowel syndrome, but many of these children must cope with setbacks, reoperations, and rehospitalizations.

Data suggest that tagged red blood cell scanning is a poor diagnostic technique for localization of gastrointestinal bleeding, and its use as a screening tool before angiography is performed is questionable.

Colon and Rectum

A small series suggests that detorsion is adequate treatment for cecal volvulus, and that resection should be reserved for patients whose cecum is necrotic. Complications and recurrences were more frequent after resectional operation than for cecopexy. The quality of life is significantly improved after resection of the colon in patients with ulcerative colitis. It did not seem to differ with the type of operation performed. Follow-up of 23 patients with carcinoid tumor of the appendix in the first 2 decades of life reveals that when metastasis is not present at the time of diagnosis in children, the tumor is clinically benign. Conservative operation is appropriate.

The long-term effects of dietary calcium on risk markers for colon cancer in patients with familial polyposis were studied. No beneficial effect for calcium on rectal mucosal proliferation was evident in these patients. Epidemiological findings of an association between beer drinking and rectal cancer focus on nitrosamine carcinogenicity. Efforts are warranted to reduce the nitrosamine content of beer. Counter to previous reports in the literature, a study indicates that cholecystectomy does not appear to be a significant risk factor for colorectal neoplasia. Patients younger than age 40 with colorectal cancer are generally symptomatic at the time of diagnosis, and survival times are similar to those in the general population.

The use of periodic serum carcinoembryonic antigen tests are justified, because these levels are elevated in 89% of patients with abdominal relapses of colorectal carcinoma. Significant number of patients with adenocarcinoma of the rectum have synchronous lesions; patients with lesions in either area should be studied preoperatively with complete colonoscopy. In patients with rectal carcinoma and poor prognosis, combined postoperative local radiation therapy plus systemic therapy with fluorouracil improves the results when compared with postoperative radiation therapy alone. A case is made for the use of loop colostomy rather than complete transection. Barium studies revealed no passage of barium into the distal colon after a loop colostomy was constructed. Significant morbidity does occur in about a third of patients after reanastomosis following a Hartmann operation. It is therefore preferable, when possible, to carry out primary resection and anastomosis. Complication rates were similar in patients having stapled or handsewn anastomoses.

The Liver and the Spleen

A warning has been issued that a fatal reaction may result from fibrin glue used for establishing hemostasis on the surface of organs. A review of an institutional experience with management of hemangiomas of the liver provides evidence that enlargement and rupture of hemangiomas smaller than 5 cm generally does not occur. Rapid tumor growth and severe symptoms should indicate surgical treatment because of the low morbidity and mortality. Intra-abdominal abscess formation remains a complication after major liver resection. Antibiotic prophylaxis does not affect the incidence. Total cystopericystectomy, separating the fibrous surface of the hydatid cysts adjacent to the hepatic parenchyma without opening the cavity, is presented as the procedure of choice for hepatic hydatidosis. Limited hepatic resection for selected cirrhotic patients with hepatocellular or cholangiocellular carcinoma can be carried out; it results in an acceptable mortality rate and a reported 5-year survival of

49%. During a 10-year period, 76 patients with hepatocellular carcinoma were treated by subtotal hepatic resection and 105 were treated by orthotopic liver transplantation. The 5-year survival rate in the group having resection was 33%, and that in the group receiving transplants, 36%. Fibrolamellar hepatocellular carcinoma and early stages of hepatocellular carcinoma were strongly represented among the long-term survivors. Hepatocellular carcinoma in children is associated with a grave prognosis. A prospective study was undertaken to evaluate the effect of continuous infusion of doxorubicin and cisplatin for the treatment of incompletely resected hepatic cancer in children. The outcome of children with hepatoblastoma was much better than that for children with hepatocellular carcinoma; the survival of children who underwent delayed hepatic resection was not statistically different from the survival of those whose hepatic tumors were removed at the initial operation. An overall actuarial 5-year survival rate of 30% has been reported for patients undergoing hepatic resection for metastatic colorectal cancer. The extent of liver involvement in the staging system may be significant, but there are no absolute indicators of outcome. Evidence is presented to support the statement that a curative operation should be considered for all patients with completely resectable metastatic neuroendocrine tumors in the liver, and that palliative surgery is also indicated.

Prophylactic sclerotherapy does not improve survival in patients with cirrhosis and esophageal varices that have not bled. The 2-year survival rates for portacaval anastomosis and sclerotherapy are essentially the same, but patients undergoing portacaval anastomosis had a lower incidence of variceal rebleeding despite a greater incidence of encephalopathy. The role of portacaval anastomosis and the elective treatment of variceal bleeding should be reassessed. The actuarial survival for patients undergoing an emergency portosystemic shunt for bleeding varices is reportedly greater than 40% and is dependent on the Child's classification. The Japanese Research Society evaluated prophylactic surgery for esophageal varices and concluded that portal nondecompression surgery is effective in preventing variceal bleeding and improving survival. A percutaneous transjugular intrahepatic portosystemic shunt is known to maintain patency for a mean of 5 months and to decompress esophagogastric varices successfully. The Sugiura procedure has managed portal hypertension secondary to extrahepatic portal vein thrombosis. In the reported series, only 2 of 27 patients rebled, and the survival rate at both 5 years and 10 years was 82%.

Splenectomy has been proved beneficial in many patients with massive splenomegaly, but the incidence of morbidity and mortality is higher than it is in other groups. That patients with immune thrombocytopenia purpura respond to steroids, IgG, or both, was highly predictive of a response to spenectomy because 97% responded to one of these regimens. By contrast, failure to respond to medical management predicted a 70% rate of failure to respond to spenectomy. The risk of postsplenectomy sepsis and its mortality has been addressed, although removal of the spleen in otherwise normal individuals does not appear to be associated with an increased incidence of infection. The presence of a coexistent disorder can increase the risk substantially. Because of the low incidence of severe late postsplenectomy infection, statistical evaluation of the effectiveness of prophylactic antibiotics, vaccination, and splenic repair is difficult.

Biliary

The use of a valved hepatic portoduodenal intestinal conduit improves the survival rate in infants with biliary atresia by preventing ascending cholangitis. Complete cyst excision is the treatment of choice for choledochal cysts. Simple anastomosis of the cyst wall to the gastrointestinal tract ultimately will result in stricture and cholangitis. Gallstone dissolution can be accomplished in almost all patients by the injection of methyl-tert-butyl ether if ursodeoxycholic acid therapy must be continued. Laparoscopic cholecystectomy is used with increasing frequency. Data suggest that it can be performed with efficacy, morbidity, and mortality rates similar to those of open cholecystectomy. Cholangiography performed via the cystic duct before any structures are divided can prevent the most serious complication—common duct injury. But in most series, fewer than 25% of patients have intraoperative cholangiography. For those who continue to champion open cholecystectomy, another series has been reported demonstrating that outpatient cholecystectomy can be performed without jeopardizing the patient's safety or comfort.

There is a difference of opinion about the usefulness of preoperative endoscopic sphincterotomy in patients undergoing elective surgery. One series reports data that do not support peroperative endoscopic sphincterotomy as a technique for clearance of common duct stones on the basis of efficacy, morbidity, or cost. Another group suggests that combined preoperative endoscopic sphincterotomy and laparoscopic cholecystectomy in treatment of patients with simultaneous cholecystolithiasis and choledocholithiasis is a safe and effective approach. Complications are associated with endoscopic sphincterotomy. Radiographic evidence of free retroperitoneal or intraperitoneal air was the most important determinant of perforation. Operative intervention is recommended for all patients with clinical evidence of perforation after endoscopic sphincterotomy. Bleeding following endoscopic sphincterotomy is an underestimated entity. Early detection of bleeding and its aggressive management limit morbidity and mortality. A technique for transduodenal exploration of the common bile duct in patients with nondilated ducts is reported. Use of a biliary catheter, inserted through the cystic duct into the duodenum, followed by inflation of the balloon and withdrawing it snuggly against the ampulla, localizes the ampulla and permits duodenotomy and standard sphincteroplasty. In patients with complicated high benign biliary strictures, use of a Roux-en-Y hepaticojejunostomy and an extended limb of the jejunum brought to the abdominal wall to allow access for a later radiologic intervention avoids the subsequent need for surgical intervention, although choledochoduodenostomy is a safe and effective method of treatment of choledocholithiasis.

Combined portal vein and liver resection for carcinoma of the biliary tract has improved the median survival rate, but the number of 5-year cures remains anecdotal. Radiation therapy does play a role after operative palliation in cancer of the proximal bile ducts. Cholangiocarcinoma may develop in patients with primary sclerosing cholangitis. But for this reason, liver transplantation may be considered earlier in the course of the disease. An improved 1-year survival has been reported after tumor resection compared with palliative surgery for patients with carcinoma of the extrahepatic bile ducts. Extended survivals rarely occur. The best prognosis among malignant tumors of the extrahepatic bile duct and pancreas is associated with tumors of the ampulla. Radical resection for ampullary carcinoma can be performed with low morbidity and mortality and should be the procedure of choice for this lesion.

Pancreas

Two distinct processes are associated with pancreatic stone formation: one is the precipitation of calcium carbonate, an important feature of chronic alcoholic pancreatitis, and the other is the precipitation of insoluble forms of lithostathine. Acute edematous pancreatitis impairs pancreatic secretion in rats. Patients with acute necrotizing pancreatitis treated with staged necrosectomy and delayed primary closures had significant long-term morbidity and a mortality rate of 17%. This method of closure, however, minimizes the incidence of recurrent intra-abdominal abscess related to persistent necrosis and undrained fluid.

Total pancreatectomy with preservation of the duodenum and pylorus can be accomplished in patients with chronic pancreatitis. The risk of stenosis can be reduced by retaining a narrow rim of pancreas between the bile duct and duodenum. An antiulcer regimen is required indefinitely.

Octreotide-induced suppression of pancreatic secretions can aid in the resolution of painful pseudocysts in some patients with chronic pancreatitis. Nonoperative invasive methods are effective in treating pancreatic fluid collections, especially in patients in whom the fluid collections are unrelated to alcoholism or biliary tract disease. Endogenous cholecystokinin stimulates pancreatic regeneration after partial removal of the organ. FOY-305 may provide useful treatment for patients with pancreatic insufficiency after either subtotal pancreatectomy or chronic pancreatitis. Bladder drainage of the transplanted pancreas normalizes peripheral insulin levels and improves the glucose response to an oral challenge, but recipients may remain insensitive to endogenous insulin. It is proposed that glucagonomas are not as rare as previously thought, and partial pancreatectomy is recommended for patients with localized lesions, whereas aggressive, cytoreductive surgery is indicated for patients with more aggressive disease.

Endocrine

Follow-up for an average of 12 years of more than 250 patients with papillary thyroid carcinoma indicates that patients with intrathyroidal disease and cervical node involvement whose tumors are larger than 1 cm should undergo lobectomy and subtotal lobectomy contralaterally, followed by radioiodine ablation of the residual thyroid disease. Treatment of smaller tumors remains uncertain. The results associated with therapy for anaplastic giant cell carcinoma remain poor. Gross removal of the tumor is indicated whenever possible, but it should not delay chemotherapy and radiation therapy. For patients with primary lymphoma of the thyroid, multidrug chemotherapy and irradiation are the chief measures of therapy. Selected patients may undergo operation if the tumor can be resected safety. Total parathyroidectomy without an autograft may be the treatment of choice in patients unlikely to receive a renal transplant. Total parathyroidectomy with autografting is appropriate after successful transplantation and in dialysis patients who are likely to receive a transplant. Adrenalectomy should be bilateral unless a truly functioning tumor can be identified in patients with Cushing's syndrome. Complete remission is achieved in more than 90% of patients. Computed tomography is the most sensitive localizing investigation for all categories of adrenal pathology, with a sensitivity of more than 90%. Supplementing CT with meta-iodobenzylguanidine may be helpful in selected cases. Gastrinomas associated with the multiple endocrine neoplasia type I syndrome tend to occur in the duodenum and to be multicentric. Solitary gastrinomas are seen mainly in sporadic Zollinger-Ellison syndrome in either the pancreas or the duodenum. When operating on these patients, it is always wise to study the duodenum carefully. This can be accomplished by endoscopy or by opening the duodenum, because the number of small intramural gastrinomas is high and they are often multiple.

1 General Considerations

Surgery in HIV-Positive and AIDS Patients: Indications and Outcomes
Vipond MN, Ralph DJ, Stotter AT (St Mary's Hosp, London; The Middlesex
Hosp, London, Glenfield Gen Hosp, Leicester, England)
J R Coll Surg Edinb 36:254–258, 1991   1–1

Background.—Many surgeons have expressed concern about operating on patients infected with HIV both because of the risk of HIV transmission and the uncertainty of healing after surgery. At 1 center a surgical service was established in conjunction with other departments that routinely care for HIV-infected patients. The types of procedures performed and the outcomes of surgery in HIV patients were reviewed.

Methods.—Findings were analyzed in 147 patients who were seropositive for HIV. Of these patients, 100 subsequently received a diagnosis of AIDS. There were 256 operations.

Findings.—The most common indications for surgery were anorectal conditions, present in 34% of the patients; placement of central venous access devices, 21%; lymph node and soft tissue biopsy, 15%; and laparotomy, 4%. Of the operations, 20% were associated with complications; 35 patients needed repeat procedures. Both the complications and the repeat procedures occurred with equal frequency in the HIV and AIDS populations. Most of the surgical procedures were minor, and the results were satisfactory, with acceptable morbidity (table).

Conclusions.—Surgery in AIDS patients can be useful to alleviate symptoms and morbidity is acceptable. In the future, more HIV-seropositive patients will be seen with common surgical conditions unrelated to their underlying infection. The morbidity of such conditions must be considered; surgery should not be denied to patients with troublesome symptoms that can be alleviated operatively. In addition, there will be an increasing need for facilities for routine surgery on such patients.

Indications and Outcome of Laparotomy in 10 Patients

Patient	Operation	Indication	Status	Outcome
1	Lavage and drainage	Primary peritonitis	HIV-positive	Dead, postoperative myocardial infarction
2	Appendicectomy	Appendicitis	AIDS	Alive at 26 months
3	Diagnostic biopsy	Tuberculosis	AIDS	Dead, 1 month, AIDS
4	Right hemicolectomy	Kaposi sarcoma, cytomegalovirus, cryptosporidia	AIDS	Dead, 5 months, AIDS
5	Defunctioning colostomy	Severe perianal sepsis	HIV-positive	
	Closure of colostomy	Sepsis resolved		Dead, 1 year, AIDS
6	Diagnostic biopsy	Small bowel lymphoma	AIDS	Dead, 1 month, AIDS
7	Small bowel resection	Small bowel volvulus	AIDS	Dead, 4 months, AIDS
8	Right hemicolectomy	B cell lymphoma	AIDS	Alive at 7 months
9	Small bowel bypass	Disseminated adenocarcinoma	AIDS	Dead, 2 months
10	Small bowel resection	Intussusception of lymphoma	AIDS	Alive at 1 month

(Courtesy of Vipond MN, Ralph DJ, Stotter AT: J R Coll Surg Edinb 36:254–258, 1991.)

A Growing Spectrum of Surgical Disease in Patients With Human Immunodeficiency Virus/Acquired Immunodeficiency Syndrome: Experience With 120 Major Cases

Diettrich NA, Cacioppo JC, Kaplan G, Cohen SM (Illinois Masonic Med Ctr, Chicago; Columbus-Cabrini Med Ctr, Chicago)
Arch Surg 126:860–866, 1991
1–2

Background.—Many patients with HIV infection have surgically correctable abnormalities. The records of all adults with HIV infection who were treated on the general surgical services of several teaching community hospitals were reviewed to evaluate the types of major surgical procedures performed and to identify factors that may affect prognosis.

Patients.—Between 1986 and 1990, 88 patients aged 22–67 years (mean, 41.6 years), with HIV infection underwent major surgery. Most of the patients were men (94.3%). The majority had recognized risk factors (93.2%), including homosexuality (73%), intravenous drug abuse (8%), and previous blood transfusion (8%). Risk factors were denied by 7%.

Findings.—Of the 120 major surgical procedures performed, 48% were in patients who fulfilled the criteria for AIDS. Further, 54 procedures were performed on an emergency basis (group A) and 66 were performed electively (group B). Overall, the surgical conditions that rarely affected the population without HIV infection presented diagnostic challenges; altered physiologic responses were observed even with routine conditions. Also, the HIV status was not always known at the time emergency procedures were undertaken. The latter included treatment of traumatic rectosigmoid perforation, shattered spleen, acute cholecystitis, and acute appendicitis. Etiologic features of intra-abdominal sepsis that are rarely seen in noninfected patients included multiple perforations resulting from cytomegalovirus enteritis, mesenteric lymphadenitis supprativum (atypical *Mycobactrium*), and primary peritonitis. The indications and spectrum of the elective procedures performed on infected patients reflected those performed in the noninfected population. Thirty-day morbidity rates were 19% in group A and 9% in group B; surgical mortality rates were 13% and 2%, respectively. Follow-up was avail-

Follow-Up of General Surgical Procedures Performed on Patients With HIV/AIDS

Surgical Survivors

Group	No. of Procedures	Surgical Mortality, No. (%)	No. of Procedures	Follow-up, No. (%)	AIDS Mortality			Alive	
					No. (%)	Mean Survival, wk	No. (%)	Mean Survival, wk
A	54	7 (13)	47	45 (80)	14 (35)	19	26 (65)	85
B	66	1 (2)	65	52 (80)	19 (37)	21	33 (63)	87

(Courtesy of Diettrich NA, Cacioppo JC, Kaplan G, et al: *Arch Surg* 126:860–866, 1991.)

able for the 92 surgical procedures (82%) not associated with mortality (table). For patients who were dead at follow-up, mean procedure-survivals were 19 weeks (group A) and 21 weeks (group B) for 33 procedures. For those who remained alive, the mean procedure-survival was 86 weeks for 59 procedures. No single preoperative factor significantly correlated with prognosis, although the combination of hypoalbuminemia and a history of opportunistic infection(s) was associated with short survival.

Implications.—Emergency and elective surgical procedures can be performed in patients with HIV/AIDS with acceptable morbidity and mortality. With the exception of tracheostomy, all procedures appear to provide, improve, or extend productivity and quality of life as defined by the patient.

▶ These articles are representative of a growing surgical literature related to patients with AIDS. LaRaja et al. (1) reported 36 patients with documented AIDS undergoing intra-abdominal surgery. Of 12 patients who underwent cholecystectomy, 9 had a calculus cholecystitis. Overall, 58% of the 36 patients had documented pathologic conditions that were secondary to AIDS. One third of the patients with cholecystitis died postoperatively. Miller et al. (2) reported 38 patients who underwent procedures for thoracic disease related to AIDS; here, the operative mortality was 26%.—S.I. Schwartz, M.D.

References

1. LaRaja RD, et al: *Surgery* 105:175, 1989.
2. Miller JI, et al: *J Thorac Cardiovasc Surg* 92:977, 1986.

2 Fluids, Electrolytes, and Nutrition

Colloids Versus Crystalloids in Fluid Resuscitation: An Analysis of Randomized Controlled Trials
Bisonni RS, Holtgrave DR, Lawler F, Marley DS (Univ of Oklahoma)
J Fam Pract 32:387–390, 1991   2–1

Introduction.—After 3 decades of controversy, it remains uncertain whether colloids or crystalloids are preferable for use in fluid resuscitation. Difficulty in predicting the effects of these fluids may be attributable in part to the fact that fluid behavior at the level of the pulmonary capillary membrane can vary with each patient's particular pathology.

Objective.—Mortality rates from randomized controlled trials comparing colloid with crystalloid fluid resuscitation were examined. Data were taken from studies of patients having major surgery on the abdominal aorta; injured, hypovolemic patients who underwent surgery; and patients with severe pulmonary failure, as evidenced by an intrapulmonary shunt exceeding 20% and x-ray findings of interstitial and intra-alveolar edema.

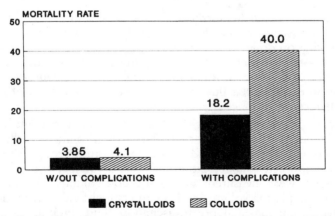

Fig 2–1.—Combined mortality rates in patients with and without complications receiving crystalloid and colloid resuscitation treatments. Those patients with complications had more severe conditions before treatment. (Courtesy of Bisonni RS. Holtgrave DR, Lawler F, et al: *J Fam Pract* 32:387–390, 1991.)

Findings.—There were no significant differences overall in mortality rates related to the use of colloids (21.25%) or crystalloids (13.4%) for resuscitation (Fig 2–1). The cost of each life saved was substantially lower when crystalloids were used instead of colloids ($45 vs. $1,493).

Recommendation.—Because colloid therapy confers no significant survival advantage, and because it is so much more expensive than crystalloid, the latter is preferred for use in fluid resuscitation.

▶ This is an interesting clinical study evaluating crystalloids and colloids in fluid resuscitation in a randomized, controlled trial of patients who sustained operative trauma, were hypovolemic, and had severe pulmonary failure. The results are very similar to the outcome of Velanovich's trials (1) on unrandomized injured patients, i.e., in this particular setting, no significant advantage could be seen for colloid over crystalloid. Because colloid is so much more expensive than crystalloid, the conclusion is that crystalloid therapy is preferable.—G.T. Shires, M.D.

Reference

1. Velanovich V: *Surgery* 105:65, 1989.

Colloid Oncotic Pressure and Body Water Dynamics in Septic and Injured Patients
Lucas CE, Ledgerwood AM, Rachwal WJ, Grabow D, Saxe JM (Wayne State Univ)
J Trauma 31:927–933, 1991   2–2

Introduction.—Both hemorrhagic shock (HS) and septic shock (SS) lead to extravascular relocation of large fluid volumes in response to fluid resuscitation designed to restore circulatory volume, vital signs, and organ function. This therapeutic fluid overload response often results in a 15% to 35% increase in total body weight. The physiology of postresuscitation extravascular fluid sequestration after treatment of HS and SS was characterized.

Patients and Methods.—Thirty-three severely injured patients with HS and 43 patients with severe SS secondary to peritonitis who had been resuscitated with blood and fluids made up the study group. Plasma volume, red blood cell volume, extracellular fluid volume, and colloid oncotic pressure were measured; and total blood volume, interstitial fluid space, and the plasma volume; and the interstitial fluid space ratio were calculated during maximal postresuscitation fluid retention as judged clinically by fluid retention, edema, positive fluid balance, and weight gain. A subgroup of 22 patients with SS and 22 with HS of equal body weight also were compared.

Results.—Both groups of patients had marked fluid retention in response to fluid resuscitation, resulting in weight gains ranging from 5 kg to 17 kg. Patients with SS had greater interstitial fluid space expansion than did patients with HS, who by inference had more intracellular expansion. Interstitial fluid space expansion correlated with reduced plasma colloid oncotic pressure in patients with SS, but not in patients with HS. In contrast, plasma colloid oncotic pressure correlated with plasma volume in patients with HS but not in those with SS. Thus the latter patients with greater interstitial fluid space expansion, which correlated with reduced plasma colloid oncotic pressure, more likely had increased capillary permeability, whereas patients with HS who had less interstitial fluid space expansion, which did not correlate with reduced plasma colloid oncotic pressure, probably had maintained capillary permeability with an altered interstitial fluid space matrix configuration that caused a reduction in protein exclusion.

Conclusion.—Although both groups of patients responded similarly to fluid resuscitation designed to restore circulatory effectiveness, the altered physiology in the extravascular spaces was highly dissimilar in that a septic insult appeared to have a greater effect on capillary membranes than did a traumatic insult.

▶ This fascinating study examined the fluid and electrolyte response to fluid resuscitation after either HS or SS. As expected, both groups of patients had marked fluid retention in response to fluid resuscitation, which was necessary to maintain hemodynamic stability. All patients gained weight immediately after resuscitation. Patients with SS had greater interstitial fluid space expansion. The latter correlated with reduced plasma colloid oncotic pressure in patients with SS but not in patients with HS. In contrast, plasma colloid oncotic pressure correlated with plasma volume only in those with HS. Consequently, the patients with SS probably had increased capillary permeability.

This study provides quantitative data that indicate a greater effect on capillary membrane leakage of protein (e.g., albumin) in sepsis than is seen in HS.—G.T. Shires, M.D.

Effects of Bicarbonate Therapy on Hemodynamics and Tissue Oxygenation in Patients With Lactic Acidosis: A Prospective, Controlled Clinical Study

Mathieu D, Neviere R, Billard V, Fleyfel M, Wattel F (Hôpital Calmette, Lille, France)
Crit Care Med 19:1352–1356, 1991   2–3

Background.—Although sodium bicarbonate therapy has been used to treat lactic acidosis for at least 30 years, increasing evidence suggests that bicarbonate may be of no benefit or may even be harmful in such cases. A prospective, randomized, placebo-controlled trial tested whether sodium bicarbonate therapy has negative hemodynamic effects in patients with lactic acidosis.

Methods.—The 8 men and 2 women studied were medical patients with acute circulatory problems and no severe renal failure. All of the patients had metabolic acidosis and increased arterial plasma lactate concentrations. At the beginning of 2 successive 1-hour study periods, the patients randomly received an intravenous injection of either 1 mmol of sodium bicarbonate per kg or an equal volume of sodium chloride. Hemodynamics and tissue oxygenation were monitored before and repeatedly during the 1-hour postinjection periods.

Results.—In these 10 critically ill patients, sodium bicarbonate increased arterial and venous pH, the serum bicarbonate concentration, and the partial pressure of CO_2 in arterial and venous blood. Sodium bicarbonate and sodium chloride produced similar hemodynamic responses. No changes were noted in tissue oxygenation, serum sodium concentration, osmolality, arterial and venous lactate, red blood cell 2,3-diphosphoglycerate, or hemoglobin affinity for oxygen.

Conclusion.—Previous research on the effects of sodium bicarbonate on lactic acidosis appears to be confirmed. Although the bicarbonate did not improve the hemodynamic variables, it did not worsen tissue oxygenation.

▶ This is another clinical trial using sodium bicarbonate as therapy in patients with lactic acidosis. This study, as many others, demonstrated that sodium chloride produces similar hemodynamic responses to sodium bicarbonate. In this particular study with relatively isotonic sodium bicarbonate, no changes were noted in tissue oxygenation, serum sodium concentration, osmolality, arterial venous lactate, red blood cell 2,3-DPG, or hemoglobin affinity for oxygen. Consequently, these studies, like many others, indicate that additional sodium bicarbonate in the treatment of lactic acidosis, presumably caused by a low-flow state, has no distinct advantage. Because all of the individuals studied were patients with low-flow problems, it is not surprising that no significant differences were found.—G.T. Shires, M.D.

Perioperative Total Parenteral Nutrition in Surgical Patients
Williford WO, for the Veterans Affairs Total Parenteral Nutrition Cooperative Study Group (DVA Med Ctr, Perry Point, Md)
N Engl J Med 325:525–532, 1991   2–4

Introduction.—Malnourished patients undergoing surgery are at greater risk for postoperative complications than are well-nourished patients. To determine the efficacy of perioperative total parenteral nutrition (TPN) in malnourished patients undergoing major intrathoracic or intraperitoneal operations, 395 such patients scheduled for laparotomy or noncardiac thoracotomy were studied.

Methods.—All patients underwent nutritional screening to confirm the baseline nutritional status; 192 were randomly assigned to receive TPN and 203 served as controls. The patients were given TPN for 7–15 days before operation and for 72 hours afterward. Patients in the control group did not receive perioperative TPN during the study period but were given it starting 72 hours after operation if indicated. Postoperative complications were monitored for 90 days, either by chart review in the hospital or by telephone interview after discharge home. Complications were classified as major or minor, and as infectious or noninfectious.

Results.—The 90-day mortality rates attributable to postoperative complications were 10.9% in the TPN group and 9.4% in controls. An additional 8 TPN patients and 3 controls died of disease progression during the 90-day follow-up period. The differences in mortality were statistically not significant. There were major complications during the first 30 days after surgery in 49 (25.5%) patients given TPN and in 50 (24.6%) controls. The overall complication rates after 30 days were 37% for patients given TPN and 36.5% for controls. The differences in major and overall complication rates were also not statistically significant. Controls, however, had slightly more noninfectious complications, whereas patients given TPN had slightly more infectious complications. When patients were subclassified as borderline, mildly, or severely malnourished, borderline and mildly malnourished patients had no demonstrable benefit from TPN, but severely malnourished TPN patients had fewer noninfectious complications than controls, with no concomitant increase in infectious complications.

Conclusion.—In the absence of other specific indications, the use of perioperative TPN to reduce postoperative complications should be limited to severely malnourished patients.

▶ This large cooperative study attempted to assess the benefits of TPN perioperatively in surgical patients. Nearly 400 patients undergoing laparotomy or noncardiac thoracotomy were studied. Roughly half of the group received TPN and the other half served as controls. Basically, the difference in the 90-day follow-up period in terms of complications was not significant. If one breaks down the groups further, however, the severely malnourished patients did have fewer noninfectious complications than the controls without a concomitant increase in infectious complications.

This study shows what many have thought, i.e., that a week to 10 days of perioperative TPN may be beneficial only in a very severely malnourished patient, not in most patients undergoing operative procedures.—G.T. Shires, M.D.

Polymyxin B Reduces Cecal Flora, TNF Production, and Hepatic Steatosis During Total Parental Nutrition in the Rat

Pappo I, Becovier H, Berry EM, Freund HR (Hebrew Univ-Hadassah Med School, Jerusalem)

J Surg Res 51:106–112, 1991   2–5

Background.—Hepatic complications frequently occur in patients without underlying liver disease who receive total parenteral nutrition (TPN). The range of abnormalities extends from a transient rise in liver enzymes to changes of portal fibrosis and periportal inflammation, and even fatal liver failure. Because intestinal bacteria have a role in various potentially hepatotoxic biochemical events, an attempt was made to learn whether endotoxin derived from the overgrowth of gram-negative organisms can produce TPN-related hepatic steatosis.

Methods.—Rats underwent jugular vein cannulation and then were assigned to receive an infusion of normal saline or a TPN formula containing 25% dextrose and 4.25% amino acids, totaling 36 calories and 3 g of protein per 100 g daily. Groups of animals received orally administered polymyxin B; a combination of neomycin, metronidazole, and vancomycin; or both treatments. After 1 week the animals were sacrificed and peritoneal macrophages were examined for spontaneous production of tumor necrosis factor (TNF). In addition, bacterial translocation to mesenteric nodes was quantified.

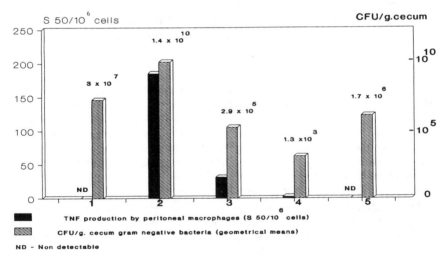

Fig 2–2.—Spontaneous production of tumor necrosis factor by peritoneal macrophages ($S_{50}/10^6$ cells ± SEM); and colony-forming units per gram (CFU/g) cecum of gram-negative bacteria (lactose positive and negative) of catheterized free feeding rats (1); total parenteral nutrition rats (2); and total parenteral nutrition rats receiving various combinations of orally administered antibiotics; polymyxin B (3); polymyxin B + neomycin + vancomycin + metronidazole (4); neomycin + vancomycin + metronidazole (5), $P < .005$: group 2 vs. groups 1, 4, 5; $P < .03$: group 2 vs. groups 3 and 4. (Courtesy of Pappo I, Becovier H, Berry EM, et al: *J Surg Res* 51:106–112, 1991.)

Findings.—Fat levels in the liver increased consistently after infusion of TPN solution, but significantly lower levels of total fat and triglycerides occurred when bowel decontamination was carried out. Polymyxin B alone was most effective. All antibiotic-treated groups had lower counts of gram-negative bacteria in the cecum than did control animals. Bacterial translocation to the mesenteric nodes was similar in all groups. Macrophage production of TNF was higher in TPN-treated rats than in either control animals or those given TPN with antimicrobial therapy (Fig 2–2).

Conclusions.—In addition to an effective antibacterial action in the gut, polymyxin B counters the adverse effects of endotoxin and the production of TNF in response to endotoxin. These effects may help to explain the protection provided by polymyxin B against endotoxin-associated hepatic toxicity and steatosis.

▶ This is another study evaluating the value of polymyxin B as a bowel sterilizer to reduce the production of TNF in the bowel as well as bacterial translocation to mesenteric lymph nodes. Fat levels in the liver increased consistently after infusion of TPN solution, but significantly lower levels of total fat and triglycerides occurred when bowel decontamination was carried out with polymyxin B. The bacteria count in the cecum was lower whether polymyxin B or some other combination of drugs (e.g., neomycin, metronidazole, or vancomycin) was used. Interestingly, bacterial translocation to mesenteric lymph nodes was similar in all groups. However, macrophage production of TNF was higher in the TPN-treated animals than in control animals or those given TPN with antimicrobial therapy.

Although this does not resolve the controversy concerning the significance of bacterial translocation and its relation to bowel flora, it does corroborate several other studies indicating that TNF production can be reduced by bowel sterilization.—G.T. Shires, M.D.

Length of Care in Patients With Severe Burns With or Without Early Enteral Nutritional Support: A Retrospective Study
Garrel DR, Davignon I, Lopez D (Univ of Montreal)
J Burn Care Rehabil 12:85–90, 1991   2–6

Introduction.—The question of how early enteral nutrition influences the length of needed care in burn-injured patients was examined in 25 patients having burns involving more than 20% of the total body surface.

Study Plan.—Twelve patients received nutritional support starting after the third postinjury day, when there was evidence of intestinal peristalsis. Eight patients treated at a later time, who were clinically similar to the others received planned nutritional support starting within 48 hours after injury. Feedings were given through a nasoduodenal or

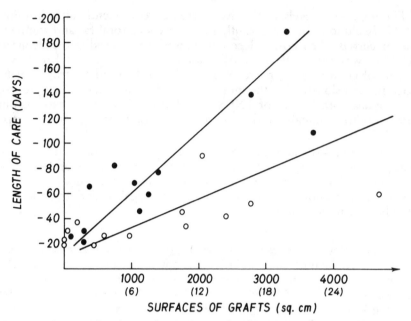

Fig 2–3.—Regression lines between length of care and surfaces of skin grafts in both groups (group 1: *filled circles*; group 2: *open circles*). Numbers in parentheses are percent of body surface area used for grafting. (Courtesy of Garrel DR, Davignon I, Lopez D: *J Burn Care Rehabil* 12:85–90, 1991.)

nasogastric tube. These patients received a protein supplement when the formula failed to provide 2 g of protein per kg daily.

Observations.—The patients given earlier nutritional support received more energy and nitrogen in the first 2 weeks. The length of care was much shorter in this group, and it correlated significantly with age and with the intakes of energy and nitrogen. The relationship between the surface grafted and the length of care differed significantly in the 2 treatment groups (Fig 2–3); only surfaces grafted were independently related to the length of care.

Conclusions.—Early enteral nutritional support may significantly enhance wound healing in burn-injured patients and shorten the length of care. Intraduodenal feeding within 48 hours of injury may be indicated in severely burned patients.

▶ This is another study of early enteral nutritional support in patients with severe burns. In this particular series, it appeared that the hospital stay was shorter because wound healing was enhanced in burn-injured patients. Intraduodenal feeding was begun within 48 hours of injury in patients with more than 20% of the total body surface area burn.—G.T. Shires, M.D.

Immediate Enteral Feeding in Burn Patients Is Safe and Effective

McDonald WS, Sharp CW Jr, Deitch EA (Louisiana State Univ, Shreveport)
Ann Surg 213:177–183, 1991   2–7

Background.—The hypermetabolic state characteristic of the postburn period can lead to visceral protein loss, impaired host antibacterial defenses, and delayed wound healing. There is increasing experimental evidence that enteral alimentation is helpful, but immediate enteral feeding has not been widely accepted clinically. Usually, enteral feedings are not begun until after the phase of acute fluid resuscitation, when gastrointestinal function has returned to normal.

Study Design.—A review was made of 106 consecutive patients with burns over at least 20% of their total body surface in whom enteral feeding began within 6 hours of injury. The primary formula used was Ensure-Plus (1.5 kcal/mL), but infant formula was given to some of the youngest patients. Feeds were given by nasogastric tube at 2-hour intervals. Older children and adults received feedings in an initial volume of 60 mL.

Results.—More than 80% of patients absorbed at least some of their tube feedings on the day of injury; 15% vomited. By day 4 the mean amount of enterally absorbed calories exceeded 1,800 kcal. Patients with more extensive burn injuries tended to absorb fewer enteral calories (Fig

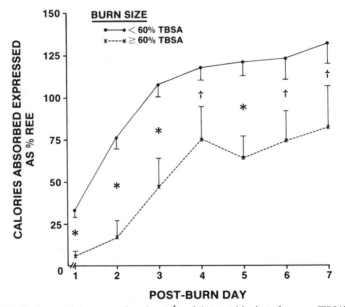

Fig 2–4.—Patients with burns over less than 60% of their total body surface area (TBSA) absorbed more calories than patients with more extensive burns. Data expressed as mean ± SEM % resting energy expenditure * $P < .01$; † $P \leq .05$. (Courtesy of McDonald WS. Sharp CW Jr. Deitch EA: *Ann Surg* 213 177–183, 1991.)

2–4). Mortality correlated inversely with the amount of enteral calories absorbed, especially in the first 3 days after injury.

Conclusions.—Immediate enteral feeding appears to be an effective and safe means of delivering nutritional support to patients with major burn injuries. This finding is consistent with observations in trauma victims that significant infectious complications are less frequent when immediate postoperative enteral nutrition is given rather than parenteral nutrition.

▶ This treatment approach is an attempt to minimize cytokine activation and bacterial invasion by immediate enteric feeding after a defined injury such as a burn. In this study, patients with total body surface area burns of more than 20% were given enteral feeding beginning within 6 hours of injury. These feedings were delivered by nasogastric tube, and about 80% of the patients absorbed at least some of their tube feedings on the day of injury. Vomiting occurred in 15% of the patients, but by the fourth postburn day the amount of enterally absorbed calories exceeded 1,800 kcal.

Obviously, early enteric feeding is coming to be seen as clinically more advantageous, with more series being published such as that reported here. It would appear, however, that defined elemental diets should be replaced with whole food as quickly as possible in terms of reduction of activation of tumor necrosis factor and bacterial translocation.—G.T. Shires, M.D.

3 Shock

A Circulating Factor(s) Mediates Cell Depolarization in Hemorrhagic Shock
Evans JA, Darlington DN, Gann DS (Univ of Maryland)
Ann Surg 213:549–557, 1991   3–1

Background.—Hypoperfusion appears to lead to cell depolarization in hemorrhagic shock; however, the mechanism is unclear. A bioassay for 1 or more presumptive circulating factors was used to demonstrate a high-molecular-weight substance that depolarizes cells after hemorrhage in rats.

Methods.—The bioassay involved loading suspensions of single cell lines with the potential-sensitive fluorescent dye bis-(1,3-dibutylbarbituric acid) trimethine oxonal. The suspensions were then exposed for 30 minutes to rat plasma drawn either before or after the rats were bled 20 mL/kg. The rats' mean arterial pressure was less than 40 mm Hg. The cell types tested included various rat cells; blood cells from cats, dogs, and pigs; mouse skeletal muscle; and human intestinal smooth muscle.

Results.—Partial depolarization was seen in plasma drawn after, but not before, hemorrhage. This was the case regardless of cell type (including skeletal and smooth muscle, liver, adrenal, kidney, and red blood cell) or species. The circulating factor appeared to have a molecular weight of more than 10,000 daltons, because it was not removed by dialysis; it appeared within 5 minutes of shock. The depolarization amplitude increased as a function of the plasma concentration and demonstrated saturation kinetics indicating specific receptor binding. Neither tumor necrosis factor nor platelet-activating factor, together or alone, was effective in this system.

Conclusions.—This sensitive in vitro bioassay appears to allow identification of the plasma factors that mediate cell depolarization, as well as definition of the intracellular mechanisms responsible for depolarization. The system is noninvasive, avoiding the cell injury caused by impalement with electrodes; it also provides stable measurements. These techniques are being used to monitor chromatographic purification of the active principle.

▶ This fascinating study uses an entirely new technique to demonstrate a circulating factor that is operative in depolarizing membranes in a variety of organs after hemorrhagic shock. These authors developed a sensitive in vitro bioassay to allow identification of plasma factors that mediate cell depolarization in hemorrhagic shock. The system is appealing in that it is noninvasive. This technique has the added advantage in that the depolarization occurred when the substance was identified in a variety of cell types, including skeletal and smooth muscle, liver, adrenal, kidney, and even a red blood cell. The assay appears to be sensitive because the factor appeared within 5 minutes of actual development of significant hypotension. Interestingly, neither tumor necrosis factor nor platelet-activating factor, together or alone, was effective in causing the polarization measured by this sensitive new technique.—G.T. Shires, M.D.

Tumor Necrosis Factor (Cachectin) in the Biology of Septic Shock Syndrome
Tracey KJ (New York Hosp-Cornell Med Ctr)
Circ Shock 35:123–128, 1991   3–2

Background.—The mortality associated with the septic shock syndrome remains high despite the availability of broad-spectrum antibiotics for 3 decades. The principal mediators of septic shock are toxic host-derived factors such as cachectin or tumor necrosis factor (TNF). The biology of TNF in septic shock syndrome, and the potential for inhibiting this cytokine, were reviewed.

Biochemistry and Biosynthesis.—Human TNF is a 17-kD polypeptide cytokine composed of 157 amino acids. Within minutes after exposure to a variety of invasive stimuli, macrophages and other immunocompetent cells synthesize large quantities of mature TNF. When released into the circulation or tissues, the biologically active form of TNF mediates a diverse range of inflammatory and metabolic effects on body tissues by interaction via 1 of 2 specific membrane receptors.

Inhibition of TNF.—In a model of lethal gram-negative bacteremia in baboons, TNF was neutralized with monoclonal anti-TNF antibodies. The development of shock was dependent on TNF activity and not bacteremia. The anti-TNF antibodies completely protected the animals when given 2 hours before exposure to bacteria. The protective effect of the antibodies may be attributable to the combined effects of inhibiting the direct toxicity of TNF and of preventing the induction of other cytokines. In a patient with septic shock, the complications of TNF toxicity may result from the effects of TNF in the tissues, even though the TNF remains undetected or is neutralized in the circulation.

Conclusion.—Although TNF appears to have been conserved throughout evolution because of its activities in host defense, overproduction can trigger the septic shock syndrome. Anti-TNF therapy is being investigated in clinical trials; it offers promise in reducing the high risk of death in patients with septic shock.

▶ This invited review article traces the evolution of TNF in the biology of the septic shock syndrome. As indicated in this paper, inhibition of TNF by pretreatment with monoclonal antibody prevents not only the consequences of septic shock as known clinically, but also the induction of other cytokines. It is clearly pointed out that the toxicity from TNF may well be caused by its effects in tissues, therefore making it a paracrine substance. The potential of anti-TNF therapy is being investigated in many centers, and even in clinical trials, in an attempt to reduce the high mortality rate associated with septic shock.—G.T. Shires, M.D.

Anti-TNF Monoclonal Antibodies Prevent Haemorrhage-Induced Suppression of Kupffer Cell Antigen Presentation and MHC Class II Antigen Expression

Ertel W, Morrison MH, Ayala A, Perrin MM, Chaudry IH (Michigan State Univ)
Immunology 74:290–297, 1991   3–3

Background.—Hemorrhage not accompanied by significant tissue injury can produce serious disturbances in immune function, increasing vulnerability to sepsis. The uptake, processing, and presentation of antigens by Kupffer cells and the expression of major histocompatibility complex (MHC) class II antigen (Ia) both are much reduced after hemorrhage, at the same time as plasma levels of tumor necrosis factor (TNF) and interleukins 1 and 6 are increased.

Study Design.—Mice were pretreated intraperitoneally with either antimurine TNF antibody or saline, and 20 minutes later were bled to a mean blood pressure of 35 mm Hg for 1 hour. Fluid resuscitation followed Kupffer cells were isolated from plasma 2 hours and 24 hours later and co-cultured with a cell clone to measure antigen presentation. Expression of MHC class Ia was determined by direct immunofluorescence.

Observations.—Hemorrhage increased circulating levels of TNF by more than 200% at 2 hours and by 76% at 24 hours. Treatment with anti-TNF antibody prevented this effect. The hemorrhage-induced rise in interleukin-6 also was abolished by pretreatment with antibody at 2 hours but not at 24 hours. The effects of hemorrhage in suppressing antigen presentation by Kupffer cells and the expression of Ia were lessened in antibody-pretreated mice. The production of interleukin-1 and TNF by Kupffer cells was further increased.

Implications.—These findings suggest that TNF has a critical role in initiating and regulating antigen presentation by Kupffer cells, the expression of MHC class II antigen, and cytokine production following hemorrhage.

▶ This study describing pretreatment with anti-TNF antibody demonstrated that the downstream effects of an increase in TNF induced by hemorrhage can be prevented. Interleukins 1 and 6, as well as TNF production, were abrogated by pretreatment with TNF antibody. It is not surprising then that the effects of hemorrhage and suppressing antigen presentation by Kupffer cells and expression of MHC class II antigens also were lessened by pretreatment with TNF antibody. This is another study showing the proximal role of TNF in immunosuppressive effects after hemorrhage, sepsis, and trauma.—G.T. Shires, M.D.

Diltiazem Restores IL-2, IL-3, IL-6, and IFN-γ Synthesis and Decreases Host Susceptibility to Sepsis Following Hemorrhage

Meldrum DR, Ayala A, Perrin MM, Ertel W, Chaudry IH (Michigan State Univ)
J Surg Res 51:158–164, 1991   3–4

Background.—Calcium channel blockers reportedly have beneficial effects on cell and organ function after endotoxic shock, organ ischemia, and reperfusion; however, their effects on immune responses after a low-flow condition are unknown. Whether diltiazem, a water-soluble calcium channel blocker, influences the production of lymphokines or alters host susceptibility to sepsis after hemorrhage was examined.

Methods.—Mice were bled to a mean blood pressure of 35 mm Hg for 1 hour, after which the shed blood was reinfused along with Ringer's lactate. Diltiazem in doses of 400 µg/kg, 800 µg/kg, and 2,400 µg/kg was given intravenously after return of the shed blood.

Observations.—Hemorrhage significantly decreased the ability of splenic lymphocytes to produce interleukins 2 (IL-2), 3 (IL-3), and 6 (IL-6), as well as interferon-γ (IFN-γ). The administration of diltiazem, 400 µg/kg, but not 2,400 µg/kg, restored the ability of the lymphocytes to produce IL-2, IL-3, IL-6, and IFN-γ. The lower dose of diltiazem also significantly improved survival after hemorrhage and subsequent exposure to septic insult.

Implications.—Calcium influx appears to be important in the lymphocyte depression and subsequent immunosuppression associated with a low-flow state. Diltiazem may offer a new means of reducing vulnerability to sepsis after trauma and shock.

▶ The role of the calcium channel blockers was investigated in preventing cell and organ damage following endotoxic shock, organ ischemia, and reperfusion. The calcium channel blocker diltiazem, given intravenously in moderate doses, restored the ability of the lymphocytes to produce IL-2, -3, and -6, as well as IFN-γ. These changes also were accompanied by significantly improved survival after hemorrhage and subsequent exposure to septic insult. The authors therefore suggest that calcium channel blockers may offer new means of reducing vulnerability to sepsis after trauma and shock.—G.T. Shires, M.D.

Interferon γ Increases Sensitivity to Endotoxin
Jurkovich GJ, Mileski WJ, Maier RV, Winn RK, Rice CL (Univ of Washington)
J Surg Res 51:197–203, 1991   3–5

Background.—A number of immune alterations are associated with severe injury, including depressed interferon-γ (IFN-γ) production. The use of IFN-γ to reverse depressed macrophage function after severe trauma has been proposed, but an inappropriate inflammatory response to an otherwise minor insult is a possible adverse effect of using IFN-γ to enhance the immune system.

Study Design.—Studies were carried out in rabbits to determine whether IFN-γ disposes normal animals to a pathophysiologic response to endotoxin infusion. Groups of animals received a subclinical dose of E *Scherichia coli* lipopolysaccharide alone, recombinant rabbit interferon in a dose of 5 μg/kg subcutaneously for 3 days, or IFN-γ followed by endotoxin. Radioiodinated albumin was given before sacrifice and bronchoalveolar lavage carried out.

Findings.—Animals given both IFN and endotoxin had significantly lower cardiac output, PO_2, and white blood cell counts than the others had, as well as an increased ratio of ^{125}I-albumin in lavage fluid and plasma. In contrast to immunosuppressed animals, pretreatment of normal animals with IFN-γ increased the pathophysiologic responses to endotoxin.

Conclusions.—Overstimulation of the normal immune system can exaggerate the immunoinflammatory response to what otherwise would be an inconsequential stimulus. This effect must be kept in mind when the use of immunomodulating agents such as IFN-γ is considered.

▶ This interesting study suggests that IFN-γ itself may have a modulating effect on the immunodepression associated with significant injury. However, as the authors point out, an inappropriate inflammatory response to an otherwise minor insult is a possible adverse effect of using IFN-γ to enhance the immune system. It is obvious from this article and others like it that the role of the downstream cascade eicosanoids and other cytokines must be carefully evaluated because one is treating the downstream effects of the proximal mediators tumor necrosis factor and platelet-activating factor.—G.T. Shires, M.D.

Nitrogen Oxide Levels in Patients After Trauma and During Sepsis

Ochoa JB, Udekwu AO, Billiar TR, Curran RD, Cerra FB, Simmons RL, Peitzman AB (Univ of Pittsburgh; Univ of Minnesota)
Ann Surg 214:621–626, 1991
                                                                        3–6

Introduction.—During the 1980s, researchers discovered some of the endogenous sources of nitrates and nitrites (NO_2^-/NO_3^-). One important source is through the conversion of L-arginine to L-citrulline and nitric oxide. The latter is a mediator having numerous functions, including the regulation of vascular tone. Nitric oxide also has a role in macrophage-mediated cytostasis and microbiostasis. A group of 39 critically ill injured and septic patients was studied to determine the relationship between nitric oxide production and the hyperdynamic state.

Methods.—The patients were divided into 3 groups according to diagnosis and clinical course. On admission, the 17 surgical patients in group I (average age, 60 years) were either clinically septic or had severe inflammatory processes. Group II (average age, 45 years) included 14 trauma victims who had uneventful recoveries after injury. The 8 trauma patients (average age, 47 years) in group III became clinically septic during their stay in the intensive care unit. All of the patients were assessed daily, and blood samples were obtained for NO_2^-/NO_3^- and endotoxin assay.

Results.—High plasma levels of NO_2^-/NO_3^-, the stable end products of nitric oxide, were seen in general surgery patients with clinical sepsis; this finding correlated with the severity of disease. The high NO_2^-/NO_3^- levels were associated with low systemic vascular resistance and high endotoxin levels. Trauma patients, even when they had clinical sepsis, had levels of nitrogen oxide lower than those found in normal controls.

Conclusion.—Nitric oxide levels may mediate the vasodilation seen in sepsis. It is unknown which cells are the main sources of nitric oxide in humans.

▶ This interesting study sought the final common denominator in cellular injury in critically ill and septic patients. In addition to free oxygen radicals and hydroxyl radicals, it is clear that high plasma levels of nitrogen oxide, the stable end products of nitric oxide, may also be part of the final common denominator correlating with disease severity. The high nitric oxide level may mediate the vasodilation seen in sepsis. The source of nitric oxide generation was not specifically described or discovered in these particular studies.—G.T. Shires, M.D.

Plasma Lipid Peroxides and Antioxidants in Human Septic Shock

Ogilvie AC, Groeneveld ABJ, Straub JP, Thijs LG (Free Univ Hosp, Amsterdam)
Intens Care Med 17:40–44, 1991
                                                                        3–7

Introduction.—Oxygen free radicals may have an important role in septic shock and the resultant tissue injury. Free radical activity is described in a wide range of disorders that may relate to septic shock, including adult respiratory distress syndrome and multiple organ system failure.

Study Plan.—Plasma levels of the lipid peroxides malondialdehyde (MDA), conjugated dienes, and fluorescent products, as well as the antioxidants α-tocopherol and glutathione peroxidase (GSH-Px) activity and its cofactor selenium, were measured in 12 patients in septic shock; 7 patients survived.

Findings.—Initially, levels of MDA and fluorescent products were elevated, whereas α-tocopherol and selenium were depressed compared with control values. Levels of conjugated dienes and GSH-Px activity were in the normal range. Patients who died had higher initial levels of MDA and fluorescent products and lower initial selenium levels than those who survived. The last measured value for GSH-Px activity was lower in nonsurvivors than survivors.

Conclusions.—Plasma levels of lipid peroxides are increased early in the course of septic shock whereas levels of the antioxidant α-tocopherol are depressed at the same time. Apparently, oxygen free radicals form in human septic shock. Antioxidant treatment (e.g., vitamin E supplementation) might limit tissue injury during septic shock by countering lipid peroxidation.

▶ This is another of the many articles stating that lipid peroxidation in human septic shock is apparent with the generation of oxygen free radicals, which in turn cause tissue injury. These authors actually measured the levels of lipid peroxidation products and found them to be elevated. They therefore suggest that the antioxidants such as vitamin E may well limit tissue injury during septic shock by countering lipid peroxidation. This inference was made by a number of authors in the past year.—G.T. Shires, M.D.

Gastric Mucosal Cytoprotection in the Rat by Scavenging Oxygen-Derived Free Radicals
Salim AS (The Royal Infirmary, Glasgow)
Am J Med Sci 302:287–291, 1991   3–8

Introduction.—Oxygen-derived free radicals have been implicated in the pathogenesis of ischemic injury to the gastrointestinal mucosa. Whether scavenging oxygen-derived free radicals would act as cytoprotective agents, preventing or minimizing ischemic injury in the rat gastric mucosa, was investigated.

Methods.—Ischemic mucosal injury was produced in rats by the intraperitoneal administration of 5 mg of reserpine per kg or 50 mg of serotonin per kg. The potentially cytoprotective agents investigated were allopurinol and dimethyl sulfoxide (DMSO); both are scavengers of hydroxyl radicals. Allopurinol is also an inhibitor of xanthine oxidase, the enzyme responsible for the formation of superoxide anions. The rats underwent pretreatment with the scavengers (at different concentrations) for 2 days before the induced ischemic mucosal injury.

Results.—The animals were significantly protected against both reserpine and serotonin injury by 2 days of pretreatment with either 1 mL of 1% allopurinol per day or DMSO. More effective, however, were the 2% solutions of each agent. With the 2% concentration, injury was limited to 40% of the rats injected with respirine and 20% of the rats that received serotonin. In addition, the 5% solutions completely protected the rat stomach without significantly influencing the H+ output.

Conclusion.—Oxygen-derived free radicals are directly implicated in the development of ischemia-induced acute gastric mucosal injury. Scavenging of these radicals offers protection against such injury without affecting acid secretion.

▶ This is another article indicating that oxygen-derived free radicals are implicated in ischemic injury, in this instance, in the gastrointestinal mucosa. In this experimental study, ischemic mucosal injury was produced by the use of reserpine and/or serotonin. The cytoprotective agents used were allopurinol and DMSO, both of which are scavengers of hydroxyl radicals. Allopurinol is also an inhibitor of xanthine oxidase, the enzyme responsible for the formation of superoxide anions.

Without question, the oxygen free radical and hydroxyl radical scavengers did significantly influence the development of ischemia-induced acute gastric mucosal injury. The problem with this study, as with so many oxygen free radical scavenger studies, is that the substances used for scavenging had to be given before the ischemic injury, suggesting that the oxygen free radical formations could have been influenced at the time of its original generation. This form of therapy will certainly need improving if the scavengers are to be used after ischemic injury occurs.—G.T. Shires, M.D.

Effect of Oxygen-Free Radical Scavengers on Survival in Sepsis
Powell RJ, Machiedo GW, Rush BF Jr, Dikdan GS (Univ of Medicine and Dentistry of New Jersey–New Jersey Med School)
Am Surg 57:86–88, 1991   3–9

Introduction.—Studies have shown that the oxygen-free radicals generated during sepsis have immunologic and hemodynamic implications in the pathophysiology of this condition. The development of oxygen free radical scavengers offers a possible treatment for life-threatening episodes of endotoxic shock and sepsis. The effects of oxygen free radical scavengers on survival were examined in an animal model of intraperitoneal sepsis.

Methods.—A group of 85 male Sprague-Dawley rats was evaluated. After cecal ligation and puncture (CLP), the 85 rats were randomized into 1 of 5 groups: 32 served as controls; 10 underwent pretreatment with α-tocopherol (PRE-AT); 12 were treated with intravenous AT at the time of CLP and again at 4 hours after CLP; 13 were treated with 3 mg of intravenous U78517F per kg at the time of CLP and again 4 hours later; and 18 received 3 mg of U74006F per kg, also administered at the time of CLP and 4 hours later. Survival was determined at 24, 36, 48, and 72 hours.

Results.—Only the groups given PRE-AT and U78517 had significant improvement in survival at 24 hours. When compared with the controls, the groups given PRE-AT, U78517F, and U74006F had a significantly higher rate of survival from 36 hours to completion of the study at 72 hours.

Conclusion.—Oxygen free radical scavengers appear to improve survival in sepsis. The scavengers U78517F and U74006F were effective without pretreatment, whereas AT was effective only as pretreatment.

▶ The authors studying red blood cell deformability in response to sepsis have extended this study to measure the effectiveness of various oxygen free radical scavengers on survival from sepsis. The findings indicate that oxygen free radical scavengers that improve survival in sepsis can experimentally be more effective that the use of AT, which is also an oxygen free radical scavenger. These experimental antioxidants appear to have more potent oxygen free radical scavenging properties than AT.—G.T. Shires, M.D.

Oxygen Free Radicals: Effect on Red Cell Deformability in Sepsis
Powell RJ, Machiedo GW, Rush BF Jr, Dikdan G (Univ of Medicine and Dentistry of New Jersey–New Jersey Med School)
Crit Care Med 19:732–735, 1991   3–10

Background.—Recent work suggests that organ failure during sepsis follows a decline in nutrient blood flow. Red blood cell deformability is reduced in the septic state, and this may have the effect of impeding microcirculatory flow. Because oxygen free radicals, which are generated during sepsis, compromise red blood cell deformability, the effects of the free radical scavenger α-tocopherol on red blood cell deformability, organ perfusion, and survival during experimental sepsis were examined.

Methods.—Rats were subjected to a sham procedure or cecal ligation and puncture. Some animals were pretreated with α-tocopherol before cecal ligation and puncture.

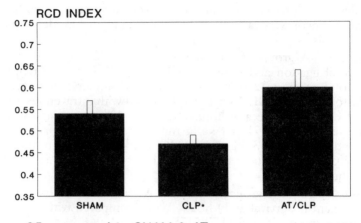

* p‹.05 compared to SHAM & AT groups

Fig 3–1.—Comparison of red blood cell deformability (RCD) index measurements between sham group (n = 13), cecal ligation and puncture group (CLP) (n = 13), and α-tocopherol/cecal ligation and puncture group (AT/CLP) (n = 8). Data are presented as mean ± SD. *P < .05 compared with sham and α-tocopherol groups. (Courtesy of Powell RJ, Machiedo CW, Rush BF Jr, et al: *Crit Care Med* 19:732–735, 1991.)

Findings.—Red blood cell deformability was significantly less after cecal ligation and puncture than after a sham procedure. Pretreatment with α-tocopherol prevented the reduction in deformability (Fig 3–1). There were no differences in arterial pH, but animals treated with α-tocopherol had a relatively high mixed venous pH and arterial-venous oxygen content difference. Animals treated with α-tocopherol survived significantly better than untreated animals undergoing cecal ligation and puncture.

Conclusions.—An oxygen free radical scavenger can prevent altered red blood cell deformability in sepsis. Normal red blood cell deformability is associated with a lack of significant peripheral shunting, improved perfusion, and better survival.

▶ This study took as a given that organ failure following sepsis is associated with the generation of oxygen free radicals. These oxygen free radicals can come from many sources, but most likely they are generated by cytokine activity. This study measured the effect of oxygen free radicals on red blood cell deformability, therefore potentially impeding microcirculatory flow. Red blood cell deformability was significantly less after sepsis compared to a sham procedure, and pretreatment with the antioxidant α-tocopherol prevented a reduction in deformability. Furthermore, there was increased survival among α-tocopherol-treated animals. Consequently, these authors believe that an antioxidant oxygen free radical scavenger such as α-tocopherol may be advantageous in the treatment of sepsis.—G.T. Shires, M.D.

Differential Pathophysiology of Bacterial Translocation After Thermal Injury and Sepsis

Jones WG II, Barber AE, Minei JP, Fahey TJ III, Shires GT III, Shires GT (Cornell Univ)

Ann Surg 214:24–30, 1991   3–11

Introduction.—Gut barrier failure after an uncomplicated injury is resolved within several days. In a chronic injury state (e.g., infection after burns), however, gut barrier dysfunction is more pronounced. Bacterial translocation occurs transiently after thermal injury and may result from an ischemic intestinal insult. Continued intestinal ischemia was evaluated in the ongoing bacterial translocation associated with sepsis after injury.

Methods.—Male Wistar rats were randomized to 1 of 4 groups; 30% burn injury with *Pseudomonas aeruginosa* wound infections (BI); BI plus fluid resuscitation (BI + Fluid); BI after pretreatment with allopurinol to inhibit xanthine oxidase (BI + Allo); or BI after azapropazone pretreatment to inhibit neutrophil degranulation (BI + Aza). The rats were studied on postburn days 1, 4, and 7 for evidence of bacterial translocation and intestinal lipid peroxidation.

Results.—As expected, the combination of burn injury and infection resulted in cachexia. The wasting associated with burn wound sepsis was not significantly prevented by treatment with either allopurinol or azapropazone; however, fluid resuscitation lessened weight loss versus all other groups on postburn days 4 and 7. Compared with the BI groups, the other 3 treatment groups had significantly reduced rates of bacterial translocation and ileal lipid peroxidation. All 4 of the groups had equally high rates of bacterial translocation associated with onset of sepsis on postburn days 4 and 7, without evidence of further intestinal lipid peroxidation.

Conclusion.—The chronic gut barrier failure associated with sepsis after injury appears to occur independently of continued intestinal ischemia. The systemic progression of bacterial translocation probably reflects changes in host responses associated with the development of sepsis.

▶ This study clearly indicates that bacterial translocation from the bowel occurs transiently after thermal injury. The investigation looked into whether this was from an ischemic intestinal insult. To produce continued translocation, the burn injury was compounded by *Pseudomonas* wound infection.

With prolonged bacterial translocation, it appeared that the initial translocation occurring in the burn injury alone could be lessened by reducing oxygen free radical formation through the use of allopurinol pretreatment to inhibit xanthine oxidase or azapropazone to inhibit neutrophil degranulation. The infected burn animals resuscitated with fluids, allopurinol, or azapropazone all had reduced rates of bacterial translocation and ileal lipid peroxidation acutely after thermal injury, but all groups had equally high rates of translocation associated with onset of sepsis without evidence of further intestinal lipid peroxidation.

These data indicate that the chronic gut barrier failure associated with sepsis after injury occurs independently of continued intestinal ischemia.—G.T. Shires, M.D.

Endotoxin-Induced Bacterial Translocation and Mucosal Permeability: Role of Xanthine Oxidase, Complement Activation, and Macrophage Products

Deitch EA, Specian RD, Berg RD (Louisiana State Univ, Shreveport)
Crit Care Med 19:785–791, 1991
3–12

Introduction.—Nonlethal doses of endotoxin can injure the intestinal mucosal barrier and promote bacterial translocation from the gut to systemic organs. The role of cytokines and complement activation in the pathogenesis of endotoxin-induced mucosal injury and bacterial translocation was investigated in normal outbred mice, complement-deficient mice, macrophage-hyporesponsive mice, and Sprague-Dawley rats.

Methods.—Mice of all 3 strains were killed 24 hours after either endotoxin or saline challenge and their organs were cultured for translocating bacteria. The intestinal mucosal structure of the ileum was analyzed by light microscopy. Outbred mice were used as positive controls as these animals are endotoxin responsive and have an intact complement system. In the next set of experiments, the ability of a polycolonal antitumor necrosis factor (TNF) antibody to prevent endotoxin-induced bacterial translocation was tested in outbred mice. In the last set of experiments, jejunal and ileal intestinal permeability was examined in Sprague-Dawley rats 2–4 hours after endotoxin or saline challenge. The ability of pretreatment with the competitive xanthine oxidase inhibitor allopurinol to prevent endotoxin-induced increased intestinal permeability also was tested.

Results.—In all 3 mouse strains, endotoxin challenge caused bacteria to translocate from the gut to a significant percentage of mesenteric lymph nodes, whereas mesenteric lymph nodes in saline-challenged controls were sterile. There was no significant difference between the 3 strains in the frequency of endotoxin-induced bacterial translocation. Thus neither complement nor macrophage activation is required for endotoxin-induced bacterial translocation to occur. Most mice killed 24 hours after endotoxin challenge had villous edema compared with saline-challenged controls. Pretreatment with anti-TNF antibody did not prevent endotoxin-induced bacterial translocation, mucosal injury, or disruption of the gut flora. Endotoxin-induced ileal permeability but not jejunal permeability was increased after pretreatment with allopurinol, indicating that endotoxin promotes bacterial translocation primarily by altering intestinal permeability.

Conclusion.—Endotoxin-induced bacterial translocation, mucosal injury, and ileal permeability are mediated by xanthine oxidase activation and not by complement activation or the release of macrophage products.

▶ This interesting study attempted to differentiate endotoxin-induced bacterial translocation and mucosal permeability etiologically. Its conclusions indicate that the role of xanthine oxidase, rather than complement activation or macrophage products, is the important one. This fits with a number of other recent studies indicating that the generation of oxygen free radicals at the cell level, as a result of lipid peroxidation brought about via the xanthine oxidate pathway, is the critical final common denominator in septic injury. Although it is true that this pathway is probably turned on by cytokines, it nevertheless appears that the final injury is at the cell membrane level.—G.T. Shires, M.D.

Effect of Ibuprofen in Patients With Severe Sepsis: A Randomized, Double-Blind, Multicenter Study

Haupt MT, Jastremski MS, Clemmer TP, Metz CA, Goris GB, and the Ibuprofen Study Group (Detroit Receiving Hosp)
Crit Care Med 19:1339–1347, 1991   3–13

Introduction.—Both laboratory and clinical studies suggest that ibuprofen may be of value in treating sepsis and septic shock. The drug reduces fever, increases blood pressure, and decreases the heart rate. The absorption, safety, and physiologic actions of ibuprofen were assessed in patients with severe sepsis.

Methods.—A total of 29 patients from 4 medical centers were studied. The patients received an initial intravenous dose of 600 mg of ibuprofen (Motrin) or placebo within 4 hours of diagnosis. This dose was given during a 20-minute interval and was followed by three 800-mg doses administered as a rectal solution every 6 hours. Ibuprofen was given in addition to the standard treatment for sepsis. Two thirds of the way through the study, the initial intravenous dose was increased to 800 mg.

Results.—Those patients who received ibuprofen had a significantly decreased temperature after infusion of the drug. The treatment and placebo groups both had significant reductions in heart rate, increases in mean arterial pressure and mean pulmonary artery pressure, and decreases in the arterial/alveolar PO_2 ratio; however, the differences between the groups were not significant. Nor did the larger initial dose of ibuprofen yield additional significant results. Both routes of ibuprofen administration were well tolerated; however, drug absorption was poor with the rectal route. The overall mortality rate was 45%.

Conclusion.—Although ibuprofen had significant antipyretic effects in patients with severe sepsis, significant changes in hemodynamic, respiratory, and metabolic variables were not observed. Larger clinical trials of ibuprofen in patients with sepsis are recommended.

▶ This investigation studied the laboratory and clinical effects of ibuprofen in treating sepsis and septic shock. Those patients who received ibuprofen had a significant decrease in temperature after administration of the drug, as well as a reduction in heart rate, an increase in mean arterial and pulmonary artery pressures, and a decrease in the alveolar-arterial PO$_2$ ratio. Ibuprofen administration was well tolerated; the previously measured changes were not statistically significant. Unlike other reports, this study did not from a clinical standpoint support the use of ibuprofen in patients. One cannot help but wonder however, whether the doses were adequate. Also, it is disappointing that none of the antioxidant properties was investigated in these patients.—G.T. Shires, M.D.

Ibuprofen Prevents Deterioration in Static Transpulmonary Compliance and Transalveolar Protein Flux in Septic Porcine Acute Lung Injury
Byrne K, Carey PD, Sielaff TD, Jenkins JK, Blocher CR, Cooper KR, Fowler AA, Sugerman HJ (Virginia Commonwealth Univ)
J Trauma 32:155–156, 1991   3–14

Background.—By promoting neutrophil adhesiveness, thromboxane A$_2$ may increase the number of neutrophils sequestered in the pulmonary microvasculature and, in this way, augment the septic response to lung injury. Release of elastase from degranulated neutrophils can make the alveolar capillary membrane more permeable to protein.

Objective and Methods.—Because the effects of the cyclooxygenase inhibitor ibuprofen in the setting of microvascular lung injury are uncertain, the effects of ibuprofen in young swine given an infusion of live *Pseudomonas aeruginosa* were evaluated. Ibuprofen was administered just before and 2 hours after onset of *Pseudomonas* infusion in a dose of 12.5 mg/kg. Static lung compliance was measured by the thermal cardiogreen technique, and the protein content of the bronchoalveolar lavage fluid was determined.

Observations.—Infusion of *P. aeruginosa* significantly reduced static lung compliance, the cardiac index, arterial oxygen pressure, and systemic arterial pressure. Pulmonary artery pressure and extravascular lung water increased, as did the protein content of lavage fluid. Treatment with ibuprofen prevented the early rise in pulmonary artery pressure and lessened the later increase in extravascular lung water seen after bacterial infusion. It also maintained lung compliance, arterial oxygen pressure, and lavage-fluid protein content (Fig 3–2) at baseline levels. The proportion of polymorphonuclear leukocytes in the lavage fluid remained at baseline after ibuprofen treatment, but peripheral leukopenia was unchanged.

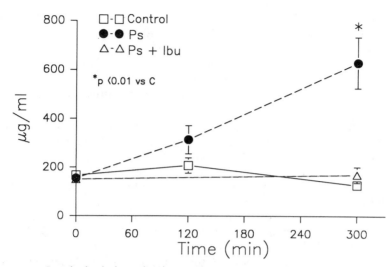

Fig 3–2.—Bronchoalveolar lavage (BAL) protein became significantly higher in the group with *Pseudomonas* (PS) infection compared to controls 5 hours after *Pseudomonas* infusion. Ibuprofen prevented the increase in BAL protein. (Courtesy of Byrne K, Carey PD, Sielaff TD, et al: *J Trauma* 31:155–166, 1991.)

Implication.—Pretreatment with ibuprofen appears to produce cyclooxygenase blockade and thereby substantially alters the pulmonary vascular response to sepsis. This type of treatment may affect neutrophil function so as to lessen many of the physiologic derangements consequent to sepsis.

▶ This is another study looking at the effects of ibuprofen on the septic state, in this case from the standpoint of inhibition of cyclooxygenase in the setting of microvascular lung injury. In animals treated with ibuprofen the early rise of pulmonary artery pressure was prevented and the later increase in extravascular lung water lessened after bacterial infusion with live *P. aeruginosa* organisms. Ibuprofen also maintained lung compliance, arterial oxygen pressure, and the lavage fluid protein content at baseline levels. These authors believe that this use of ibuprofen may affect neutrophil function so as to lessen some of the physiologic derangement secondary to sepsis.—G.T. Shires, M.D.

Experience With Phenylephrine as a Component of the Pharmacologic Support of Septic Shock
Gregory JS, Bonfiglio MF, Dasta JF, Reilley TE, Townsend MC, Flancbaum L (Ohio State Univ)
Crit Care Med 19:1395–1400, 1991   3–15

Background.—Patients with septic shock are at risk for multisystem organ failure. The goal of hemodynamic support in these patients is to maintain effective tissue perfusion. Although vasopressor agents may improve perfusion and preserve organ function, the use of such agents in hemodynamic support is controversial. The safety and effectiveness of phenylephrine, a selective α_1-adrenergic receptor agonist, were evaluated in patients with septic shock.

Methods.—The study group included 13 surgical intensive care unit patients; the mean age was 67 years. All of the patients were treated with phenylephrine, in addition to standard therapy for septic shock. They also underwent invasive hemodynamic monitoring. A dosage of .5–9 μg of phenylephrine per kg per minute was administered intravenously to maintain a mean arterial pressure (MAP) > 70 mm Hg.

Results.—Significant increases in MAP, systemic vascular resistance index, left ventricular stroke work index, and stroke volume index occurred after administration of phenylephrine and at the time of the greatest oxygen consumption. Although the cardiac index was unchanged initially, it increased at the time of greatest oxygen consumption. No changes were observed in the pulmonary artery occlusion pressure or heart rate. During phenylephrine therapy, the average baseline oxygen consumption increased from 145 mL/min·m² to 200 mL/min·m² and the oxygen delivery increased from 44 mL/min·m² to 597 mL/min·m². The serum creatinine concentrations remained unchanged, whereas the blood lactate concentrations decreased and the urine output increased significantly.

Conclusion.—Phenylephrine rapidly stabilized MAP at > 70 mm Hg with no detrimental effects on cardiac output. Use of the drug in hemodynamic support contributed to the maintenance of perfusion pressure and the optimization of oxygen delivery and consumption.

▶ This clinical study measured the ability of a pure α-adrenergic agonist, phenylephrine, to increase peripheral vascular resistance in the septic patient. As the authors point out, phenylephrine could be used in septic shock patients to increase blood pressure during vasodilation without detrimental effects on oxygen transport or organ function. The clinical effectiveness of such an approach was studied in hemodynamic support of 13 patients with septic shock and vasodilation. It would appear from the clincal results that this drug could be used as a pure α-adrenergic agonist with maintenance of perfusion pressure and optimazation of oxygen delivery and consumption while restoring the arterial blood pressure.—G.T. Shires, M.D.

Comparative Evaluation of the Effects of Felodipine, Hydralazine and Naloxone on the Survival Rate in Rats Subjected to a "Fixed Volume" Model of Hemorrhagic Shock

Chintala MS, Jandhyala BS (Univ of Houston)
Circ Shock 32:219–229, 1990

3–16

Introduction.—In a previous study, the calcium antagonist felodipine effectively restored renal and mesenteric blood flow and prevented renal failure in the Wiggers' fixed pressure model of hemorrhagic shock in which shed blood is reinfused. Whether felodipine would also promote survival in a fixed volume loss model of hemorrhagic shock in which shed blood is not reinfused was investigated. The findings were compared with those of hydralazine, an arteriolar dilator but not a calcium antagonist, and naloxone, which was shown to promote survival in both models of hemorrhagic shock.

Methods.—Anesthetized Sprague-Dawley rats were subjected to acute withdrawal of 40% of their blood volume during a 10-minute period. The shed blood was not reinfused. Felodipine, hydralazine, or naloxone was administered intra-arterially 10 minutes before the hemorrhage or immediately thereafter. Felodipine was given at 3 different doses. Control animals were given either saline or felodipine vehicle. All animals were observed for survival during the next 72 hours. Blood pressure and heart rate were measured in all animals that were alive 72 hours after hemorrhage.

Results.—Survival in saline-treated rats was the same as that in vehicle-treated rats, and the data from these 2 groups were pooled. Felodipine given at 3 different doses resulted in dose-dependent survival rates ranging from 50% to 90% when administered before hemorrhage and from 40% to 100% when given immediately after hemorrhage. Survival in the vehicle-treated control group was 33%. Hydralazine and naloxone both enhanced survival. However, the overall efficacy of the 2 higher doses of felodipine in enhancing survival was significantly greater than that of equihypotensive doses of hydralazine, and it was comparable to that of naloxone.

Conclusion.—Felodipine effectively promotes survival in a model of hemorrhagic shock in which shed blood is not reinfused.

▶ Previous studies have shown that calcium antagonists such as felodipine may restore renal and mesenteric blood flow and prevent renal failure in a Wiggers' fixed pressure model of hemorrhagic shock after reinfusion of shed blood. The current study sought to determine whether the same results would occur if shed blood was not reinfused.

The results indicated improvement in survival when felodipine was administered before or immediately after hemorrhagic shock. Similar results, but of lesser efficacy, occurred when hydralazine or naloxone was given. These data indicate that the salutary effects of the calcium blocker can be related to its calcium antagonistic effect as well as to its arterial or dilator properties.—G.T. Shires, M.D.

Acute Release of Cytokines Is Proportional to Tissue Injury Induced by Surgical Trauma and Shock in Rats

Bitterman H, Kinarty A, Lazarovich H, Lahat N (Technion-Israel Inst of Technology, Haifa)

J Clin Immunol 11:184–192, 1991   3–17

Introduction.—Recent animal and human studies have demonstrated increased serum levels of interleukin-1 (IL-1), IL-6, and tumor necrosis factor (TNF) after tissue injury. Although these studies suggested an important role for cytokines in the early mediation of surgical trauma and shock, the effects of cytokines and their serum levels in septic shock are poorly understood. The acute sequential serum profile of cytokines was defined in a rat model of splanchnic artery occlusion shock and the effects of graded tissue injury imposed by ischemia compared.

Methods.—Splanchnic artery occlusion shock was induced in anesthetized Sprague-Dawley rats by totally occluding the celiac and superior mesenteric arteries for 40 minutes, after which the rats with splanchnic artery occlusion shock were subjected to reperfusion. Two groups of rats had sham operations. One sham-shock group underwent all surgical procedures performed in the animals with splanchnic artery occlusion shock except that the splanchnic arteries were not clamped. The second sham-shock group underwent only carotid artery cannulation and tracheostomy. In a fourth group of rats only 1 blood sample was withdrawn from the carotid artery immediately after anesthesia. Serum IL-1, IL-2, IL-6, and TNF levels were measured at the end of the stabilization period and at 40, 50, 70, and 190 minutes later. No individual rat had more than 3 blood samples taken. All removed blood was replaced with an equal amount of normal saline solution.

Results.—No IL-1 activity was detected throughout the 190-minute experiment in any of the 4 groups. Increased IL-2 activity was detected only in the rats with splanchnic artery occlusion shock. Graded increases in serum TNF and IL-6 activities proportional to the surgical trauma were detected, and these increases were highest in the group with splanchnic artery occlusion shock. Serum TNF and IL-6 levels were highest at 30 minutes after reperfusion.

Conclusion.—Cytokines have a role in the early mediation of surgical trauma and shock.

▶ This interesting study examined the sequential profile of serum cytokine appearances in an experimental model of splanchnic ischemia reperfusion producing shock in control models of surgical trauma. The study detected graded increases in serum TNF and IL-6 activity that were proportional to the surgical trauma and ischemia, with peak levels occurring 30 minutes after reperfusion. Serum IL-1 and IL-2 levels were not reflective of the increase in surgical trauma.

The acute appearance of IL-6 and TNF in plasma immediately after ischemia and trauma is not surprising. However, because most of these substances are produced and have their effects locally, carrying out these studies over a longer period of time would probably not show a relationship between the degree of trauma and the actual serum level of cytokines.—G.T. Shires, M.D.

Inhibition of Macrophage-Activating Cytokines Is Beneficial in the Acute Septic Response

Redmond HP, Chavin KD, Bromberg JS, Daly JM (Univ of Pennsylvania; Med Univ of South Carolina)
Ann Surg 214:502–508, 1991   3–18

Background.—Bacterial infection remains a frequent cause of death in critically ill patients despite many advances in management. Several studies have reported an increased occurrence of gram-negative septicemia associated with a mortality rate as high as 35%. Whereas interferon-γ (IFN-γ) and other cytokines enhance the antimicrobial actions of macrophages, the systemic implications of activating macrophages are uncertain.

Objective and Methods.—The effects of IFN-γ and interleukin-4 (IL-4), as well as monoclonal antibodies directed against these cytokines, were examined in mice treated with lipopolysaccharide. Groups of animals received IFN-γ, IL-4, IgG_1 isotype antibody, anti–IFN-γ, or anti–IL-4, at the same time as endotoxin or 2 hours afterward. The release of superoxide anion by macrophages was determined 6 hours after endo-

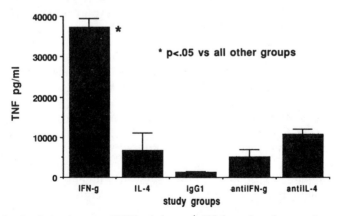

Fig 3—3.—Graph showing serum TNF levels (mean ± SD) for each study group. Serum was harvested (n = 3 mice per group) 2 hours after simultaneous lipopolysaccharide challenge (60 mg/kg) and cytokine/monoclonal antibody administration. (Courtesy of Redmond HP, Chavin KD, Bromberg JS, et al: *Ann Surg* 214:502–508, 1991.)

toxin treatment, as well as tumor necrosis factor (TNF) and IL-6 production.

Observations.—Interferon-γ synergized with endotoxin to induce a high level of macrophage activation, as reflected by O²-production. Both anti–IFN-γ and anti–IL-4 inhibited the primary effect of endotoxin. Both IFN-γ and IL-4 were associated with increased cellular TNF release from peritoneal macrophages. The highest TNF levels occurred when IFN-γ was given at the same time as endotoxin (Fig 3–3). Serum IL-6 levels were highest in animals given IFN-γ and IL-4. Treatment with either of these agents lowered survival compared with control animals, whereas anti–IFN-γ significantly enhanced survival.

Conclusions.—Antibody against IFN-γ may have a useful role in modulating the acute septic response. It might be helpful to combine such monoclonal antibodies with antimicrobial agents.

▶ This study examines the role of the downstream cytokines after TNF activation in sepsis. These authors found that IFN-γ and IL-4, as well as monoclonal antibodies directed against these cytokines, were useful after the induction of endotoxin sepsis. They suggest that antibodies against IFN-γ may prove to have a useful role in modulating the acute septic response.—G.T. Shires, M.D.

Survival After Hypertonic Saline Resuscitation From Hemorrhage
Soliman MH, Ragab H, Waxman K (Univ of California-Irvine Med Ctr, Orange)
Am Surg 56:749–751, 1990   3–19

Introduction.—Hypertonic saline can increase the plasma and interstitial volumes in hemorrhagic shock by recruiting intracellular water and may help to restore normal circulation to vital organs. Whereas resuscitation with hypertonic saline compares favorably with normal saline or Ringer's lactate, hypernatremia and hyperosmolarity are possible complications. In addition, a shift of fluid from the intracellular to the intravascular compartment may lead to cellular dehydration.

Methods.—Halothane-anesthetized rats were bled of 21 mL/kg over 5 minutes and, 10 minutes after hemorrhage, were infused with either 42 mL of Ringer's lactate solution per kg or 10.6 mL of 3% saline per kg. The 2 treatments provided equal amounts of sodium.

Results.—Only 36% of animals given hypertonic saline survived at 72 hours compared with 64% of those given Ringer's lactate (Fig 3–4). Serum sodium and chloride levels were significantly higher in the group given hypertonic saline at the end of infusion. There were no significant differences in serum potassium or bicarbonate levels.

Conclusions.—Lower survival after resuscitation with hypertonic saline may relate to intracellular dehydration, leading to impaired cell and organ recovery. Both the time and amount of such resuscitation should be

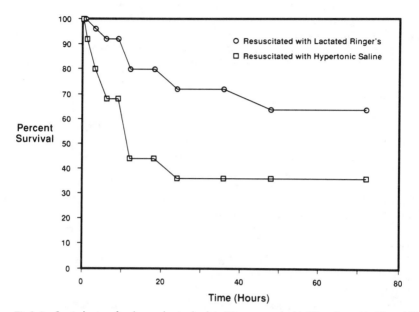

Fig 3–4.—Survival rates after hemorrhagic shock in 25 rats treated with 3% sodium chloride and 25 rats treated with lactated Ringer's injection. (Courtesy of Soliman MH, Ragab H, Waxman K: *Am Surg* 56:749–751, 1990.)

limited, and it seems wise to replace free water aggressively as soon as possible.

▶ This experimental study showed a significantly lower survival after resuscitation with hypertonic saline as compared to normal saline or Ringer's lactate. The authors point out that there was significant hypernatremia and hyperosmolarity associated with the reduced survival associated with hypertonic saline.—G.T. Shires, M.D.

Effect of Injured Vessel Size on Bleeding Following Hypertonic Saline Infusion in "Uncontrolled" Hemorrhagic Shock in Anesthetized Rats

Krausz MM, Kablan M, Rabinovici R, Klin B, Sherman Y, Gross D (Hadassah Univ Hosp, Jerusalem)
Circ Shock 35:9–13, 1991   3–20

Background.—In an experimental model of "uncontrolled" hemorrhagic shock (UCHS), hypertonic saline (HTS) infusion was shown to increase bleeding from injured vessels, decrease mean arterial pressure (MAP), and hasten death. The effect of injured vessel size on the bleeding response to HTS in UCHS was studied in rats.

Methods.—The experiments were done in male Hebrew University strain rats. The rats were anesthetized and then randomized into 4 groups. In group I, 8 rats had UCHS induced by resection of 8% of the end of the tail; they received no treatment. Group II consisted of 8 rats who had undergone the same resection of the tail followed by treatment with 7.5% NaCl, 5 mL/kg (HTS). The 9 rats in group III had 50% of the tail resected and received no treatment, whereas the 12 rats in group IV also had the 50% resection but were given treatment with 5 mL of NaCl (HTS) per kg.

Results.—In group I, 2.6 mL of bleeding and a decrease in the MAP from 107 mm Hg to 80 mm Hg occurred within 5 minutes after resection. In group II, blood loss and the decrease in MAP were not significantly different from group I. After HTS in group II, the blood loss progressed to 4.9 mL after 4 hours, compared with a loss of only 3.4 mL in group I. There was no change in MAP and no mortality. Group III had a blood loss of 4.3 mL and a decrease in MAP to 41 mm Hg after 5 minutes; group IV had similar findings. In group IV, HTS treatment increased blood loss to 8.3 mL after 4 hours, compared with a loss of 5.7 mL in group III. In addition, group IV had a decrease in MAP to 22 mm Hg and a 58.3% mortality rate, compared with an increase in MAP to 78 mm Hg and no mortality in group III.

Conclusions.—Resection of large-caliber vessels appears to increase early blood loss in rats. In the larger vessels, HTS treatment increases blood loss, decreases MAP markedly, and also increases mortality. Thus HTS treatment may be dangerous in trauma patients with UCHS.

▶ This interesting experimental study measured the effect of HTS resuscitation in uncontrolled hemorrhagic shock in animals with small- and large-size vessel injury producing the hemorrhage. Resection of the larger caliber vessel increased early blood loss, and HTS treatment further increased the blood loss, decreased the MAP, and increased mortality significantly. The authors therefore again make the plea that the use of HTS as a form of fluid resuscitation should be considered carefully before being given to a traumatized patient.—G.T. Shires, M.D.

Hypertonic Saline Alters Plasma Clotting Times and Platelet Aggregation
Reed RL II, Johnston TD, Chen Y, Fischer RP (Univ of Texas, Houston)
J Trauma 31:8–14, 1991   3–21

Introduction.—Hypertonic saline has been recommended for use in resuscitating patients from hypovolemic shock and burn injury, but recent studies suggest that it may exacerbate bleeding. Hypertonic saline has the property of dilating blood vessels. In addition, it may have anticoagulant effects on both plasma clotting factors and platelets.

Methods.—Normal human plasma was serially diluted with hypertonic (7.5%) saline or physiologic .9% saline. Prothrombin time and activated

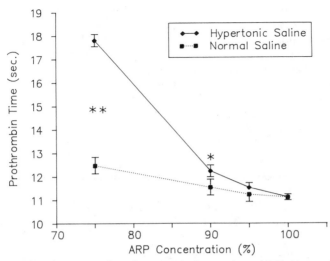

Fig 3–5.—Prothrombin times performed on assayed reference plasma *(ARP)* dilutions, using either normal (.9%) or hypertonic (7.5%) saline as the diluent. Data are presented as mean ± 1 SD for each dilution tested. *Asterisk* indicates *P* < .01, hypertonic saline vs. normal saline; *double asterisk, P* < .001, hypertonic saline vs. normal saline (by Student's *t*-test using Bonferroni's modification). (Courtesy of Reed RL II, Johnston TD, Chen Y, et al: *J Trauma* 31:8–14, 1991.)

partial thromboplastin time were measured and platelet aggregation studies were performed.

Results.—Hypertonic saline significantly prolonged the activated partial thromoboplastin times and prothrombin time at 10% dilution (Fig 3-5). Clinically significant lengthening of the prothrombin time did not occur until dilution with hypertonic saline exceeded 10%. Platelet aggregation with either adenosine diphosphate or collagen was impaired by hypertonic saline.

Conclusion.—Replacement of 10% or more of the plasma volume by hypertonic saline has definite anticoagulant effects. Clinically significant effects, however, are not likely with a standard resuscitation load of 5 mL/kg.

▶ These authors point out that hypertonic saline may compound the clotting difficulties in patients with preexisting injury such as shock or burn injury. This study was purposely done with hypertonic saline, only omitting dextran. Studies have already shown that with any significant volume of administration of dextran, clotting abnormalities inevitably occur.

The present study showed that with normal human plasma diluted with hypertonic saline only, the activated partial thromboplastin time and prothrombin time were significantly prolonged. As the authors point out, the clinical significance of this prolongation did not occur until approximately 10% dilution of normal plasma had occurred. In addition, platelet aggregation was impaired by hypertonic saline adding another anticoagulant effect.

The question was raised of whether a transient alteration in clotting ability might occur from rapid infusion of even smaller volumes of hypertonic saline as well as dextran solutions, even though the clinical uses of hypertonic saline and dextran have been less than 10% of plasma volume. As the authors point out, other alterations in blood coagulation that occur in trauma patients (e.g., hypothermia, acidosis, hypoperfusion, tissue trauma, and consumptive coagulopathy) could also contribute to a clotting defect. An infusion of dextran solutions or hypertonic saline, when added to these other factors, might well aggravate a coagulopathy.—G.T. Shires, M.D.

Acute Hypotension Caused by Rapid Hypertonic Saline Infusion in Anesthetized Dogs
Kien ND, Kramer GC, White DA (Univ of California, Davis)
Anesth Analg 73:597–602, 1991   3–22

Introduction.—Animal studies have shown that resuscitation from severe hemorrhagic shock is possible with a small bolus infusion of 7.5% hypertonic saline solution (HTS). The infusion rapidly improves cardiovascular and metabolic function by increasing plasma volume, inducing vasodilation, and augmenting myocardial performance. The safety and efficacy of rapid infusions of HTS were assessed.

Methods.—Experiments were performed in 10 mongrel dogs to evaluate the immediate cardiovascular effects of HTS. Left ventricular pressure and wall motions were measured simultaneously in the anesthetized dogs for assessment of cardiac contractility.

Results.—The mean arterial blood pressure was significantly decreased (from 95 mm Hg to 51 mm Hg) at 45 seconds after onset of an infusion of HTS (3 mL/kg/min). This decrease, however, was abrupt and transient. At the same time, there were significant increases in cardiac output (from 2.8 L/min to 3.9 L/min) and coronary blood flow (from 23.7 mL/min to 49.8 mL/min). The heart rate remained constant, but increases occurred in both systolic shortening of left ventricular diameter and wall thickening, suggesting improvement in cardiac contractility. The decreases in systemic and pulmonary vascular resistance were 60% and 27%, respectively.

Conclusion.—The acute hypotension that occurs after a rapid infusion of HTS is secondary to decreased systemic vascular resistance. Whereas a brief period of hypotension is well tolerated when circulatory function is normal, adverse consequences may occur in some patients. It is recommended that HTS be given slowly to avoid or minimize an acute hypotensive response.

▶ This experimental study from the home of the resurgent interest in hypertonic fluids demonstrates a remarkable decrease in systemic vascular resistance when the HTS is given rapidly intravenously. This adds to the weight of evidence indicating that even a small bolus of HTS produces remarkable vasodilation with a decrease in systemic vascular resistance. As the authors point out, this results in transient hypotension in normal animals. However, they also caution that adverse consequences may well occur in a patient who is already hypovolemic.—G.T. Shires, M.D.

Prehospital Hypertonic Saline/Dextran Infusion for Posttraumatic Hypotension: The USA Multicenter Trial
Mattox KL, Maningas PA, Moore EE, Mateer JR, Marx JA, Aprahamian C, Burch JM, Pepe PE (Baylor College of Medicine; Black Hills Inst for Prehosp Care, Rapid City, SD; Denver Gen Hosp; Med College of Wisconsin; City of Houston Emergency Med Services)
Ann Surg 213:482–491, 1991   3–23

Introduction.—The safety and efficacy of prehospital fluid resuscitation with a small volume of 7.5% sodium chloride in 6% dextran 70 in posttraumatic hypotension was assessed in a prospective, multicenter, double-blind, randomized clinical trial.

Methods.—During a 13-month period, 424 patients with posttraumatic hypotension were randomly allocated to receive hypertonic saline/dextran (HSD), 250 mL, or lactated Ringer's solution, 250 mL, administered after initial vital signs were obtained but before routine prehospital and emergency center resuscitation. Patients were followed for 24 hours or until death. Of the 424 patients, 359 (84.7%) met the criteria for efficacy analysis, and 51% of them were treated with HSD.

Results.—Of the patients, 77 died; 65 (84%) died within the first 24 hours and 3 died after 7 days. There was an apparent but not significantly different trend for better survival among patients treated with HSD. Of the 77 deaths, 35 occurred in HSD-treated patients and 42 in those treated with standard lactated Ringer's solution. There was no difference between groups in mean injury severity score, the mean Trauma Score plus Injury Severity Score, probability of survival, revised trauma scores, age, ambulance times, preinfusion blood pressure, and etiology distribution. Although there was no significant difference in overall survival between the groups, HSD-treated patients requiring operation had enhanced survival. The HSD-treated patients had fewer complications than did those treated with lactated Ringer's solution.

Conclusion.—Prehospital administration of HSD for posttraumatic hypotension is safe and appears to have some advantage over lactated Ringer's solution in patients requiring surgical treatment.

▶ This multi-institutional trial tested the efficacy and safety of prehospital fluid resuscitation with a small volume of 7.5% sodium chloride and 6% dextran 70. There was essentially no difference in the use of HSD compared with a balanced saline solution, lactated Ringer's. It should be pointed out, however, that the volume of lactated Ringer's was far less than is generally used in patient fluid resuscitation and, in fact, was no greater than the HSD solution that was used. It should be further pointed out that all of the patients were resuscitated in an urban center where transport time was rapid, and previous authors have shown that, in any event, the difference in overall survival in this setting is probably not influenced by what fluid therapy is administered. Consequently, it would seem that no conclusions can be drawn from this trial.—G.T. Shires, M.D.

Cross-Linked Hemoglobin Solution as a Resuscitative Fluid After Hemorrhage in the Rat
Przybelski RJ, Malcolm DS, Burris DG, Winslow RM (Walter Reed Army Inst of Research, Washington, DC; Uniformed Services Univ of the Health Sciences, Bethesda, Md; Walter Reed Army Med Ctr, Washington, DC; Letterman Army Inst of Research, San Francisco)
J Lab Clin Med 117:143–151, 1991   3–24

Introduction.—Previous studies demonstrated that a new hemoglobin derivative that is cross-linked intramolecularly between its α chains has oxygen transport properties similar to those of whole blood. The efficacy of a 14% cross-linked hemoglobin solution as a resuscitation fluid was evaluated in a rat model having relevance to military combat or civilian prehospital care settings.

Methods.—Anesthetized rats were bled at 20 mL/kg or approximately one third of their total blood volume. On completion of the bleed, control animals were observed, but not resuscitated. The other animals were resuscitated with heparinized shed blood, lactated Ringer's solution, or 14% hemoglobin solution administered at half volume of 10 mL/kg or whole volume of 20 mL/kg. The heart rate, mean arterial pressure (MAP), and transcutaneous oxygen tension were monitored throughout the study.

Results.—Animals resuscitated with either half-volume or whole-volume hemoglobin solution responded quickly and positively to the infusions. Animals treated with the hemoglobin solution had significantly higher MAPs than did those resuscitated with either autologous blood or lactated Ringer's solution. The heart rate and transcutaneous oxygen tension responses in hemoglobin-treated animals were not significantly different from those in animals given autologous blood throughout the observation period. Thus resuscitation with 10 mL/kg of 14% hemoglobin solution was as effective as nearly twice that volume of whole blood in restoring cardiovascular parameters and tissue oxygenation.

Conclusion.—Resuscitation with a 14% cross-linked hemoglobin solution promptly restores the heart rate, MAP, and transcutaneous oxygen tension after an acute nonlethal hemorrhage. Because the MAP returned to baseline before the hemoglobin solution was completely infused, even a lower dose of this solution might be effective.

▶ This is an additional study on the potential value of red blood cell free hemoglobin solutions as a blood substitute. As many authors have shown previously, the oxygen dissociation desirability of stroma free hemoglobin is feasible as a blood substitute. In this particular instance, the cross-linking of hemoglobin was accomplished clinically and, with additional sterilization, purification, and modification, the material was effective in resuscitating rats depleted of red blood cells.

The problem with this study and so many others is that the experimental animal was the rat, which is notoriously insensitive to endotoxin contamination of hemoglobin. Because the affinity of endotoxin for hemoglobin is enormous, further studies on this solution in higher species of animals are necessary to determine its safety from the standpoint of endotoxin involvement as well as its production of oxygen free radicals when the solution leaks out of capillaries.—G.T. Shires, M.D.

4 Trauma

Functional Scoring of Multi-Trauma Patients: Who Ends Up Where?
Emhoff TA, McCarthy M, Cushman M, Garb JL, Valenziano C (Baystate Med
Ctr, Springfield, Mass; Tufts Univ)
J Trauma 31:1227–1232, 1991   4–1

Introduction.—Standard trauma scoring systems, such as the Glasgow
Coma Scale and the Injury Severity Score, are based on anatomical and
physiologic variables that are predictive of mortality. A more useful system would be one based on function, the true measure of trauma morbidity. Such a system, the Functional Independence Measure (FIM), was
assessed in 109 patients.

Patients.—The patients were adults admitted consecutively to a level I
trauma center between May 1988 and June 1989. All of the patients required the services of a multidisciplinary trauma team. The function
scores were assigned on a consensus basis and covered 5 general categories: self-care, sphincter control, mobility, locomotion, and communica-
tion/social skills. The patients were assessed over a period of 13 months
for admission/discharge scores and discharge disposition.

Results.—Of the 109 patients, 42 were discharged home and 67 entered rehabilitation facilities. For those who returned home, the average
FIM score on admission was 63 (50% of normal function). In contrast,
the average admission score for those who went to a rehabilitation facil-
ity was 31 (25%) of normal. The average discharge scores were 108 (86%
of normal) for those who went home and 52 (41% of normal) for patients who entered rehabilitation facilities. Patients with musculoskeletal
injuries had a higher rate of discharge to the home (57%) than did the
patients with head injuries (9%). Of the 5 general areas scored, 4 showed
highly significant differences between groups of patients who went
home and those who entered rehabilitation.

Conclusion.—The FIM appears to be a useful tool for measuring a
patient's total function. It tracked progress through the period of acute
hospitalization and correctly categorized both cognitive and physical dysfunction as discharge planning was being done.

▶ This is another attempt to devise a reliable trauma scoring technique. This
particular system, the FIM, was used in the functional scoring of multiple
trauma patients. Patients sustaining trauma, admitted consecutively over a
1-year period, were assessed. Functional scores were assigned on a consen-

sus basis in 5 categories—self-care, sphincter control, mobility, locomotion, and communication skills.

The FIM appeared to be a very useful tool for measuring a patient's total function. It was used to track progress through the period of hospitalization and correctly categorize cognitive and physical dysfunction as discharge planning was being done. This interesting approach bears further study.—G.T. Shires, M.D.

Do Trauma Centers Improve Outcome Over Non-Trauma Centers: The Evaluation of Regional Trauma Care Using Discharge Abstract Data and Patient Management Categories

Smith JS, Martin LF, Young WW, Macioce DP (Milton S Hershey Med Ctr, Hershey, Pa; Pittsburgh Research Inst)
J Trauma 30:1533–1538, 1990   4–2

Background.—Evaluations of trauma care have confirmed that survival rates are improved when definitive treatment is received quickly; however, few data exist concerning the outcome of injured survivors treated at trauma as opposed to nontrauma centers. With the development of patient management categories (PMCs), a computerized patient classification system, such as outcome study is now possible. A comparison was undertaken of trauma center treatment and nontrauma center treatment of femoral shaft fractures requiring open reduction and internal fixation (ORIF).

Methods.—Data were obtained from 15 trauma centers and 120 nontrauma hospitals in the western third of Pennsylvania and the entire state of Maryland. During the study period, the PMC software identified 1,332 patients with fractures of the shaft of the femur who underwent ORIF. The outcome was compared for the 2 types of institutions according to the following criteria: time to the operating room, patient age, associated injuries, and the development of complications and death.

Results.—More patients with multiple injuries were taken to trauma centers, except in the older age group (despite its higher risk for complications and death). There were significantly fewer complications and lower mortality rates among those treated at trauma centers. In both types of centers, associated injuries, age, complications, and/or delay in time to the operating room significantly increased a patient's length of stay.

Conclusion.—Examining discharge abstract data using the PMC methodology appears to confirm that trauma center care lowers mortality and significantly decreases the morbidity rates for patients who have been severely injured in accidents.

▶ This interesting study uses a new approach to examine the question concerning the efficacy of trauma centers over nontrauma centers in the care of the severely injured patient. Using the PMC approach, i.e., a computerized patient classification system, an outcome study was possible. Data were obtained concerning a comparable injury—in this case, a femoral shaft fracture requiring surgery—from 15 trauma centers and 120 nontrauma hospitals in a defined geographic region. The outcome was compared for the 2 types of institutions based on a number of criteria, including time to operating room, patient age, associated injury, the development of complications, and death. As expected, in both types of centers, associated injuries, age, complications, or delay in going to the operating room significantly increased the patient's length of stay in the hospital.

The major conclusion, obtained from examining discharge abstract data, revealed that trauma center care significantly lowered mortality as well as morbidity for patients with comparably severe injuries. This kind of comparison has previously been assumed to be true, but these new data prove the point.—G.T. Shires, M.D.

Continuous Arteriovenous Hemofiltration With Dialysis (CAVH-D): An Alternative to Hemodialysis in the Mass Casualty Situation
Omert L, Reynolds HN, Wiles CE (Maryland Inst for Emergency Med Services Systems, Baltimore)
J Emerg Med 9:51–56, 1991   4–3

Introduction.—Dialysis equipment may be inaccessible or inoperable in a disaster situation, and a large number of patients with acute renal failure secondary to crush syndrome could overwhelm an existing functional dialysis program. An alternative is continuous arteriovenous hemofiltration with dialysis (CAVH-D). This smaller device is an effective means of dialysis and may be substantially independent of indigenous supplies.

Technique.—The CAVH-D system was designed to improve solute clearance over that achievable with CAVH alone by using the patient's arterial pressure to pump blood through a circuit. Although CAVH effectively removes large volumes of fluid, its convective clearance does not clear large amounts of solute such as urea. In CAVH-D a dialysate port is added that permits countercurrent flow of dialysate (Fig 4–1). Either normal saline or Dianeal may be used as dialysate.

Advantages.—Vascular access is readily obtained with this technique, most often using polyurethane catheters in the femoral vessels. Heparinization may not be necessary, especially in patients with preexisting coagulopathy. All of the equipment can be managed by the nursing staff, and it might be possible for a single nurse to manage several CAVH-D patients at the same time. Hemodynamic stability is not a problem with this treatment. The needed equipment is considerably lighter and less bulky than that used for traditional hemodialysis.

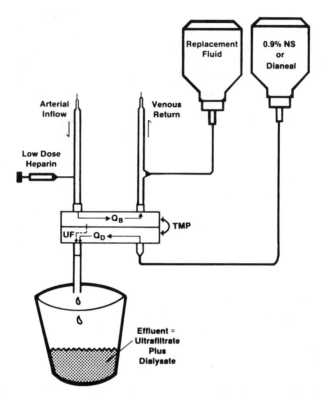

Fig 4–1—Basic configuration of CAVH-D *Abbreviations:* UF ultrafiltrate; Q_B blood flow; Q_D dialysate flow; *TMP* transmembrane pressure (Courtesy of Omert L, Reynolds HN, Wiles CE, *J Emerg Med* 9:51–56, 1991.)

Disadvantages.—The CAVH-D patient is restricted to bed during treatment, which may last for several days. Both arterial and venous access sites are required.

Conclusion.—It seems likely that the CAVH-D system could be useful in settings other than the mass casualty situation. Whether early institution of this treatment can prevent renal failure secondary to rhabdomyolysis remains to be determined.

▶ This is an interesting new dialysis device for continuous arterial venous hemofiltration with a dialysis membrane. The remarkable advantages of this equipment are that it is extremely lightweight and mobile and also apparently very effective. The disadvantage is the patient must stay in bed during the entire sequence of hemodialysis. The only difference in terms of access is that in this system, there needs to be an arterial cannula in addition to the venous cannula.

Nevertheless, it would appear that in the mass casualty situation this might be a remarkable advantage in terms of immediately available and lightweight mobile dialysis equipment.—G.T. Shires, M.D.

Continuous Arteriovenous Rewarming: Report of a New Technique for Treating Hypothermia
Gentilello LM, Rifley WJ (Univ of Washington; Univ of Nevada)
J Trauma 31:1151–1154, 1991   4–4

Introduction.—Prolonged cold water submersion with complete neurologic recovery may occur in children, but the survival of adults whose core temperature falls below 32°C is rare. Conventional warming techniques to treat hypothermia include the use of heating blankets, radiant warmers, body cavity lavage, and airway rewarming, but none of these techniques increases the body temperature by more than 1°C per hour. Cardiac bypass is an effective treatment for hypothermia, but the need for systemic heparinization precludes its use in trauma victims. Continuous arteriovenous rewarming (CAVR) was used in an adult victim of severe hypothermia that was refractory to other rewarming techniques.

Case Report.—Man, 28, landed upside down in a gully containing a torrent of icy water after driving his car into a wall and veering down an embankment. Paramedics arrived several minutes later, but it was another 20 minutes before the victim could be extricated from the submerged car. On arrival at the hospital, the patient was apneic and pulseless; his pupils were fixed and dilated. His initial core temperature was 31.5°C by bladder thermistor. When after 1 hour of conventional warming methods his core temperature had dropped another 2 degrees, CAVR with a modified commercially available rapid fluid warmer was instituted. The initial core temperature gain was 2°C at 15 minutes, 3°C at 30 minutes, and 4.5°C at 1 hour. The time to resolution of the hypothermia was 1 hour and 25 minutes, or 1°C every 15.4 minutes. Spontaneous respirations resumed and the patient's movements became purposeful toward the end of the procedure. Although the early hospital course was complicated by adult respiratory distress syndrome and acute renal failure, the patient recovered and was discharged with intact memory, association, and other cognitive skills.

Conclusions.—Although CAVR is analogous to cardiac bypass in that it infuses warm blood directly into the heart, it does not require a blood pump, membrane oxygenator, or systemic heparinization. The hypothermia, associated coagulopathy, and myocardial depression were rapidly corrected by CAVR. This report describes the longest period of submersion ever tolerated by an adult in which full neurologic recovery ensued.

▶ This is an interesting new technique for more rapid restoration of body temperature to normal after severe hypothermia, as occurs in cold water submersion. The technique basically uses a new rapid fluid warmer without cardiopulmonary bypass simply as a fast way to warm the endogenous blood volume. There is little doubt that normothermia was reached much more quickly and, furthermore, the patient survived without sequelae. This will probably prove to be a true advance in the treatment of total body hypothermia that is severe.—G.T. Shires, M.D.

Trauma During Pregnancy: A Review of 79 Cases

Esposito TJ, Gens DR, Smith LG, Scorpio R, Buchman T (Maryland Inst for Emergency Med Services Systems, Baltimore)
Arch Surg 126:1073–1078, 1991   4–5

Introduction.—Insufficient data are available to allow direct decisions on the management of pregnant women who are injured. A review was made of 79 such patients seen at a trauma center over a 9-year period. These patients constituted fewer than 1% of all acute admissions during the review period, and 2.6% of females aged 14–45 years.

Findings.—The women were fairly evenly distributed over the 3 trimesters of pregnancy. Most were injured in an auto collision. Eight patients (10%) died. Of 53 known pregnancy outcomes, 34% were unsuccessful. All 3 fetuses that sustained direct injuries died. Seven women underwent emergency cesarean section; 4 of the infants were delivered alive, and 3 were discharged. The outcome was much poorer in women who were in shock or hypoxic at the time of admission. Diagnostic peritoneal lavage was 95% accurate in the 21 patients examined.

Seat Belt Use.—Injury severity scores did not vary significantly as a function of the use of a seat belt. Comparable proportions of belted and unbelted occupants had a successful pregnancy outcome. The 1 death was in an unrestrained patient.

Conclusions.—Pregnancy does not increase maternal mortality from trauma, and pregnant women should use seat belts. In the setting of trauma during pregnancy, the blood pressure, pulse, and PO_2 are not reliable indicators of adequate maternal resuscitation or a normal fetus.

▶ This is one of the few articles written on the effectiveness or danger associated with wearing seatbelts during pregnancy. The review indicated that wearing a seatbelt did not increase fetal damage, nor did it increase the rate of fetal loss.

This is interesting because it has been speculated that wearing a seatbelt could be detrimental in that the fetus might be extruded through the anterior abdominal wall. It would appear, at least from this review, that wearing seatbelts is still desirable, even during pregnancy. Industry efforts are currently being expended to promote the use of a webbing between the lap and shoulder belt, perhaps increasing fetal protection when a seatbelt is worn by a pregnant woman.—G.T. Shires, M.D.

Peritoneal Lavage Enzyme Determinations Following Blunt and Penetrating Abdominal Trauma

McAnena OJ, Marx JA, Moore EE (Univ of Colorado)
J Trauma 31:1161–1164, 1991   4–6

Introduction.—Diagnostic peritoneal lavage (DPL) is limited in its ability to identify isolated hollow viscus injury at an early stage. These structures tend not to bleed much, and a lag of at least 3 hours is needed to provoke an inflammatory peritoneal reaction.

Objective and Methods.—The value of estimating lavage amylase (LAM) and lavage alkaline phosphatase (LAP) levels was examined in a series of 1,969 DPL studies carried out in injured patients during a 4-year period. Whereas LAM was determined in 96% of the patients, LAP was determined in 88%. The series included 1,536 patients with blunt injury and 433 with penetrating trauma.

Findings.—A total of 67 patients (3.6%) had negative lavage findings when red blood cells were counted; however, they had a LAM level of at least 10 IU/L. Of these patients, 55 had blunt injuries. The mean LAM level was 122 IU/L. A group of 13 patients had an LAP level of at least 3 IU/L; of these, 7 had significant intra-abdominal injuries. Ten of the 13 patients who had an LAM level of at least 20 IU/L and an LAP level of at least 3 IU/L had small bowel injuries; the other 3 had pancreaticoduodenal injuries.

Recommendations.—It makes sense to estimate enzyme levels in lavage fluid. An LAM level of 20 IU/L or greater and an LAP level of at least 3 IU/L mandate laparotomy when the history is consistent with small bowel injury. An increase in level of either LAM or LAP warrants close observation.

▶ These authors attempted to extend the ability of diagnostic peritoneal lavage to identify hollow viscus injury. As pointed out, the hollow viscus structures tend not to bleed much and a lag of several hours is needed to provoke an inflammatory peritoneal reaction. Consequently, the authors measured the lavage amylase and lavage alkaline phosphatase levels in a series of nearly 2,000 diagnostic peritoneal lavage studies carried out in injured patients. Interestingly, half of the patients who had a negative lavage for red blood cells but an elevated lavage level of amylase had clinically significant injuries requiring laparotomy, which usually showed injury to the small bowel. Consequently, it looks like the sensitivity of 87%, specificity of 75%, and positive predicted value of 46% for significant intra-abdominal injury may well indicate that these tests should be added to the diagnostic peritoneal lavage studies in injured patients in whom the red blood cell recovery with lavage is either absent or not diagnostic.—G.T. Shires, M.D.

Triple-Contrast CT Scans in Penetrating Back and Flank Trauma
Himmelman RG, Martin M, Gilkey S, Barrett JA (Cook County Hosp, Chicago)
J Trauma 31:852–855, 1991   4–7

Introduction.—Triple-contrast CT (3-CT) has recently been introduced for evaluation of penetrating wounds to the back and flank. This technique involves the oral, intravenous, and rectal administration of contrast medium. To date, few studies have described the use of this specific technique.

Methods.—To determine whether 3-CT is an accurate predictor of the absence of retroperitoneal injury requiring surgical repair, 88 patients with penetrating wounds to the flank or back were evaluated by 3-CT. Stab wounds were present in 67 patients and gunshot wounds in 21. Patients with clinical or radiologic indications for emergency laparotomy were excluded. All patients were advised to undergo diagnostic peritoneal lavage (DPL) before 3-CT. Patients with positive DPL findings for penetration of the peritoneal cavity underwent exploratory laparotomy. Those with a negative DPL underwent 3-CT. Patients with low- or moderate-risk CT scans were observed for 48 hours, whereas those with high-risk CT scans were either taken to the operating suite or were observed at the discretion of the trauma surgeon.

Results.—All 88 patients underwent 3-CT scanning, and 78 had DPL; the other 10 patients refused DPL. Nine patients had CT scans indicating high risk, and 5 of them underwent exploratory laparotomy. Significant injuries were found in 2 of these 5 patients. Of the 79 patients with non–high-risk scans, 77 were observed without complication and 2 underwent surgical exploration for positive DPL, but no significant lesion was found.

Conclusion.—A 3-CT scan is highly effective in predicting the absence of significant retroperitoneal injuries in patients with penetrating wounds to the flank or back. Its negative predictive value for low or moderate risk of retroperitoneal injury is 100%.

▶ In this study, CT was used in the assessment of penetrating wounds of the back and flank. The authors used oral, intravenous, and rectal contrast media in combination. All of the patients had a negative DPL before undergoing 3-mode CT. The authors believe that CT results can be expressed as high risk and low risk. In the high-risk group, 5 of the 9 patients underwent exploratory laparotomy and 2 such patients had significant injuries. In the low-risk scan group, 77 patients were observed without complication, but 2 underwent surgical exploration because of positive DPL but no significant lesion was found. In summary, these authors believe that a 3-mode CT scan is more effective than conventional CT scan in predicting the absence of significant retroperitoneal or intraperitoneal injuries in patients with penetrating wounds of the flank or back.—G.T. Shires, M.D.

A Prospective, Randomized Comparison of Computed Tomography With Conventional Diagnostic Methods in the Evaluation of Penetrating Injuries to the Back and Flank

Easter DW, Shackford SR, Mattrey RF (Univ of California, San Diego; Univ of Vermont)
Arch Surg 126:1115–1119, 1991   4–8

| | Accuracy of Evaluation Methods | | |
Result	Immediate Operation*	CT Evaluation	Conventional Evaluation
True-positive	15	2	1
False-positive	9	1	2
True-negative	58†	28	27
False-negative	3†	0	0
Total	**85**	**31**	**30**
Predictive value, %			
Positive	63	67	33
Negative	95	97	100
Sensitivity, %	83	100	100
Specificity, %	86	96	93
Accuracy, %	86	97	93

* Number of patients.
† By design, those with negative immediate assessment findings were randomized into conventional or CT evaluation.
(Courtesy of Easter DW, Shackford SR, Mattrey RF *Arch Surg* 126 1115–1119, 1991.)

Introduction.—Penetrating injuries to the back and flank remain difficult to assess and manage, but recent reports suggest that CT is an accurate means of evaluating such injuries.

Study Design.—Computed tomography was compared with conventional diagnostic methods in a prospective series of 85 patients aged 18 years or older who had sustained penetrating injuries to the back or posterior aspect of the abdomen. Twenty-four patients underwent immediate laparotomy and were not randomized. Thirty-one of the remaining patients had CT assessment with intragastric contrast medium, and 30 patients were evaluated conventionally.

Outcome.—Nine of the 24 immediate operations proved to be unnecessary. Hospital costs were significantly higher for these patients than for those in either randomized group. In the randomized group there were 3 true positive and 3 false positive findings. Both CT assessment and conventional evaluation were highly accurate and specific in patients whose injuries necessitated operation (table). It took longer to make a hospital disposition in the CT group, but these patients required fewer diagnostic tests.

Conclusions.—When severe visceral injury is present in a patient with penetrating injury of the back or flank, it probably will be recognized by either conventional assessment or CT examination. In this series, patients in either group whose findings were normal could have been safely discharged.

▶ This is another attempt to resolve the dilemma concerning penetrating injuries to the back and flank with regard to the need for operative intervention. In the present study, conventional diagnostic methods or CT assessment were both used. The conclusion was that when visceral injury is present in a patient with penetrating injury to the back and flank, it can be recognized by either conventional assessment or CT examination. More importantly, patients in either group whose findings were normal could have been safely discharged. Therefore, the belief that CT is useful in assessment of damage done by penetrating injuries of the back or flank is supported.—G.T. Shires, M.D.

Emergency Arteriography in the Assessment of Penetrating Trauma to the Lower Limbs

Jebara VA, Haddad SN, Ghossain MA, Nehmé D, Aoun N, Tabet G, Ashoush R, Atallah NG, Boustany FN, Saade B (St Joseph Univ Hosp, Beirut, Lebanon)
Angiology 42:527–532, 1991   4–9

Introduction.—Vascular trauma to the extremities is a true emergency often requiring active resuscitation, rapid decision making, and early surgical intervention, especially in patients who have sustained high-velocity wounds and have associated multiple organ injuries. Although it is generally agreed that hemodynamically unstable patients need to be operated on immediately without emergency arteriography (EA), the role of EA in hemodynamically stable patients remains controversial. Emergency arteriography in patients with penetrating wounds to the lower extremities was studied.

Patients.—The arteriograms were reviewed of 80 males and 7 females aged 13–56 years who were injured in 100 lower limbs by high-velocity missiles. Thirteen patients had bilateral lower limb injuries. Indications for arteriography included proximity to a major vessel in 90 patients, multiple injuries in 19, and severe bone fractures or dislocations in 10. In most patients, EA was performed within 30 minutes after admission to the emergency room while the patient was still being resuscitated. Patients with an abnormality considered indicative of an arterial lesion on the arteriogram underwent emergency operation. Patients with a negative arteriogram, but in whom arterial trauma was strongly suspected on clinical grounds, underwent immediate surgical exploration. The remaining patients were admitted for observation and followed by echo-Doppler studies.

Results.—Of 79 limbs with positive EA findings, an arterial injury was found and treated in 76; no arterial lesion was found in the other 3 limbs. Of the 21 patients with normal arteriograms, 10 underwent surgical exploration because of a high clinical suspicion of vascular injury; 2 of these patients actually had an arterial injury. In 8 patients arteriographic findings led to modification of the surgical procedure. The 11 remaining patients had normal findings on clinical and echo-Doppler follow-up. Thus EA had a sensitivity of 97%, a specificity of 86%, a positive predictive value of 96%, a negative predictive value of 90%, and an accuracy of 95%.

Conclusion.—Emergency arteriography is a safe, accurate, and efficient method for diagnosing vascular injuries in hemodynamically stable patients. It avoids unnecessary surgical exploration and optimizes the surgical procedure by showing which artery is involved and the exact level of the vascular injury.

▶ This study reemphasizes the value of EA in patients who have sustained penetrating trauma to the lower extremities from high-velocity missiles. In this vast experience in Lebanon, unstable patients were operated on without EA. However, the role of EA in hemodynamically stable patients was extremely useful. In 76 of 79 patients with positive arteriography findings, a significant arterial injury was found. Interestingly, of 21 patients with normal arteriograms, 10 underwent surgical exploration because of a high clinical suspicion of vascular injury. Two of the 21 actually had an arterial injury. This led to a remarkable sensitivity of 97%, specificity of 86%, positive predicted value of 96%, negative predictive value of 90%, and an accuracy of 95%—truly remarkable results.—G.T. Shires, M.D.

The Management of Large Soft-Tissue Defects Following Close-Range Shotgun Injury
Hoekstra SM, Bender JS, Levison MA (Wayne State Univ)
J Trauma 130:1489–1493, 1990   4–10

Introduction.—The management of patients with large soft tissue defects caused by close-range shotgun blasts remains a major challenge to the trauma surgeon. Even if a patient survives the initial injury, the large devitalized wound areas generate a host of problems.

Patients.—Data were reviewed on 220 patients treated for shotgun wounds over an 8½-year period. Data on 43 were reviewed in depth. The average trauma score was 16 and the average injury severity score (ISS) was 12. In 22 patients there were soft tissue defects of an extremity, 18 had abdominal or chest injuries, and 3 had head or neck injuries. Of the 43 patients, 14 arrived in shock.

Management.—All patients underwent immediate surgical exploration and wide débridement of all devitalized tissue, along with repair of associated injuries. All wounds initially were left open and packed with fine-mesh gauze. Patients then underwent mandatory daily operative dressing changes with further débridement and irrigation until the wound could be closed primarily or could be safely allowed to granulate. All patients were given perioperative broad-spectrum antibiotics.

Results.—Complete débridement required a mean of 3 operating room visits. An average of 4.7 blood units was required during resuscitation and initial operation. In 4 wounds there was delayed primary closure, 8 were covered with split-thickness skin grafts, 9 were closed with myocutaneous flaps, and 19 were closed by secondary intent. Wound sepsis caused by inadequate débridement developed in 2 patients who were transferred after initial treatment elsewhere; both patients eventually underwent amputation. A third patient in whom early myonecrosis developed after a lengthy arterial repair also required amputation.

Conclusion.—Close-range shotgun blasts require a major time commitment by the trauma surgeon. Wound management by wide débridement at initial operation and mandatory reexamination with additional débridement in the operating room usually results in a satisfactory outcome.

▶ This report describes a different approach to large abdominal wall defects after a close-range shotgun injury. The authors used temporary packing with fine-mesh gauze or rayon cloth and ultimately closed all wounds with grafting, including flap closure.

This article is in contradistinction to many recent articles advocating the use of some form of mesh at the initial operative procedure. This approach has the advantage of obviating an average of 2 or 3 more dressing changes before closure with autogenous tissue.—G.T. Shires, M.D.

Analysis of Pulmonary Microvascular Permeability After Smoke Inhalation

Isago T, Noshima S, Traber LD, Herndon DN, Traber DL (Univ of Texas, Med Galveston; Shriners Burns Inst, Galveston)
J Appl Physiol 71:1403–1408, 1991   4–11

Objective.—Inhalation injury is a significant cause of death in thermally injured persons. The role of the pulmonary microvasculature in edema formation was examined in a sheep model in which pulmonary pressure was increased by pulmonary venous occluders in unanesthetized animals.

Methods.—Microvascular permeability to protein, a determinant of effective oncotic pressure, is represented in the Starling equation as the oncotic reflection coefficient (σ). A chronic sheep lung lymphatic preparation served to estimate σ and the filtration coefficient (K_f) after smoke inhalation. Animals were insufflated with either room air or cotton smoke.

Findings.—Pulmonary lymph flow rose by nearly fourfold after inhalation injury. At the same time, σ was reduced and K_f was elevated. The pulmonary capillary pressure also was increased. Both σ and K_f returned toward baseline values within 48 hours of injury, but the pulmonary capillary pressure remained elevated. Increased permeability accounted for 66% of the rise in capillary filtration 24 hours after inhalation and 25%

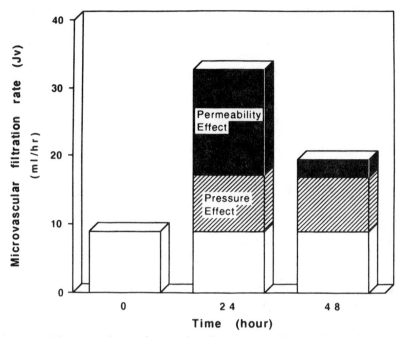

Fig 4–2—Relative contribution of increased capillary pressure and increased permeability to total capillary filtration after smoke inhalation. (Courtesy of Isago T, Noshima S, Traber LD, et al. *J Appl Physiol* 71:1403–1408, 1991.)

at 48 hours. Increased capillary pressure was responsible for 34% of the rise in capillary filtration 24 hours after infiltration and for 75% at 48 hours (Fig 4–2).

Conclusion.—The pulmonary edema that develops after smoke inhalation results from marked increases in both capillary pressure and permeability. Altered capillary permeability is especially important in the early phase of edema formation, whereas hydrostatic pressure changes predominate later in the course of inhalation injury.

▶ This interesting experimental article examined the role of the pulmonary microvasculature in edema formation in a sheep model after smoke inhalation injury. The conclusions of this study indicate that pulmonary edema developing after smoke inhalation results from marked increases in both capillary permeability and capillary pressure. It was the authors' feeling that the altered capillary permeability is especially important in the early phase of edema formation, whereas hydrostatic pressure changes predominated later in the course of inhalation injury. This experimental article tends to confirm the presence, which has been postulated, of direct alveolar capillary membrane injury with smoke inhalation.—G.T. Shires, M.D.

Management of Penetrating Colon Injuries: A Prospective Randomized Trial
Chappuis CW, Frey DJ, Dietzen CD, Panetta TP, Buechter KJ, Cohn I Jr (Louisiana State Univ)
Ann Surg 213:492–498, 1991   4–12

Introduction.—The management of colon injuries remains controversial, but most recent reviews favor an aggressive approach with primary repair. A prospective study enrolled 56 patients with penetrating colon injuries, 28 of whom underwent primary repair or resection with anastomosis. The other 28 patients were managed by diversion.

Patients and Management.—Most of the patients in both groups were young men. The average trauma score was similar in the 2 treatment groups. Twenty-four patients in the diversion group had colostomy, 3 had ileostomy, and 1 had a jejunostomy. Eleven patients in the primary repair group underwent resection with anastomosis (in 10 cases a stapled functional end-to-end anastomosis), and 17 had débridement and closure.

Outcome.—Complications were equally frequent in the 2 groups, but all dehiscences occurred in patients having diversion. Sepsis-related complications occurred in 18% of this group and in 21% of the group having primary repair. Twenty-two patients had the stoma closed.

Implications.—Virtually all civilian patients with penetrating colon trauma can be safely managed by primary repair. Primary repair or resection and anastomosis should be considered for all such patients.

▶ This remarkable study of relatively low-velocity injuries was presented as evidence based on findings in 28 patients that all colon injuries can be repaired primarily. This is probably the same as saying that when one swallow comes back to Capistrano, summer is in full bloom.

Certainly, many surgeons would agree that frequently a primary colon repair can be done safely, particularly in civilians who sustain low-velocity injuries. However, to say on the basis of this very limited experience that primary repair of the colon is consistently and uniformly safe seems to be stretching the rubber band beyond its tolerance.—G.T. Shires, M.D.

Nonoperative Management of Splenic Injuries
Oller B, Armengol M, Camps I, Rodriguez N, Montero A, Inaraja L, Salvia MD, Salva JA (Autonomous Univ of Barcelona, Spain)
Am Surg 57:409–413, 1991   4–13

Introduction.—Increasing awareness of the physiologic importance of the spleen has raised interest in the nonoperative management of splenic injury. Such management has proved effective in children with both splenic and renal lesions. Nonoperative management was assessed in 49 adults and 7 children older than 7 years who had splenic injuries confirmed by ultrasonography or CT.

Criteria for Selection.—Only patients with massive bleeding, associated abdominal injury requiring surgery, or blood dyscrasia underwent operation. Surgery was indicated if bleeding persisted after the patient received up to 4 units of packed red blood cells in the acute phase, or if bleeding recurred. During observation, patients were at total rest for 48 hours in the emergency department. A nasogastric tube was placed for continuous aspiration, and antibiotics were given to avoid infection.

Outcome.—Twelve of the 56 patients required emergency surgery because of associated lesions. Eight had massive bleeding. Fifteen of the 44 patients who were initially observed were hypotensive or had a low hematocrit. Eighty-four percent of patients did satisfactorily, the splenic lesion resolving within a mean time of $5^1/_2$ weeks. Fifteen patients required transfusion; 7 patients required surgery, but only 1 needed emergency splenectomy.

Implications.—In many patients the injured spleen heals spontaneously without complications. The view that splenic injury should always be treated surgically now is obsolete.

▶ This is another article attempting to extend indications for the nonoperative management of splenic injuries. However, the authors themselves admit that patients with massive bleeding associated with abdominal injury or blood dyscrasia should be excluded from consideration. Furthermore, surgery was required only if bleeding persisted after the patient received up to 4 units of packed red blood cells or bleeding recurred. The authors do not mention the fact that, in sustained attempts to use conservative therapy by giving additional blood, the danger of transmitted disease may well be a contraindication to such an approach. Nevertheless, the authors' major point is that frequently, if bleeding can be controlled, a spleen can be salvaged in the operating room. Nonoperative management is still fraught with far more difficulties.—G.T. Shires, M.D.

Total Mesh Wrapping for Parenchymal Liver Injuries: A Combined Experimental and Clinical Study
Stevens SL, Maull KI, Enderson BL, Meadors JN, Elkins LW Jr, Hopkins FM (Univ of Tennessee, Knoxville)
J Trauma 31:1103–1109, 1991   4–14

Introduction.—More patients who sustain severe hepatic injuries now reach the operating room alive, but existing treatments are still often inadequate. Failure to control hemorrhage remains the most critical problem. Perihepatic gauze packing was resurrected as a method of achieving hemostasis in patients with extreme liver injuries. Total mesh wrapping was developed because of complications associated with the gauze packing technique.

Patients.—Total mesh wrapping was attempted in 6 patients with blunt exsanguinating liver injuries. All patients were resuscitated but required multiple transfusions on hospital arrival. Two patients were stabilized initially with volume replenishment, and 4 were immediately taken to the operating room.

Surgical Technique.—Absorbable vicryl mesh is commercially available in 12-in. squares. Two squares are sewn together for one third of the distance, yielding a configuration resembling an inverted pair of pants. The "crotch" of the mesh pant is sutured to the diaphragm immediately anterior to the inferior vena caval diaphragmatic hiatus. Each "pant leg" is then passed over the right and left hepatic lobes and the mesh is sutured.

Outcome.—In 2 patients with bursting injuries to the liver, the mesh technique failed intraoperatively despite adequate tamponade. Postmortem examination revealed juxtacaval lacerations and hepatic vein avulsion injuries, which are not treatable by this technique. Although the hepatic wrap effectively stanched the parenchymal bleeding, the retrohepatic vein and retroperitoneal hemorrhage progressed unchecked. The other patient, who had a bilobar gunshot wound, died 38 days later of sepsis. The hepatic wrap method successfully controlled hemorrhage in the remaining 3 patients, resulting in long-term survival.

Conclusion.—The total hepatic mesh wrap technique can effectively secure hemostasis in patients with severe, diffuse, nonmechanical parenchymal bleeding. The technique is not intended to be used in place of controlling mechanical hemorrhage from discrete vessels or débriding dead hepatic parenchyma.

▶ These authors confirm that more patients with severe hepatic injury are reaching the operating room alive, but that failure to control hemorrhage remains the most critical problem in management. As a consequence, there has been a recent resurgence in the use of perihepatic gauze packing as a means of achieving emergency hemostasis in extreme liver injuries. It is also true that problems with removing the pack and sepsis in many of these patients are prohibitive unless consumptive coagulopathy has been corrected in the interim. These authors turned to total mesh wrapping because of the complications associated with the gauze packing technique.

Absorbable vicryl mesh was used to wrap the liver, both the right and left hepatic lobes, and the mesh was sutured to encapsulate the liver. In effect, the total hepatic mesh wrap technique was effective in securing hemostasis in patients with severe diffuse nonmechanical parenchymal bleeding. This is one more technique that may be used to attempt to control bleeding in patients with severe liver injuries.—G.T. Shires, M.D.

Preliminary Vascular Control for Renal Trauma
Atala A, Miller FB, Richardson JD, Bauer B, Harty J, Amin M (Univ of Louis-ville)
Surg Gynecol Obstet 172:386–390, 1991   4–15

Background.—When renal trauma has occurred and a large hematoma crosses the midline, dissection is time consuming and not always possi-ble. If a rapidly expanding renal hematoma is seen, delay in gaining vas-cular control permits continued blood loss in an unstable patient. Even control of the renal pedicle may be ineffective if more than 1 renal artery supplies the kidney, as is the case in nearly one third of the patients.

Objective.—Results were evaluated in 297 patients seen in a 10-year period with renal trauma. Sixty-three of 75 patients with penetrating in-jury and 12 of 222 patients with blunt injury underwent renal explora-tion. In 32 patients, vascular control was achieved before Gerota's fascia was entered. In the remaining 43 patients, the vascular pedicle was con-trolled manually immediately after Gerota's fascia was entered and, after brief clearing of the fascia, a clamp was placed on the pedicle. Renal in-jury was graded as shown in Figure 4-3.

Discussion.—The need for nephrectomy related to the degree of in-jury but not to the way in which vascular control was achieved. Gaining control after Gerota's fascia was opened not only failed to increase the need for nephrectomy, but it shortened the overall operating time by an average of nearly 1 hour. No complications resulted from renal explora-tion.

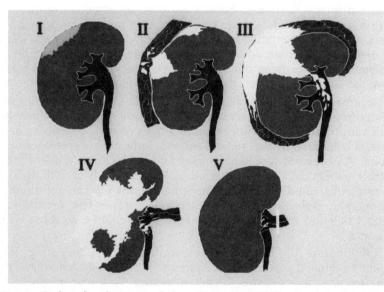

Fig 4–3.—Grading of renal injuries: grade I, renal contusion; grade II, minor laceration; grade III, major laceration; grade IV, shattered kidney, and grade V, vascular injury. (Courtesy of Atala A, Miller FB, Richardson JD, et al; *Surg Gynecol Obstet* 172:386–390, 1991.)

Recommendation.—It seems best to obtain vascular control after Gerota's fascia is entered when a large hematoma crosses the midline, and also if a rapidly expanding renal hematoma is seen or the patient is unstable. The same approach is helpful if the injury itself has opened Gerota's fascia.

▶ This is another article advocating more aggressive control of renal vasculature when there is little doubt that the kidney has been severely injured. These authors recommend proximal control of the renal vessels after opening Gerota's fascia. It is also true that the vascular control may well be done with vascular instrumentation, so that one is not committed to nephrectomy with proximal renal arterial and venous control. In this series, obtaining vascular control after opening the Gerota's fascia did not increase the nephrectomy rate and shortened the operative time by approximately an hour.—G.T. Shires, M.D.

Retroperitoneal Trauma
Frame SB, McSwain NE Jr (Univ of Tennessee, Knoxville; Tulane Univ)
Complications in Surgery February,46–50, 1991   4–16

Introduction.—Increasingly, patients arrive at emergency rooms with injuries that would have been fatal in the past. Reported mortality in patients with retroperitoneal hematoma is 20%, but it is considerably higher when a major vascular injury is present.

Mechanisms.—A knife or bullet can injure any structure in the retroperitoneal space. High-velocity projectiles may cause damage by a blast effect. Whereas penetrating injuries of the back or flank may not lead to intraperitoneal damage, structures overlying the spine are especially vulnerable to damage from blunt trauma. Deceleration injury is prone to move the kidneys and exert shearing force at points of tethering.

Diagnosis.—Peritoneal lavage is not a reliable means of detecting early isolated retroperitoneal injuries. Plain abdominal x-ray studies may help by demonstrating retroperitoneal air or a mass effect secondary to hematoma. Hematuria is the most sensitive indicator of retroperitoneal trauma. A cystogram should be obtained if bladder injury is suspected. In a stable patient, lack of visualization of 1 renal unit is an indication for arteriography, although under proper conditions CT can substitute for angiography. Reliable CT studies are highly dependent on the interpreter's skill and experience. Triple contrast should be used for CT assessment.

Exploration.—All hematomas associated with penetrating injury should be opened and explored. Assessment of the duodenum and pancreas requires an extensive Kocher maneuver. Any patient who is explored for abdominal injury might have damage to a hollow viscus and should receive antibiotic coverage for the most common enteric bacteria. Intravenous cefoxitin is suggested.

▶ This article reemphasizes that more and more patients are arriving in the emergency rooms with injuries previously reported as fatal. Certainly, in this group of patients, retroperitoneal hematoma is a potentially serious injury with overall mortalities ranging in the 20% range. This article adds credence to the previously recommended categorization of retroperitoneal injuries: zone 1, central injuries—all retroperitoneal hematomas should be explored; zone 3, pelvic rim injuries—exploration should probably be avoided unless the injuries continue to bleed massively; even then it probably is better left alone for tamponade; zone 2, lateral injuries—many believe that all be explored if the hematoma is of any significant size; certainly, an expanding or significantly bleeding hematoma in the zone 2 region demands exploration. The authors make the point that many patients are still lost because of failure of aggressive attacks on retroperitoneal hematomas, and this is probably correct.—G.T. Shires, M.D.

Gut Bacterial Translocation Via the Portal Vein: A Clinical Perspective With Major Torso Trauma
Moore FA, Moore EE, Poggetti R, McAnena OJ, Peterson VM, Abernathy CM, Parsons PE (Denver Gen Hosp)
J Trauma 31:629–638, 1991   4–17

Introduction.—Animal studies suggest that the transmural migration of viable gastrointestinal organisms may be a major factor in the development of posttrauma multiple organ failure. There also is clinical evidence that bacterial translocation is common in injured patients. The gut-portal vein-liver axis was evaluated shortly after injury to learn whether gut-derived organisms, endotoxin, or cytokines appear in the portal vein and if their presence correlates with the occurrence of multiple organ failure.

Patients and Methods.—Thirteen patients with blunt and 7 with penetrating injuries had portal venous catheters placed for blood sampling. This continued for up to 5 days postoperatively. The patients, known to be at risk of multiple organ failure, all required emergency laparotomy. Eleven patients had received massive transfusion, 6 had sustained major abdominal trauma, and 3 had multiple fractures.

Findings and Outcome.—Six patients had multiple organ failure, 5 of them more than 5 days after injury. Two of these patients had positive early portal vein cultures, and 3 of them ultimately had positive systemic blood cultures. The only positive systemic culture obtained in the first 5 days grew *Staphylococcus aureus;* the specimen was obtained from a patient with concurrent staphyloccal pneumonia. Endotoxin was not detected in either portal or systemic blood within 48 hours of surgery. Portal and systemic blood levels of C3a, tumor necrosis factor, and

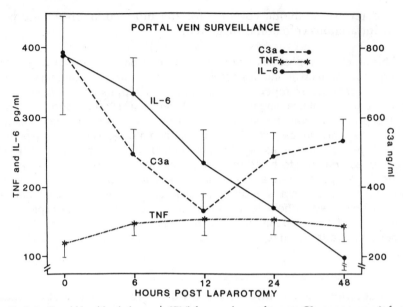

Fig 4–4.—Portal blood levels (mean ± SEM) for complement fragment C3a, tumor necrosis factor (TNF), and interleukin=6 (IL=6) obtained in the operating room (0 hour) and at 6, 12, 24, and 48 hours postoperatively. (Courtesy of Moore FA, Moore EE, Poggetti R, et al: *J Trauma* 31:629–638, 1991.)

interleukin-6 (Fig 4-4) were nearly identical and did not differ in patients who had multiple organ failure.

Further Observations.—In a later group of 31 trauma patients who required urgent laparotomy, 3 of the 11 whose systolic blood pressure was below 90 torr had positive blood cultures, and 2 of them exsanguinated. None of the 20 patients with higher blood pressure had positive blood cultures.

Interpretation.—This study failed to consistently demonstrate portal or systemic bacteria within 5 days of injury in patients in whom multiple organ failure occurs. Nevertheless, delayed bacterial translocation through a disrupted gut mucosa, induced by environmental cofactors in an immunocompromised host, may help to sustain multiple organ failure.

▶ This is the second study in traumatized patients attempting to document transmural migration of viable gastrointestinal organisms after injury as a predisposing factor in the development of multiple organ failure. Here, the bowel portal vein liver access was evaluated shortly after injury in order to learn whether bowel-derived organisms, endotoxin, or cytokines appear in the portal vein. In 6 patients multiple organ failure developed, in 5 of them more than 5 days after injury. Two of the patients had positive early portal vein cultures and 3 had systemic vein blood cultures that were positive. Portal and systemic blood levels of C3a, tumor necrosis factor, and interleukin-6 were almost identical and did not differ in the patients in whom multiple organ failure developed.

As the authors point out, this study failed to consistently demonstrate portal systemic bacteria within 5 days of injuries in patients who progressed to multiple organ failure. However, bacterial translocation through a disrupted bowel mucosa may be an environmental factor when there is concomitant mucosal injury. As the authors point out, much more work needs to be done in this area.—G.T. Shires, M.D.

Bacterial Translocation in Trauma Patients
Peitzman AB, Udekwu AO, Ochoa J, Smith S (Univ of Pittsburgh)
J Trauma 31:1083–1087, 1991   4–18

Introduction.—Sepsis is a major cause of morbidity and death in trauma patients. Bacterial translocation, which is induced by hypotension, endotoxemia, or burn injury, occurs reproducibly in the laboratory setting; however, bacteremia has not been observed consistently in trauma patients studied several days after injury.

Study Design.—Bacterial translocation to the mesenteric lymph nodes (MLNs) was studied in a prospective series of 29 patients, 25 with blunt trauma and 4 who underwent laparotomy for primary gastrointestinal disease.

Findings.—Of the 4 patients who underwent laparotomy for gastrointestinal disease, 3 had positive MLN cultures. All MLNs obtained from trauma patients were culture negative, as were all peritoneal cultures. Two trauma patients and 1 of the patients who were operated on died with *Pseudomonas aeruginosa* infection. A total of 40% of the trauma patients had complications.

Conclusions.—Bacterial translocation to the MLNs appears to be uncommon in acutely injured patients. The classic bacterial route from the gut to the MLNs and then to the liver, spleen, and circulation may require time as well as gut mucosal injury.

▶ This interesting study examined the role of bacterial translocation in injured patients. A group of patients with primary intestinal disease was used for comparison, and live organisms could be recovered from the mesenteric lymph nodes in patients with primary intestinal disease; no such recovery was possible in the injured patients.

This is fascinating in view of the frequently demonstrated phenomenon in the laboratory that translocation to mesenteric lymph nodes is a short and transient affair unless infection supervenes. The patients studied here had 2 major problems: all had received a cephalosporin before the operative procedure and the obtaining of lymph nodes for culture, and it may well be that the antibiotic coverage prevented bacterial growth in the biopsied lymph nodes; these patients, certainly immediately after surgery, did not have a significant superseding infection that, even in animal experiments, is necessary to produce significant and prolonged translocation.

There is no question that the entire issue of bacterial translocation in relation to sepsis from endogenous organisms is unclear.—G.T. Shires, M.D.

Aminoglycoside Combinations Versus Beta-Lactams Alone for Penetrating Abdominal Trauma: A Meta-Analysis

Hooker KD, DiPiro JT, Wynn JJ (Univ of Missouri-Kansas City School of Pharmacy; Univ of Georgia College of Pharmacy; Med College of Georgia, Augusta)
J Trauma 31:1155–1160, 1991   4–19

Introduction.—It remains uncertain whether single-drug treatment is as effective as combinations including an aminoglycoside in patients with penetrating abdominal injury.

Methods.—The efficacy of single β-lactam antimicrobials was compared with that of combinations containing aminoglycoside in a meta-analysis of 17 published, randomized trials that included 1,956 patients with gunshot and/or stab wounds or blunt injuries.

Results.—None of the trials demonstrated a statistically significant difference between single-agent treatment and combination treatment. When data from all 17 trials were analyzed, the risk of infection when a single drug was used was actually lower than when combination treatment was given, although the difference was not significant (Fig 4–5).

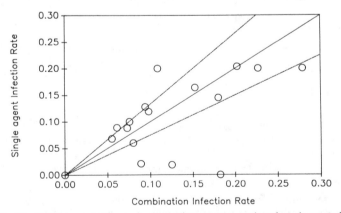

Fig 4–5.—The infection rate in the single agent β-lactam group is plotted on the *vertical axis* and the infection rate of the aminoglycoside combination group is plotted on the *horizontal axis*. Equal rates (*centerline*) and 25% risk reduction are indicated by the 3 lines. The lack of a consistent treatment effect (heterogeneity) is demonstrated. (Courtesy of Hooker KD, DiPiro JT, Wynn JJ: *J Trauma* 31:1155–1160, 1991.)

Conclusion.—A single β-lactam antimicrobial may be used in place of traditional combination treatment in patients with penetrating abdominal injury.

▶ The relatively new meta-analysis technique of comparison of multiple studies was used to predict outcome after single-drug or combination-drug treatment, including an aminoglycoside, in patients with penetrating abdominal injuries. The conclusions were that a single β-lactam antimicrobial may be used in place of traditional combination treatment in patients with penetrating abdominal injury. This same message has been voiced in several individual clinical studies, and it appears that the weight of evidence is now swinging clearly toward the use of a single broad-spectrum, effective, safe antibiotic as early therapy after penetrating abdominal injury.—G.T. Shires, M.D.

A Randomized Trial of Replacement Antioxidant Vitamin Therapy for Neutrophil Locomotory Dysfunction in Blunt Trauma
Maderazo EG, Woronick CL, Hickingbotham N, Jacobs L, Bhagavan HN (Hartford Hosp, Hartford, Conn; Univ of Connecticut; Hoffmann-La Roche, Inc, Nutley, NJ)
J Trauma 31:1142–1150, 1991   4–20

Background.—There is evidence that byproducts of oxygen reduction have a causative role in the polymorphonuclear neutrophil (PMN) dysfunction and cell damage associated with hyperactivated states such as severe injury. The serum and cellular levels of consumable antioxidants (ascorbic acid, α-tocopherol) are reduced after blunt injury.

Objective.—The effects of antioxidant vitamins on the recovery of PMN function were examined in 46 patients with serious blunt trauma; all but 1 of the 46 had been in a motor vehicle accident. In a placebo-controlled, double-blind, randomized block design, the patients received 100 mL of 5% dextrose in water or saline; 200 mg or 500 mg of ascorbic acid plus 50 mg of dl-α-tocopherol; or each antioxidant alone.

Findings.—The locomotor ability of PMNs was improved by antioxidant treatment. Although administration of both agents was much more effective than the use of either agent alone, administration of a single agent was more effective than placebo administration.

Conclusion.—Treatment with α-tocopherol and ascorbic acid significantly improves the mobility of PMNs in patients with serious blunt injuries. It is reasonable to expect improved antibacterial defense as a result.

▶ This is another in a variety of articles this year indicating that the final common denominator after cytokine release is probably lipid peroxidation by oxidants such as oxygen free radicals, hydroxyl free radicals, and the like. The current study used an antioxidant vitamin and α-tocopherol as therapy to improve locomotory function in PMLs. It was clear that in this model, both ascorbic acid and α-tocopherol were effective in improving the PMN locomotor abnormality that occurs after blunt trauma.—G.T. Shires, M.D.

5 Wound Healing

Cigarette Smoking Decreases Tissue Oxygen

Jensen JA, Goodson WH, Hopf HW, Hunt TK (Univ of California, San Francisco)

Arch Surg 126:1131–1134, 1991   5–1

Introduction.—Because rates of epithelialization, collagen deposition, and angiogenesis are clearly related to tissue oxygen tension (PO_2), evidence that smoking compromises tissue PO_2 might help to explain why it influences healing adversely.

Methods.—Subcutaneous wound PO_2 was estimated using a tonometer in 8 normal subjects who first were asked to think about smoking and take puffs from unlighted cigarettes, and then to smoke at their usual rate for 10 minutes. Measurements continued for an hour.

Findings.—A significant fall in subcutaneous PO_2 followed smoking in all subjects (Fig 5-1). A decrease of up to 48% was evident at 30 minutes, but values were within 5% of baseline 1 hour after the subjects began smoking. Skin temperature fell from 31.8°C to 31.5°C and then increased. The mean blood nicotine level peaked at 11.1 ng/mL from a baseline of 4.3 ng/mL.

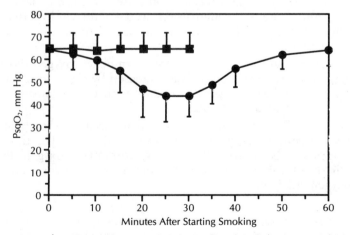

Fig 5-1.—Mean ± 1 SD wound-tissue oxygen tension ($Psqo_2$) in the upper arms of 8 volunteers during and after a 10-minute period of smoking lighted (*circles*) and unlighted (*squares*) cigarettes. (Courtesy of Jensen JA, Goodson WH, Hopf HW, et al: *Arch Surg* 126:1131–1134, 1991.)

Conclusions.—The adverse effects of cigarette smoking on wound healing may be caused in large part by activation of the adrenergic system, vasoconstriction, and a decrease in subcutaneous wound PO_2. α-adrenergic blockade might be helpful if it is necessary to ensure wound healing in a patient who is not willing to stop smoking.

▶ This is an elegant description of the effect of smoking on subcutaneous O_2 levels. It is a shame that the authors didn't perform simultaneous transcutaneous oxygen measurements because these are more universally used today and would be helpful in evaluating potential healing problems in cutaneous ulcers as well as incisional wounds. The suggestions of α-adrenergic blockers to promote healing in smokers seems sound but must await trials before being accepted as fact.—M.C. Robson, M.D.

Relationship of Oxygen Dose to Antiogenesis Induction in Irradiated Tissue
Marx RE, Ehler WJ, Tayapongsak P, Pierce LW (Univ of Miami; Wilford Hall USAF Med Ctr, Miami)
Am J Surg 160:519–524, 1990   5–2

Objective.—Hyperbaric oxygen is effective in preventing and treating osteoradionecrosis and in reconstructing tissue defects within an irradiated field, ostensibly by inducing capillary angiogenesis and fibroplasia. The degree of angiogenesis was quantified after exposure of irradiated tissue to hyperbaric oxygen.

Methods.—Anesthetized rabbits were exposed to mandibular irradiation with a ^{60}Co source and received 30 doses of 2 Gy, 5 days a week. After 6 months some of the animals received a course of hyperbaric oxygen, delivered at 2.4 ATA for 90 minutes a day, 5 times a week for a total of 20 sessions.

Observations.—Although exposure to normobaric oxygen did not alter angiogenesis, vascular density was increased by eight- to ninefold on exposure to hyperbaric oxygen, compared with both exposure to normobaric oxygen and air breathing.

Discussion.—Oxygen in hyperbaric form acts as a drug to enhance angiogenesis in chronically hypovascular irradiated tissue. The therapeutic range appears to be narrow. Presumably, normobaric oxygen does not physically dissolve enough oxygen into the tissues to form a sufficiently steep oxygen gradient.

▶ This elegantly designed study demonstrates the utility of hyperbaric oxygen to aid angiogenesis in radiated, hypoxic, poorly perfused wounds. However, if the discussion is correct, it would suggest that other wounds for which hyperbaric oxygen is continually touted would not benefit from its use.

Breathing 100% oxygen at 1 ATA should provide the necessary gradient to stimulate angiogenesis in most wounds.—M.C. Robson, M.D.

Injury Induces In Vivo Expression of Platelet-Derived Growth Factor (PDGF) and PDGF Receptor mRNAs in Skin Epithelial Cells and PDGF mRNA in Connective Tissue Fibroblasts

Antoniades HN, Galanopoulos T, Neville-Golden J, Kiritsy CP, Lynch SE (Harvard School of Public Health; Ctr for Blood Research, Boston; Inst of Molecular Biology, Boston; Harvard School of Dental Medicine)
Proc Natl Acad Sci USA 88:565–569, 1991   5–3

Background.—Platelet-derived growth factor (PDGF) is a potent mitogen, a chemoattractant for connective tissue cells, and a stimulator of collagen synthesis by fibroblasts. It may also play a role in wound healing. This hypothesis was tested by experiments involving healing of cutaneous injury in pigs.

Methods.—Skin biopsy specimens from 3 pigs were tested before and after surgically induced wounding to a depth of about 1 mm. Expression of c-*sis*/PDGF-2 and PDGF receptor mRNAs was assessed by in situ hybridization. Expression of the corresponding protein products was assessed by immunocytochemistry.

Results.—Skin epithelial cells obtained before injury showed no expression of PDGF-receptor b or c-*sis* mRNAs or protein products. In contrast, epithelial cells from wounded tissue expressed c-*sis*/PDGF-2 and PDGF receptor mRNAs and the proteins cross-reactive to the appropriate antibodies. Connective tissue fibroblasts did not express c-*sis* mRNA before injury. After injury, fibroblasts expressed c-*sis* mRNA and proteins, and significantly increased their expression of PDGF receptor mRNA and protein. Wounded tissues strongly expressed c-*sis* and PDGF receptor within 2–3 days of injury, with expression declining thereafter.

Conclusions.—Acute skin injury caused by surgical incision in swines seems to induce reversible expression of PDGF receptor b mRNA and c-*sis*/PDGF-2 in epithelial cells. Skin injury also appears to increase expression of PDGF receptors in skin fibroblasts. Platelet-derived growth factor and its receptor may function in an autocrine/paracrine fashion to regulate the normal healing process. Defects in regulation might be involved in impairment of healing or in proliferative disorders.

▶ This paper fills a void in the understanding of tissue repair. It was known that levels of growth factors such as PDGF exist ubiquitously. However, receptors were not found on normal wound healing cells such as soft tissue fibroblasts or skin keratinocytes. These authors demonstrate that the necessary receptors appear as a result of injury. They further show that the receptors disappear after healing. This observation should prevent proliferative scar formation (keloid or hypertrophic scar) or tumor formation.—M.C. Robson, M.D.

Stimulation of Healing of Chronic Wounds by Epidermal Growth Factor

Brown GL, Curtsinger L, Jurkiewicz MJ, Nahai F, Schultz G (Univ of Louisville; Emory Univ; Univ of Florida)
Plast Reconstr Surg 88:189–196, 1991
5–4

Background.—Peptide growth factors are thought to play vital roles in the natural process of wound healing in the skin. In studies of both animals and human beings, topical application of biochemically defined peptide growth factors have promoted wound healing. The effect of topically applied epidermal growth factor (EGF) on the healing of chronic wounds was evaluated in a prospective, open-label, crossover study.

Methods.—The subjects were 5 men and 4 women (average age, 57 years), all with wounds that had failed to respond to conventional medical and surgical treatments, including débridement, skin grafts, and vascular reconstruction (table). The ulcers had been present for an average of 12 months before EGF treatment was started. All wounds were treated twice a day with Silvadene for 3 weeks to 6 months. If that treatment had no effect, treatment with Silvadene containing EGF, 10 $\mu g/g$, was begun.

Results.—None of the wounds showed any evidence of healing during Silvadene treatment. With EGF-Silvadene treatment, however, 8 of 9 wounds healed completely. The average time to healing was 34 days, and there was no recurrence for 1–4 years. There was 1 treatment failure in a patient with rheumatoid arthritis, although her wound decreased in size.

Conclusions.—Results of this preliminary study suggest that EGF may promote healing of chronic wounds and that further clinical evaluation of this treatment is justified. A double-blind study of a uniform population of patients is needed. The findings imply that the wound may contain insufficient levels of EGF, or that the effectiveness of growth factors is limited by other factors.

▶ This reviewer believes that this report must be viewed very critically. The etiologies of the chronic wounds are mixed. No attributes of the wounds were described, e.g., local vascularity, oxygen tension, scarring of the wound margins, or tissue bacteriology. This was a one-way crossover study, and without bacteriology of the wounds it is difficult to interpret. The vehicle for the EGF itself has known wound healing properties (1). Despite this, the paper is one of the first clinical trials of growth factors and may predict an ability to treat the chronic, indolent wound.—M.C. Robson, M.D.

Chronic Ulcers Treated With Epidermal Growth Factor–Silvadene

Case	Age	Sex	History	Previous Treatments	Ulcer Size Before Epidermal Growth Factor Treatment	Duration of Ulcer	
						Before Epidermal Growth Factor	With Epidermal Growth Factor
1	59	M	Diabetes, metatarsal amputation	2 failed skin grafts 6 months Silvadene	8 × 3 cm	9 months	21 days
2	62	M	Diabetes, great toe amputation	1 failed skin graft 3 weeks Silvadene	4 × 3 cm	1 month	12 days
3	72	M	Diabetes, metatarsal amputation	1 failed skin graft 3 months Silvadene	1.5 × 1.5 cm	12 months	41 days
4	48	M	Diabetes, foot ulcer	1 failed skin graft 1 month Silvadene	2 × 2 cm	6 months	42 days
5	65	F	Rheumatoid arthritis, pretibial ulcer	2 failed skin grafts 2 months Silvadene	4 × 4 cm	12 months	24 days
6	54	F	Rheumatoid arthritis, medial malleolar ulcer	2 failed skin grafts 1 month Silvadene	8 × 10 cm	48 months	120 days*
7	60	M	Old burn wound, pretibial ulcer	2 failed skin grafts 4 months Silvadene	7 × 4 cm	12 months	92 days
8	58	F	Old burn wound, forearm (diabetic)	1 month Silvadene	6 × 2 cm	2 months	14 days
9	40	F	Midline abdominal incision	6 failed wound closures 1 month Silvadene	4 × 3 cm	7 months	28 days

* Wound decreased to 6 × 8 cm but failed to heal completely.
(Courtesy of Brown GL, Curtsinger L, Jurkiewicz MJ, et al: *Plast Reconstr Surg* 88:189–196, 1991.)

Reference

1. Penneys NS: *Acta Dermatol Venerol (Stockh)* 62:59, 1982.

Platelet-Derived Growth Factor-BB and Transforming Growth Factor Beta$_1$ Selective Modulate Glycosaminoglycans, Collagen, and Myofibroblasts in Excisional Wounds

Pierce GF, Vande Berg J, Rudolph R, Tarpley J, Mustoe TA (Amgen Inc, Thousand Oaks, Calif; VA Med Ctr, La Jolla; Univ of California, San Diego; Scripps Clin and Research Found, La Jolla; Washington Univ)
Am J Pathol 138:629–646, 1991   5–5

Introduction.—Both recombinant platelet-derived growth factor (PDGF) and transforming growth factor-beta$_1$ (TGF-β_1) alter the rate of extracellular matrix formation in incisional wounds. However, incisional healing is difficult to quantify. A full-thickness excisional wound model in the rabbit ear was developed to analyze growth-factor-mediated wound repair.

Methods.—The rabbit ear was subjected to a 6-mm wound made through perichondrial membrane to bare cartilage. Growth factors or buffer were applied and levels of glycosaminoglycan (GAG), collagen, myofibroblasts, and acute inflammatory cells were monitored.

Results.—A single application of either PDGF-BB or TGF-β_1 significantly increased the depth, area, and volume of new granulation tissue. Both factors augmented extracellular matrix formation and healing in 10-day wounds. Whereas PDGF had more marked effects on macrophage influx and GAG deposition, TGF-β_1 selectively induced mature collagen bundles at the leading edge of new granulation tissue. Myofibroblasts were present in control wounds but absent from early growth-factor-treated wounds.

Conclusion.—In this model, PDGF-BB augmented the acute inflammatory phase of wound healing, and TGF-β_1 had a more direct effect on collagen synthesis. Inhibition of myofibroblast formation suggests that these factors may be helpful in stimulating extracellular matrix formation when wound contraction should be minimized.

▶ Using a rabbit ear model described by Mustoe et al. (1), the authors were able to demonstrate the effect of PDGF and TGF-β_1 on extracellular matrix and granulation tissue. They also show a significant difference between these growth factors because PDGF deposits more extracellular matrix and TGF-β_1 deposits more collagen early in the wound healing scheme. This paper may give credence to the concept that myofibroblasts are skeletons of active fibroblasts. They are not present early in these proliferative wounds treated with growth factors.—M.C. Robson, M.D.

Reference

1. Mustoe TA, et al: *J Clin Invest* 87:694, 1991.

Effect of bFGF on the Inhibition of Contraction Caused by Bacteria
Stenberg BD, Phillips LG, Hokanson JA, Heggers JP, Robson MC (Univ of Texas, Galveston; Shriners Burns Inst, Galveston)
J Surg Res 50:47–50, 1991   5–6

Introduction.—Bacterial activity can inhibit wound contraction by promoting breakdown of proteins and eliminating the fibrinous elements required for healing to take place. Basic fibroblast growth factor (bFGF) is chemotactic to mesodermal cells and is mitogenic. It is a strong inducer of angiogenesis and has augmented the production of extracellular matrix components such as fibronectin and proteoglycans.

Methods.—A model of acutely contaminated injury in the rat served to evaluate bFGF for altering the inhibition of wound contraction by bacteria. Wounds measuring 1.5 cm² were excised through the skin and panniculus carnosus and were inoculated with *Escherichia coli*. The amount of bFGF applied ranged from 1 to 100 μg.

Results.—Infection significantly prolonged the time to total wound closure, but application of bFGF in any dose promoted wound closure. The lower doses appeared to be more effective than when 100 μg of bFGF was applied to a 1.5-cm² wound. Treatment with bFGF decreased the breaking strength of healed wounds.

Conclusion.—The use of bFGF shortened the time of wound healing in the presence of bacteria in this study. The factor may prove useful in the management of contaminated human wounds.

▶ The authors have presented a model of an acutely contaminated wound to test agents of wound modulation. The presence of bacteria inhibits healing by contraction. Application of the peptide growth factor bFGF overcomes the inhibition without significantly decreasing the bacterial count. Because open wounds tend to have a tissue bacterial presence, this model may be useful to predict clinical efficacy.—M.C. Robson, M.D.

Growth Factor-Induced Acceleration of Tissue Repair Through Direct and Inductive Activities in a Rabbit Dermal Ulcer Model
Mustoe TA, Pierce GF, Morishima C, Deuel TF (Washington Univ; Amgen, Inc, Thousand Oaks, Calif)
J Clin Invest 87:694–703, 1991   5–7

Introduction.—The full potential of polypeptide growth factors and the mechanisms by which they effectively initiate the time-dependent activities essential to wound healing are not established. A unique animal wound model with properties resembling the wound in human leg ulcers was used to test the influence of 4 growth factors on the rates of healing.

Methods.—Five μg of platelet-derived growth factor-B chain (PDGF-BB), epidermal growth factor, basic fibroblast growth factor, and transforming growth factor-β_1 (TGF-β_1) were applied locally to a full thickness dermal ulcer on an avascular base in a rabbit ear. The wound model precluded significant wound contraction and required new granulation tissue and epithelial cells for healing to originate centripetally.

Results.—There was a twofold increase in complete reepithelialization of wounds treated with PDGF-BB, basic fibroblast growth factor, and epidermal growth factor. Transforming growth factor-β_1 significantly inhibited reepithelialization. Platelet-derived growth factor-BB and TFG-β_1 uniquely increased the depth and area of new granulation tissue, the influx of fibroblasts, and the deposition of new matrix into wounds. Total protein synthesis (cells and media) estimated by [^{14}C]leucine incorporation in explants from 7-day-old PDGF-BB-treated wounds were 473% that of controls.

Conclusions.—Wound healing in a novel animal model was significantly augmented by a single application of PDGF-BB, epidermal growth factor, basic fibroblast growth factor, or TFG-β_1. Each growth factor induced unique responses in enhancing the healing of experimental ulcers. Platelet-derived growth factor-BB promoted wound reepithelialization to the same extent as epidermal growth factor and basic fibroblast growth factor. Only PDGF-BB and TFG-β_1 stimulated significant new granulation tissue, suggesting an important use of these growth factors in healing full-thickness dermal wounds.

▶ Animal models need to mimic human wounds to allow extrapolation of experimental results for possible clinical efficacy. Most animal wound models heal with a large degree of contraction. Lower extremity ulcers in humans heal mainly by extracellular matrix deposition and epithelialization. Therefore, the authors designed a model that heals similarly to the leg ulcer. Using this model they compared several peptide growth factors and could differentiate their effects on matrix deposition and epithelialization. This paper should signify another advance in clarifying wound healing modulation by growth factors and help in predicting clinical efficacy.—M.C. Robson, M.D.

Synthesis of Type I Collagen in Healing Wounds in Humans
Haukipuro K, Melkko J, Risteli L, Kairaluoma MI, Risteli J (Univ of Oulu, Finland)
Ann Surg 213:75–80, 1991   5–8

Introduction.—Types I and III collagens both appear in the granulation tissue of healing wounds, type III appearing in a higher proportion

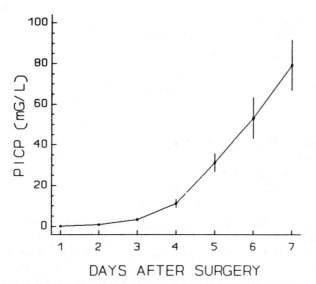

Fig 5-2.—Effect of time on the mean concentration of PICP in wound fluid of patients operated on for colorectal cancer. (Courtesy of Haukipuro K, Melkko J, Risteli L, et al: *Ann Surg* 213:75–80, 1991.)

than in the surrounding dermis. Type III procollagen synthesis has been measured in a healing wound by a radioimmunoassay for the aminoterminal propeptide of type III procollagen (PIIINP). A radioimmunoassay was developed to detect synthesis of type I procollagen by measuring the carboxyterminal propeptide of type I procollagen (PICP).

Methods.—To collect wound fluid from 20 surgical patients, 2 rubber tubes were left in the wounds after surgery. The PICP and PIIINP concentrations in the wound fluid were measured by specific radioimmunoassay for 7 days after surgery.

Results.—The mean concentration of PICP in wound fluid rose rapidly each day and achieved a mean concentration by day 7 that was 380 times the level on day 1 (Fig 5-2). The mean concentration of PIIINP rose more slowly, reaching a concentration on day 7 that was 250 times the level on day 1. The mean wound fluid concentration on day 1 was about twice as high as that in preoperative serum for PICP and 20 times as high for PIIINP.

Conclusions.—The assay for the carboxyterminal propeptide was a useful indicator of wound healing. The concentration of the PICP antigen can be considered a direct measure of collagen type I synthesis.

▶ On-line measurement of type I collagen by a simple radioimmunoassay technique aids the understanding of wound healing and provides a means of assessing modulation. It was found previously that type III collagen could be measured, and this technique has been quite useful (1). This new method may be especially helpful in understanding the proliferating literature regarding fetal wound healing.—M.C. Robson, M.D.

Reference

1. Haukipuro H, et al.: *Ann Surg* 206:752, 1987.

Alterations in Proteoglycan Synthesis Common to Healing Wounds and Tumors
Yeo T-K, Brown L, Dvorak HF (Beth Israel Hosp, Boston)
Am J Pathol 138:1437–1450, 1991   5–9

Background.—Both wound healing and the generation of tumor stroma share hyperpermeable vessels, fibrinogen extravasation, and extravascular clotting. In both cases, deposits of fibrin gel serve as an initial stroma before being replaced by granulation tissue. The role of proteoglycans in wound healing and tumor stroma generation remains uncertain.

Methods.—Immunohistochemical and biochemical methods were used to study dermatan sulfate proteoglycan (DSPG) and chondroitin sulfate proteoglycan (CSPG) in normal guinea pig and human dermis, healing skin wounds and scars, and several carcinomas. The tumors studied included guinea pig and human breast, colon, basal cell, and squamous lesions.

Findings.—Normal dermis stained weakly for CSPG and strongly for decorin, a small DSPG. The granulation tissue of healing skin wounds and scars stained weakly or not at all for decorin but intensely for CSPG. Decorin staining returned after digestion with chondroitin ABC lyase. Tumor stroma also stained strongly for CSPG and weakly, at best, for decorin. As in healing wounds, decorin staining reappeared after lyase digestion, suggesting that antigenic sites were masked by glycosaminoglycan chains.

Conclusions.—Similar abnormal patterns of proteoglycans expression are evident in healing skin wounds and the stroma of different types of carcinoma. The biological significance of these abnormalities remains uncertain, but larger and more heterogeneous proteoglycans may contribute to altered cell adhesion, migration, and proliferation.

▶ There are many similarities between the actively healing wound and the neoplastic tumor (1). Cell adhesion, migration, and proliferation are important events in both processes. In this paper, the authors found that healing wounds and stroma express a common pattern of altered proteoglycan staining. These observations may provide clues to the mechanisms responsible for both wound healing and tumor stroma generation.—M.C. Robson, M.D.

Reference

1. Dvorak HF: *N Engl J Med* 315:1650, 1986.

Studies in Fetal Wound Healing: V. A Prolonged Presence of Hyaluronic Acid Characterizes Fetal Wound Fluid
Longaker MT, Chiu ES, Adzick NS, Stern M, Harrison MR, Stern R (Univ of California, San Francisco)
Ann Surg 213:292–296, 1991   5–10

Background.—Fibrosis, scarring, and sometimes contracture characterize adult wound repair. Fetal wounds heal without fibrosis or scarring. A fetal wound extracellular matrix (ECM) rich in hyaluronic acid (HA) could permit repair without scar formation. A study was done to determine whether HA has a prolonged presence in fetal wound fluid.

Methods and Results.—A wire mesh cylinder model was used to test HA levels in fetal and adult lamb wound fluid. The HA level rose rapidly in adult wound fluid, peaked at day 3, and dropped to 0 by day 7. In fetal wound fluid, HA levels rose rapidly and remained significantly increased for 3 weeks (Fig 5–3).

Conclusions.—The prolonged presence of HA in fetal wound matrices may promote healing by regeneration instead of scarring. The prolonged application of HA or HA-protein complexes to wounds in children or adults may modulate healing in a way more like that observed in fetal wounds.

▶ Fetal wound healing experiments provide data that perhaps can be applied to other examples of wound healing. There are species differences,

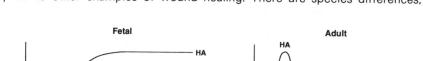

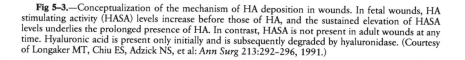

Fig 5–3.—Conceptualization of the mechanism of HA deposition in wounds. In fetal wounds, HA stimulating activity (HASA) levels increase before those of HA, and the sustained elevation of HASA levels underlies the prolonged presence of HA. In contrast, HASA is not present in adult wounds at any time. Hyaluronic acid is present only initially and is subsequently degraded by hyaluronidase. (Courtesy of Longaker MT, Chiu ES, Adzick NS, et al: *Ann Surg* 213:292–296, 1991.)

however, and all of the data are not in agreement. Nevertheless, these authors are systematically dissecting out the variables and making useful observations. The full story on HA is not in. Possibly, it is because the HA-fibrin interaction may be more important than HA alone (1).—M.C. Robson, M.D.

Reference

1. Weigel PH, et al: *J Theor Biol* 119:219, 1986.

6 Infections

Prevalence of Infection With Human Immunodeficiency Virus in Elective Surgery Patients

Charache P, Cameron JL, Maters AW, Frantz EI (Johns Hopkins Hosp and Univ)

Ann Surg 214:562–568, 1991

6-1

Introduction.—Knowing which surgical patients are most likely to be infected with HIV could lead to procedural and behavioral adjustments that would further limit the risk of infection in health care workers. An anonymous survey was made of 4,087 patients admitted for elective surgery at a large urban hospital. Both children and adults were included.

Findings.—Eighteen patients (.4%) proved to be infected with HIV, as confirmed by Western blot antibody testing (Fig 6-1). Thirteen of the 18 patients had risk factors, most often a history of a positive HIV test. Only .12% of the patients were infected without any history of a risk factor, or with a history of transfusion only.

Conclusions.—Human immunodeficiency virus infection is infrequent in patients scheduled for elective surgery. There would not seem to be substantial reason to screen all such patients for HIV antibody. Never-

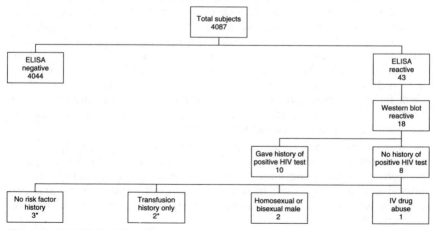

* Risk would not be identified by admission history.

Fig 6-1.—Serologic test results, number of cases of true HIV infection, and information available on admission for infected cases. (Courtesy of Charache P, Cameron JL, Maters AW, et al: *Ann Surg* 214:562–568, 1991.)

theless, there will be a small number of HIV-positive patients who cannot be identified by the admitting history, thus necessitating strict adherence to universal precautions throughout the hospital, and especially in the operating area.

Universal Precautions Are Not Universally Followed
Courington KR, Patterson SL, Howard RJ (Univ of Florida)
Arch Surg 126:93–96, 1991   6–2

Background.—Health care workers are at increased risk of infection with many pathogens transmitted by blood and body fluids, particularly HIV and hepatitis B virus. Adherence to the universal precautions of the Centers for Disease Control, which address use of barrier techniques, handwashing, handling of sharp instruments, saliva precautions, workers with exudative lesions, and pregnant workers, should be high. Adherence to the precautions was investigated in surgical patient care areas in a university hospital.

Methods.—The surgical teams of an 18-unit operating room, 3 surgical ward patient-care teams, and surgical intensive care personnel in an 18-bed unit were observed in the course of their routine patient care activities both before and after they attended educational programs specifically designed to improve compliance with universal precautions.

Results.—Infractions were observed in 57% of observed procedures in the first study and 58% of procedures in the second study. In the first study at least 1 member of the operating room team failed to wear eye protection, most commonly a surgical nurse-technician. In the second study infractions occurred in 81% of procedures and the surgical nurse-technicians were significantly less compliant than before. Plastic surgery, gynecology, otolaryngology, and urology teams consistently had at least 1 noncompliant member. The cardiothoracic team had the best total compliance. The most common offense on the surgical ward was failure to wear gloves. Medical students committed the most infractions in the first study and residents in the second. In the surgical intensive care ward, failure to wear gloves was also the most common infraction, with most offenders being residents. This was the only unit in which compliance significantly improved between studies.

Conclusions.—Lack of adherence to universal precautions appears to be common, and 1-time educational efforts appear insufficient to rectify this condition. Ongoing educational programs for personnel caring for surgical patients may result in substantial overall improvement. Services in which widespread blood loss is relatively uncommon should receive particular attention.

▶ The 2 papers reviewed in Abstracts 6–1 and 6–2 represent must reading for all surgeons. The first suggests that the diagnosis of a positive HIV state occurs in patients who have no risk factors. The only way to prevent exposure in such cases is to routinely follow the universal precautions recommended by the CDC. The second paper demonstrates quite alarmingly that such precautions are not followed. Even educational programs regarding the universal precautions did not result in compliance by surgical team members. The data are clear. We must do better or risk exposure.—M.C. Robson, M.D.

Surgical Wound Infection Rates by Wound Class, Operative Procedure, and Patient Risk Index
Culver DH, Horan TC, Gaynes RP, Martone WJ, Jarvis WR, Emori TG, Banerjee SN, Edwards JR, Tolson JS, Henderson TS, Hughes JM, and the Natl Nosocomial Infections Surveillance System
Am J Med 91 (suppl 3B):152S–157S, 1991   6–3

Background.—Measuring clinical outcomes is becoming increasingly important, but lack of an adequate means of adjusting for case mix has impeded a determination of nosocomial infection rates that can be used to make meaningful intrahospital and interhospital comparisons. The traditional classification of surgical wound infections (SWIs) into clean, clean-contaminated, contaminated, and dirty-infected cases fails to account for intrinsic patient risk.

Objective.—A simple index was developed by analyzing 10 potential risk factors using logistic regression techniques. Data from 44 National Nosocomial Infections Surveillance System hospitals were used in the study. The score on the Study on the Efficacy of Nosocomial Infection

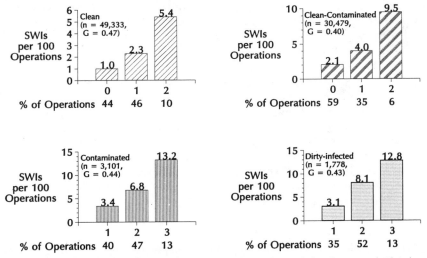

Fig 6–2.—Surgical wound infection (*SWIs*) rates, by traditional wound classification and risk index. *G*, Goodman-Kruskal correlation coefficient. (Courtesy of Culver DH, Horan TC, Gaynes RP, et al: *Am J Med* 91 (suppl 3B):152S–157S, 1991.)

Control (SENIC) index is the number of risk factors present among an American Society of Anesthesiologists (ASA) score of 3, 4, or 5; a contaminated or dirty-infected operation; and an operation lasting for more than a critical time, which depends on the particular procedure.

Findings.—Wound class remained a moderately accurate predictor of SWI risk, but the ASA score was at least as good as a single risk predictor. The composite index provided substantial improvement in predicting the risk of SWI (Fig 6–2). Infection rates rose significantly with the number of risk factors in most types of surgery.

Conclusions.—The SENIC index predicts infection risk better than the traditional system of classifying surgical wounds, and it performs well across a wide range of surgical procedures.

Effect of Surgeon's Diagnosis on Surgical Wound Infection Rates

Taylor G, McKenzie M, Kirkland T, Wiens R (Univ of Alberta Hosps, Edmonton)

Am J Infect Control 18:295–299, 1990   6–4

Background.—Rates of surgical wound infection can be reduced by reporting specific infection rates to individual surgeons. Infection control programs and even the Centers for Disease Control (CDC) have recommended surgeon-specific wound surveillance. The CDC's definition accepts a surgeon's diagnosis alone of surgical wound infection. A surgeon-specific surveillance was undertaken to determine the impact of this criterion on infection rates.

Methods.—Criteria for diagnosis of surgical wound infection were analyzed prospectively during a 6-month period. Incisions were examined by infection control practitioners (ICPs) 48 hours postoperatively and every 2 days thereafter for up to 2 weeks. Patients in general surgery, neurosurgery, orthopedics, and cardiovascular surgery were examined.

Results.—Surgical wound infection was determined by the presence of pus, erythema, or serosanguinous discharge; a positive wound culture; the presence of a deep-seated surgically related infection; or the surgeon's diagnosis alone. Of 116 diagnosed wound infections, 9% were identified by the ICP without an accompanying physician's diagnosis by the time of discharge. Surgeons alone diagnosed 16% of all wound infections and 25% of clean wound infections. There was a tendency toward early infection diagnosis in clean procedures (e.g., cardiovascular surgery and neurosurgery), perhaps because of the serious consequences of infection.

Conclusions.—The surgeon's diagnosis can have a major impact on surgical wound infection. However, the diagnosis varies by surgical service and individual surgeon. Only 4% of orthopedic infections were diagnosed by the surgeon alone, compared to 30% of cardiovascular and

40% of neurosurgical infections. It is recommended that infection control criteria not recognize surgeon's diagnosis alone.

▶ Modern surgical care necessitates that surgeons, services, and hospitals determine nosocomial infection rates, including wound infection rates. The clinical wound categories ranging from clean to dirty do not account for intrinsic patient risk. The paper by Culver et al. (Abstract 6–3) attempts to modify this to allow interservice and interhospital comparisons. This appears to be a useful advance. However, the second paper (Abstract 6–4) demonstrates that the surgeon's diagnosis of a surgical wound infection is not a valid criterion to use in compiling data.—M.C. Robson, M.D.

Correlation of APACHE II Score, Drainage Technique and Outcome in Postoperative Intra-Abdominal Abscess
Levison MA, Zeigler D (Wayne State Univ; Detroit Receiving Hosp)
Surg Gynecol Obstet 172:89–94 1991   6–5

Background.—No randomized studies have been done to compare percutaneous and surgical drainage of abdominal abscesses, and few studies have included information on physiologic scoring. Seven years' experience was reviewed to compare percutaneous and operative drainage. Although this series was not randomized, the effect of the severity of illness on outcome was studied.

Methods.—Of 91 patients who had an intra-abdominal abscess postoperatively, 45 had percutaneous drainage under CT or ultrasound guidance and 46 had operative drainage. The Acute Physiology and Chronic Health Evaluation (APACHE) II scoring system, which includes 12 physiologic variables, was used to retrospectively evaluate the severity of the illness.

Results.—The 2 groups were similar as to age, sex, location of abscess, and severity of illness as assessed by the APACHE II. The overall mortality rate was 28%. The mean age of survivors was about 50 years, compared to 67.5 years for those who died. Survivors' APACHE II scores were 8.6, compared to 22.2 for patients who died; 1.7% of patients with an APACHE II score of less than 15 died, compared to 78% of those with an APACHE II score of 15 or more. Among patients with the higher APACHE II scores, 92% of those who underwent percutaneous drainage died, compared to 70% of those who had operative drainage. The outcome clearly depended on the severity of illness.

Conclusions.—Some sort of objective severity scoring system should be used to assess the results of treatment for intra-abdominal infection. Surgical treatment should not be avoided because the patient is too ill; exploration should be done promptly if there is any question as to the adequacy of percutaneous drainage of the abscess.

Clinical Outcome of Seriously Ill Surgical Patients With Intra-Abdominal Infection Depends on Both Physiologic (APACHE II Score) and Immunologic (DTH Score) Alterations

Poenaru D, Christou NV (McGill Univ)
Ann Surg 213:130–136, 1991

6–6

Background.—Appropriate decision-making for acutely ill surgical patients requires an accurate means of predicting the outcome. For patients with serious intra-abdominal infections, it seems likely that immune function influences the final outcome. Impaired delayed-type hypersensitivity (DTH) responses are associated with increased mortality in surgical patients.

Study Design.—The Acute Physiology and Chronic Health Evaluation (APACHE) II scores and DTH responses were estimated in 118 patients with surgical infections. The findings were then related to outcome. Resultant risk assessments were compared with those made by using APACHE II scores alone in 354 other surgical patients. The DTH skin test responses to 5 recall antigens were determined.

Results.—The model derived by logistic regression analysis from APACHE II and DTH data had greater predictive capacity than APACHE II scores alone in the validation sample (Fig 6–3). The combined model exhibited significantly improved predictive power in both groups of patients.

Conclusion.—The DTH response, a broad marker of immunocompetence, is an independent prognostic factor in surgical patients. When used in conjunction with APACHE II scores, a measure of acute physiology, relatively accurate predictions of outcome are possible.

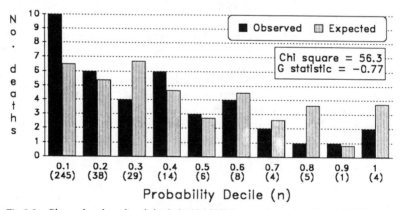

Fig 6–3.—Observed and predicted deaths by APACHE II score in conjunction with DTH score in 354 patients used to test predictive model. (Courtesy of Poenaru D, Christou NV: *Ann Surg* 213:130–136, 1991.)

▶ All available data should be used in making surgical decisions on critically ill patients. The 2 papers reviewed in Abstracts 6–5 and 6–6 show how the APACHE II score can be used in decision making in patients with intra-abdominal abscesses. The first paper suggests that it may be helpful in determining the type of intervention. The second shows that the APACHE II score combined with DTH tests is predictive of outcome. These types of tests can allow development of more homogeneous subgroups, permitting tighter specification of surgical knowledge.—M.C. Robson, M.D.

Combined Use of Topical and Systemic Antibiotics
Scher KS, Peoples JB (Wright State Univ)
Am J Surg 161:422–425, 1991   6–7

Background.—Systemically administered antibiotic agents can reduce the incidence of postoperative wound infection. The topical application of antibiotics has received less attention, but also appears to prevent surgical infection. Using an animal model, the effectiveness of topical and systemic antibiotic administration was compared with the value of combined therapy.

Methods.—Surgical incisions were made on Swiss white female mice divided into 4 treatment groups: a control group, and groups receiving 1 mg of sodium cefazolin powder placed in the wound before closure, 1 mg of sodium cefazolin by intraperitoneal injection 1 hour before surgery, and combined administration of the 2 methods. Repetitions of this basic experiment were carried out with 4 contaminating organisms.

Results.—After moderate contamination with *Staphylococcus aureus* or *Escherichia coli* (10^8 colony-forming units), topical and systemic antibiotics were equally effective in reducing wound bacterial content and infection rates. Combining the modes of antibiotic delivery offered no additional benefit. With heavy contamination (10^{12} colony-forming units), however, the combined administration of topical and systemic antibiotics significantly lowered infection rates compared with a single mode of delivery.

Conclusion.—Wound infection is an important postoperative complication. Usually, either systemic or topical antibiotics are effective in reducing infection rates. The combined regimen may be helpful in penetrating injuries or when unexpected soilage complicates an elective operation.

▶ The authors have cleared the air somewhat regarding the best route of antimicrobial delivery. Many surgeons have held strongly to their own views regarding the systemic vs. the topical route. In this experimental model, both rates were equally effective for moderately high contamination, and the 2 routes were not synergistic. However, for massive contamination, the combination of systemic and topical administration was most efficacious. This experiment would be difficult to perform clinically, so the results may have to be extrapolated to the patient.—M.C. Robson, M.D.

Studies of the Route, Magnitude, and Time Course of Bacterial Translocation in a Model of Systemic Inflammation

Mainous MR, Tso P, Berg RD, Deitch EA (Louisiana State Univ, Shreveport)
Arch Surg 126:33–37, 1991   6–8

Objective.—Intestinal mucosa does not block all bacterial translocation. Factors promoting the translocation process have been identified. The anatomical route and timing of translocating bacteria were investigated in an animal model.

Methods.—A group of 101 rats received intraperitoneal doses of normal saline solution or 1 of 2 dosages of the inflammatory agent zymosan (0.1 mg/g or .5 mg/g). Portal and systemic blood was obtained for culture, and the mesenteric lymph node (MLN) complex, spleen, liver, and cecum were harvested for bacteriologic studies at intervals.

Results.—Both the systemic effect of zymosan and its effect on bacterial translocation appeared to be dose dependent. None of the animals that received the 0.1 mg/g dose died or had signs of systemic toxic effects. In these animals, bacterial translocation was limited to the MLN complex. All rats that received .5 mg/g had signs of systemic toxicity within 24 hours and 40% died within 48 hours. Bacteria spread to the liver, spleen, and bloodstream in these rats (Fig 6–4). The MLN complex became infected as early as 2 hours in both groups, but it peaked at 6 hours and declined by 24 hours. Bacterial levels remained elevated in the MLN complexes for 24 hours in the rats given .5 mg/g.

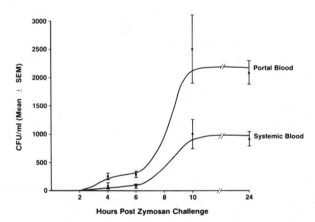

Fig 6–4.—Comparison of the magnitude of portal and systemic bacteremia after challenge with zymosan. The number of colony-forming units (CFUs) in the portal blood was significantly greater than in the systemic blood at 4,6, and 24 hours after challenge (P <.01). Plotted values are mean ± SEM. (Courtesy of Mainous MR, Tso P, Berg RD, et al: *Arch Surg* 126:33–37, 1991.)

Conclusions.—The route and extent of bacterial translocation was dependent on the degree of inflammation caused by zymosan. The rats that received .5 mg/g had systemic effects, 40% mortality, and bacterial spread to systemic organs. The major route of bacterial translocation appeared to be portal blood.

▶ Bacterial translocation has been difficult to understand for clinical surgical patients because of confusion emanating from the animal studies. One point of confusion was the apparently different rates by which the bacteria translocated to the bloodstream. The authors appear to have clarified the situation by demonstrating that the route of translocation may be dependent on the degree of inflammation in the bowel wall.—M.C. Robson, M.D.

Clostridium difficile Disease in a Department of Surgery: The Significance of Prophylactic Antibiotics
Yee J, Dixon CM, McLean APH, Meakins JL (Royal Victoria Hosp, Montreal; McGill Univ)
Arch Surg 126:241–246, 1991   6–9

Background.—*Clostridium difficile* has become increasingly recognized as an important nosocomial pathogen. It is mainly responsible for antibiotic-associated colitis. Because it has been difficult to quantify the potential complications of antibiotic therapy, this problem has received relatively little attention. Characteristics of an outbreak of *C. difficile* in a large university hospital were reviewed.

Patients.—Fifty patients with diarrhea and *C. difficile* toxin-positive stool were identified in a 1-year period. This disease occurred during hospitalization in 36 cases. The patients received 102 courses of antibiotics before the development of diarrhea, with 70% receiving more than 1 agent. Twenty-five patients had 37 courses of prophylactic antibiotics, with 12 patients receiving these agents for 24 hours or less. Cephalosporins were most commonly prescribed. Among 36 patients admitted to surgical wards, 22 had received only prophylactic antibiotics. Perioperative prophylaxis was the only indication for antibiotics in 20 of 33 surgical patients; 12 had such prophylaxis for 24 hours or less.

Outcome.—Patients with *C. difficile* cultures initially received either metronidazole, 500 mg orally every 8 hours, or vancomycin, 125–500 mg every 6 hours. Metronidazole was used in 33 of 50 cases (66%); 9 of these patients had relapses and required vancomycin. Vancomycin was the initial therapy in 7 of 50 patients (14%), usually the most seriously ill. Seven patients died in the hospital; *C. difficile* was responsible for death in 1 case and contributory to 3 others.

Conclusions.—*Clostridium difficile* disease may occur as a nosocomial infection associated with short courses of prophylactic antibiotics. It should be recognized as a significant potential complication. In some institutions this risk may outweigh the advantage of reductions in already low rates of wound infection after clean surgery.

▶ The indications for perioperative prophylactic antibiotics must be carefully satisfied before routine usage. More and more complications attributable to unwarranted antibiotic usage are being reported. Superinfection with C. difficile is one of the emerging severe complications. This series in a single hospital documents the danger. This article makes a plea for judicious use of prophylactic antibiotics only when justified by a known risk of infection if antibiotics are not used. Because most surgeons and surgical services do not have adequate data regarding infection rates for any single operation, it is difficult to justify prophylactic antibiotics based on a known incidence. However, complications such as those caused by C. difficile demand that such data be kept concurrently and applied to treatment decisions, e.g., when to use prophylactic antibiotics and the agent of choice.—M.C. Robson, M.D.

Impact of Magnetic Resonance Imaging on the Management of Diabetic Foot Infections
Durham JR, Lukens ML, Campanini DS, Wright JG, Smead WL (Ohio State Univ)
Am J Surg 162:150–154, 1991   6–10

Objective.—The influence of MRI on management of the infected feet of patients with diabetes was examined in 18 individuals with clinically apparent foot infections that seemed to be salvageable. No patient was clinically unstable because of systemic sepsis. Magnetic resonance imaging was done initially in 12 patients and postoperatively in 6 others who remained febrile after débridement and drainage of a foot abscess.

Findings.—Magnetic resonance images served to rapidly and reliably localize unsuspected or poorly localized abscess cavities, promoting thorough drainage while avoiding the need for wide exploration. It was possible to distinguish abscesses from cellulitis and osteomyelitis. In the group that had postoperative studies, all 4 patients who lacked MRI evidence of undrained pus or residual necrotic tissue recovered uneventfully. Two others had undrained pockets of infection and did well when drainage was repeated.

Advantages.—Magnetic resonance imaging can rapidly localize infection in the feet of patients with diabetes and pinpoint clinically unsuspected, or poorly localized, abscess cavities. It provides a noninvasive means of assessing patients who continue to be febrile after drainage of a foot abscess, and it may avoid unnecessary reoperation.

Unsuspected Osteomyelitis in Diabetic Foot Ulcers: Diagnosis and Monitoring by Leukocyte Scanning With Indium In 111 Oxyquinoline
Newman LG, Waller J, Palestro CJ, Schwartz M, Klein MJ, Hermann G, Har-

rington E, Harrington M, Roman SH, Stagnaro-Green A (Mount Sinai Med Ctr, New York)
JAMA 266:1246–1251, 1991   6–11

Background.—The prevalence of osteomyelitis in diabetic foot ulcers has not been established. Diagnosing this infection early is critical, because prompt antibiotic therapy reduces the rate of amputation.

Methods.—The prevalence of osteomyelitis was studied in 35 patients with 41 foot ulcers. The results of radiographs, leukocyte scans with ^{111}In-labeled oxyquinoline, and bone scans were compared with the diagnostic criteria standards of bone histologic and culture findings. Leukocyte scans were done every 2–3 weeks during antibiotic therapy.

Results.—Bone biopsy and culture showed that osteomyelitis underlay 68% of the foot ulcers. Only 32% of the 28 cases of osteomyelitis were clinically diagnosed by the referring physician (Fig 6–5). Osteomyelitis occurred in 68% of the outpatients and in 68% of ulcers not exposing bone. No evidence of inflammation was seen in 64% of the patients on physical examination. All patients with exposed bone had osteomyelitis. Leukocyte scanning had the highest sensitivity (89%) of all imaging tests. The leukocyte scan image intensity in patients with osteomyelitis decreased after 16–34 days of antibiotic treatment and normalized within 36–54 days.

Conclusions.—Most diabetic foot ulcers have clinically unsuspected underlying osteomyelitis. Leukocyte scans are highly sensitive for diagnosing osteomyelitis and may be valuable for monitoring the effectiveness of antibiotic therapy. Diabetic patients with foot ulcers that expose

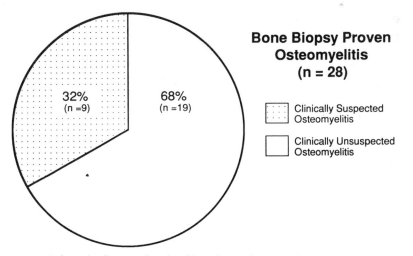

Fig 6–5.—Relationship between clinical and bone biopsy diagnoses of osteomyelitis. (Courtesy of Newman LG, Waller J, Palestro CJ, et al: *JAMA* 266:1246–1251, 1991.)

bone should be treated for osteomyelitis, and those without exposed bone should have leukocyte scanning.

▶ Foot ulcers and infections in the diabetic patient are receiving added attention with the advent of new wound healing agents such as peptide growth factors. What has become readily apparent is that our ability to clinically diagnose the extent of the disease process has been limited. The 2 papers reviewed in Abstracts 6–10 and 6–11 show how more sophisticated tests can help to delineate the process. Whereas MRI appears to be extremely sensitive for finding hidden unsuspected abscesses, ^{111}In-labeled oxyquinoline leukocyte scans diagnose osteomyelitis. Adding these tests to the surgeon's diagnostic methods will define the extent of disease and help in treatment, classification, and comparison of results.—M.C. Robson, M.D.

7 Burns

Fluid Resuscitation With Deferoxamine Prevents Systemic Burn-Induced Oxidant Injury
Demling R, LaLonde C, Knox J, Youn Y-K, Zhu D, Daryani R (Brigham and Women's Hosp; Beth Israel Hosp; Children's Hosp, Boston)
J Trauma 31:538–544, 1991   7-1

Background.—Oxidants released after burn injury produce local burn wound and systemic injury in experimental animals and patients. The effect on hemodynamic stability of deferoxamine (DFO) infused after burn injury, as well as local and systemic inflammation and oxidant-induced lipid peroxidation, were investigated.

Methods.—Eighteen sheep were anesthetized and given a 40% total body surface burn. They were fluid resuscitated to restore oxygen delivery and filling pressures to baseline levels. The sheep were resuscitated with lactated Ringer's (LR) solution alone, 5% hetastarch and LR, or 5% hetastarch complexed with DFO, 8 mg/mL. All sheep were killed 6 hours after the burns were inflicted.

Results.—The sheep that were resuscitated with LR and LR plus hetastarch had significant lung inflammation and increases in lung and liver malondialdehyde (MDA) compared with controls. Those sheep that were resuscitated with hetastarch alone needed 15% less fluid. In both groups, the VO_2 returned to baseline levels within 2 hours. Resuscitation with hetastarch-DFO reduced total fluids by 30% over LR and prevented the lung and liver MDA increases. Postburn VO_2 increased by 25% above baseline levels. Animals given DFO had significantly increased burn tissue edema compared with animals in the other groups.

Conclusions.—The use of DFO for burn resuscitation prevents systemic lipid peroxidation and reduces the vascular leak in nonburn tissues while also increasing O_2 utilization. Hetastarch-DFO resuscitation may increase burn tissue edema, possibly by increasing burn tissue perfusion.

▶ Various inflammatory mediators are released by the insult of thermal trauma. Neutralizing these mediators or preventing their formation and/or release should result in therapeutic advances. These investigators serially investigated the mediators and in this work demonstrated a beneficial effect of an iron chelator, DFO, as an antioxidant. The interesting thing is that burn wound edema was increased in this study. This may be an unwanted side effect. Other antioxidants decrease burn wound edema (1,2). Possibly combining DFO with an arachidonic acid inhibitor would give the beneficial effect of an antioxidant, without increasing detrimental burn wound edema.—M.C. Robson, M.D.

References

1. Demling RH, LaLonde C: *Surgery* 107:85, 1990.
2. Till G, et al: *Am J Pathol* 135:195, 1989.

Thermal Skin Injury: Effect of Fluid Therapy on the Transcapillary Colloid Osmotic Gradient

Onarheim H, Reed RK (Univ of Bergen, Norway)
J Surg Res 50:272–278, 1991   7–2

Introduction.—Thermal injury rapidly increases vascular permeability and promotes edema formation. Markedly negative interstitial hydrostatic pressure (P_{if}) has been observed after injury. Postburn changes in interstitial pressure were examined by determining how infusions of Ringer's lactate and plasma influence the P_{if}.

Methods.—Rats subjected to full-thickness scald burns over 40% of the body surface were resuscitated for 3 hours using either Ringer's lactate solution or plasma. Interstitial fluid was collected with nylon wicks,

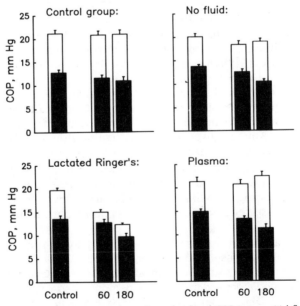

Fig 7–1.—Colloid osmotic pressure in plasma (*open bars*) and COP in interstitial fluid (*filled bars*) in control and 60 and 180 minutes after burn injury. Colloid osmotic gradient corresponds to the difference between COP in plasma and COP in interstitial fluid. Means ± SEM, = 8. (Courtesy of Onarheim H, Reed RK: *J Surg Res* 50:272–278, 1991.)

and colloid osmotic pressure (COP) was measured in both serum and wick fluid. The P_{if} was measured using micropipettes.

Observations.—The P_{if} decreased from -2 mm Hg to -20 to -40 mm Hg after burn injury and rose to slightly positive values after fluid therapy began. The plasma COP was 20.6 mm Hg, whereas the interstitial fluid COP was 13.7 mm Hg, producing a baseline transcapillary oncotic pressure gradient of 6.9 mm Hg. After burn injury, the COP in plasma fell to 18–19 mm Hg and that in interstitial fluid fell to 10.4 mm Hg. Ringer's lactate markedly lowered the COP in plasma and nearly abolished the gradient. Plasma, in contrast, maintained COP in plasma and the gradient rose significantly (Fig 7–1).

Implications.—The use of noncolloid saline solution for initial fluid therapy can be expected to favor edema formation. Plasma, in contrast, maintained or increased the COP gradient in this study.

▶ Protein is being administered earlier during resuscitation of large burns than in the past. Some centers now maintain serum albumin levels above 2.5 at all times. The experimental studies described in this paper by Onarheim and Reed present evidence to support that practice. By directly measuring colloid osmotic pressure in interstitial fluid, they demonstrated that plasma resuscitation increases the COP gradient, whereas Ringer's lactate practically annihilates it.—M.C. Robson, M.D.

Alveolar Macrophage Chemotaxis in Fire Victims With Smoke Inhalation and Burns Injury
Riyami BMS, Kinsella J, Pollok AJ, Clark C, Stevenson RD, Reid WH, Campbell D, Gemmell CG (Glasgow Royal Infirmary)
Eur J Clin Invest 21:485–489, 1991   7–3

Background.—Most deaths of fire victims are caused by respiratory complications. Smoke inhalation is now recognized as the single most prominent risk factor. Patients with both smoke inhalation and cutaneous burns often die of complications resembling adult respiratory distress syndrome.

Study Plan.—Migration of alveolar macrophages was studied in vitro in bronchoalveolar lavage samples from 24 fire victims and 19 controls, all cigarette smokers.

Findings.—Both unstimulated and stimulated migration of macrophages toward casein- and zymosan-activated serum were increased when samples from smoke inhalation victims were compared with those from controls. Such an effect was not evident when cells from burn-injured patients lacking smoke inhalation were studied. Lavage fluid from fire victims exhibited chemotactic activity for normal human neutrophils and contained complement components.

Implications.—Activation of alveolar macrophages may contribute to pathophysiologic changes in patients with smoke inhalation, particularly those who also have surface burns. Initial treatment of these patients should focus on reducing activation of phagocytic cells in the lungs.

▶ Demonstration of macrophage activation may lead to further observations in the pathophysiology of inhalation injury. One wonders what mediators or growth factors these activated macrophages might produce. Activated wound macrophages produce growth factors that, in the lung, could lead to increased fibrosis, a condition simulating adult respiratory distress syndrome. Studying explanted alveolar macrophages in tissue culture might yield such information.—M.C. Robson, M.D.

Differential Effects of Three Enteral Dietary Regimens on Selected Outcome Variables in Burn Patients
Gottschlich MM, Jenkins M, Warden GD, Baumer T, Havens P, Snook JT, Alexander JW (Shriners Burns Inst, Cincinnati; Univ of Cincinnati; The Ohio State Univ)
J Parenteral Enteral Nutrition 14:225–236, 1990   7–4

Introduction.—Nutritional support is an integral component of a burn care regimen. Studies have suggested that current high-fat, high-linoleic acid, low-protein commercial enteral products fail to meet the unique nutritional needs of patients with severe thermal injury. A new modular tube feeding (MTF) recipe was developed to meet the extraordinary needs of burn patients, applying the nutritional principles documented in a burned guinea pig model. The MTF is a high-protein, low-fat, linoleic-acid restricted formulation enriched with omega-3 fatty acids, arginine, cysteine, histidine, vitamin A, zinc, and ascorbic acid.

Study Design.—In a prospective, double-blind study, 50 patients aged 3–76 years with burns ranging from 10% to 89% total body surface area were randomized into 3 groups comparing MTF to 2 popular enteral dietary regimens for burn patients, Osmolite/Promix and Traumacal. Age, percent total and third-degree burns, resting energy expenditure, and calorie and protein intake were similar in all groups.

Findings.—Patients given the MTF dietary regimen had a significantly reduced incidence of wound infection and a shortened length of hospital stay/percent burn, compared with the other 2 groups. In addition, patients who received MTF had a reduced incidence of diarrhea, improved glucose tolerance, lower serum triglycerides, reduced total number of infectious episodes, and trends toward improved preservation of muscle mass, although these were not statistically significant. The overall mortality rate was 20%, and 7 of 10 deaths occurred among patients receiving the high-fat, high-linoleic acid feeding.

Conclusion.—These findings suggest that burn patients require more than a high-calorie, high-protein diet. It appears that MTF is effective in modulating an improved response to burn injury.

▶ These investigators systematically studied nutritional requirements following burning. Having perfected the requirements in a detailed series of animal experiments, they formulated a recipe and have now tested it clinically. Their rigorous evaluation demonstrated the superiority of the new recipe. It is now necessary to see whether other burn centers can demonstrate the same improvements using this dietary supplement. Often, when a new methodology is introduced into a burn treatment regimen, other subtle changes are made that could contribute to improved statistics.—M.C. Robson, M.D.

Effects of Topical Antimicrobial Agents on the Human Neutrophil Respiratory Burst
Hansbrough JF, Zapata-Sirvent RL, Cooper ML (Univ of California, San Diego)
Arch Surg 126:603–608, 1991   7–5

Introduction.—Some antimicrobial agents, when applied to wounds, appear to be effective in chemically débriding the wound as well as in controlling microbial growth. Few studies have evaluated the effects of topical antimicrobial agents on the functions of host defense cells. The respiratory burst of human peripheral blood polymorphonuclear leukocytes (PMNs) was examined after exposure of cells to a number of topical antimicrobial agents.

Methods.—In blood samples obtained from normal volunteers, PMNs were separated and prepared for exposure to the antimicrobial agents. A flow cytometric assay was used to study the effects of these agents.

Results.—Mafenide acetate, sulfadiazine silver, gentamicin sulfate, acetic acid, and providone-iodine were highly inhibitory to the neutrophil oxidative burst at or below clinical concentrations and after short (30-minute) exposure to cells. Modified Dakin's solution (.25% diluted sodium hypochlorite) caused extensive death of PMNs, as confirmed by a vital dye assay that also employs flow cytometry. Exposure to Polysporin appeared to stimulate PMN oxidative burst activity at the clinical dosage. Diluted gentamicin and acetic acid augmented intracellular hydrogen peroxide production, but to a lesser extent than Polysporin.

Conclusion.—The effects of antimicrobial agents on PMNs may have clinical application, but further studies on the mechanisms involved are required. Future studies may determine which topical agents will effectively control microorganism growth while minimally affecting host defense functions.

▶ Topical antimicrobials used to treat burns do more than control bacterial growth. Some have been demonstrated to be cytotoxic to keratinocytes (1) and some injurious to fibroblasts (2). In this study, the authors examined the respiratory burst of the neutrophil and found a spectrum of effects of various clinically used topical antimicrobials. This emerging information requires that the burn surgeon be aware of the multiple effects of the topical antimicrobial and choose the drug for the specific indication. The timing of use is important, as is the bacterial specificity. Add to that the effect the antimicrobial has on host defense and wound healing.—M.C. Robson, M.D.

References

1. Cooper ML, et al: *J Surg Res* 48:190, 1990.
2. McCauley RL, et al: *J Surg Res* 46:267, 1989.

Pain Control in Paediatric Burns: The Use of Patient-Controlled Analgesia
Gaukroger PB, Chapman MJ, Davey RB (Adelaide Children's Hosp, Adelaide, South Australia)
Burns 17:396–399, 1991   7–6

Introduction.—Pain relief often is a problem in burn-injured children, and inadequate relief may contribute to psychological difficulties. Patient-controlled analgesia (PCA) has been used in both children and adults to relieve postoperative pain; it has also been used in burn-injured adults. Patient-controlled analgesia was assessed in 11 children with burns.

Methods.—Patient-controlled analgesia usually began in the recovery room after initial débridement. Morphine was used in all patients and was administered intravenously using a Graseby PCAS device. Boluses consisted of .016 mg of morphine per kg with a minimum of 5 minutes between boluses. Supplemental pain relief during dressing changes and physiotherapy was provided by self-administration of 50% nitrous oxide in oxygen.

Observations.—Morphine requirements varied widely and were unrelated to the extent of burn injury. Three children had evidence of tolerance to opiates. Morphine use declined when skin coverage was complete in all but 1 patient, who weaned themselves from opiate therapy. There were few problems. One patient with upper limb burns had trouble activating the device and was given a foot-operated pneumatic trigger. Nurses reported that PCA reduced their workload and enhanced pain control, with psychological benefit to the patients.

Conclusions.—Patient-controlled analgesia provides analgesia of good quality to school-aged children who undergo débridement and grafting of burn injuries. The patients treated have required intravenous access for other reasons.

▶ Pain management in burned children is a big problem. The psychological and humanitarian aspects of pain control have been well demonstrated. The drawbacks of the technique described may be intermittent ileus and somnolence to the degree of inability to participate in physical therapy. These variables are not recorded in this paper. If the necessary feeding can continue uninterrupted and physical therapy can be unimpeded, then the method may prove to be beneficial. A more difficult problem to measure may be an increase in bacterial translocation from the intestine in patients with very large burns if transit time is significantly delayed.—M.C. Robson, M.D.

Donor-Specific Tolerance Permits Burn Allografting Without Increased Sepsis
Garrison JL, Cunningham PR, Lust RM, Thomas FT (East Carolina Univ, Greenville, NC)
J Surg Res 49:390–393, 1990   7-7

Background.—Early excision and grafting in burn victims is desirable. The removal of the eschar restores immunocompetence, eliminates the rich milieu in which bacteria grow, and reduces infectious complications. When little native uninjured tissue is available for autografting, skin allografting permits massive burn excision. The functional survival of skin allografts relies on frequent allograft replacement or chronic immunosuppression; however, chronic immunosuppression puts the patient at risk for infection. Host resistance to infection after induction of donor-specific tolerance was assessed.

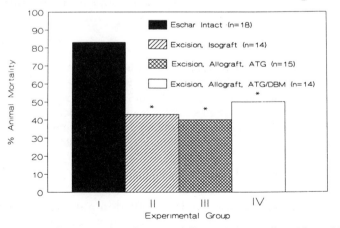

Fig 7–2.—Mortality by group, 8 days after septic challenge. No statistically significant difference in mortality was seen among the excision and grafted groups (II, III, IV). Compared to eschar intact animals, groups II, III, and IV had significantly decreased mortality (* $P \leq .05$). (Courtesy of Garrison JL, Cunningham PR, Lust RM, et al: *J Surg Res* 49:390–393, 1990.)

Methods.—Resistance to a septic challenge produced by cecal ligation and puncture 10 days after a 30% total body surface area burn was determined in 4 groups of mice. In group 1 the eschar was left intact. Group 2 had burn excision and isograft. Group 3 had burn excision, allograft, and antithymocyte globulin (ATG). Group 4 had burn excision, allograft, ATG, and donor bone marrow infusion.

Results.—The 8-day mortality in each of the 4 groups was 83%, 43%, 40%, and 50%, respectively. Ninety-seven percent of the mice that died had positive blood cultures. Mortality was significantly lower in the mice undergoing burn excision and grafting. However, allografted mice that were given ATG or ATG and donor bone marrow infusion did not have higher death rates than the isografted mice that received no immunosuppression (Fig 7–2).

Conclusions.—Skin allografting with donor-specific tolerance induction may provide the benefits of burn excision without the risks of infection that occur in chronic immunosuppression. Further research to define the mechanism for improved outcomes with early excision and grafting is being done.

▶ Although the authors have shown that skin allograft survival can be prolonged by donor-specific tolerance without increasing the septic complications, this observation may not be clinically relevant. In massive human burns, natural immunosuppression allows prolongation of allograft survival without rejection. With staged early excision and use of widely meshed autografts from unburned areas beginning on the day of burning, 90% to 95% of burn injuries can be covered before allograft rejection becomes a clinical problem. Therefore, these observations in mice would have to be investigated clinically before they are applicable to the burn surgeon's approach to treatment.—M.C. Robson, M.D.

Burned Children From the Bashkir Train-Gas Pipeline Disaster: II. Follow-Up Experience at Children's Hospital 9, Moscow
Remensnyder JP, Ackroyd FP, Astrozjnikova S, Budkevitch LG, Buletova AA, Creedon CM, Lankina N, Lybarger PM, Okatyev V, Prodeus PP, Ruslan K, Salvo PM, Shopova L, Tuohy CB, Vasileva L, Vozdvidzensky S (Children's Hosp 9, Moscow; Shriners Burns Inst, Boston; Massachusetts Gen Hosp, Boston)
Burns 16:333–336, 1990   7–8

Background.—Twenty-five children burned in a train-gas pipeline accident in 1989 were treated in Moscow by a team of Soviet and United States surgeons and nurses. After 7 months the United States team was invited to return to Moscow to participate in status evaluation and surgery for the children.

Findings.—The sequelae observed included major scarring, posttraumatic stress syndrome, hepatitis, and myocardial damage. The excellent healing observed in some of the children's scars was attributed to a regimen of daily electrophoresis with hyaluronidase to the scars, alternating on a monthly basis with daily ultrasound and application of hydrocortisone cream. These scars had healed flat, were pale pink, and were not pruritic. No elastic compression, the recommended burn care at most United States centers, was used in these children. Reconstructive surgery included scar revision, Z-plasties, local flaps, or the use of full- or split-thickness grafts after scar excision or release.

▶ Follow-up of children treated by the United States–Russian team has provided exciting and provocative information. If the treatment used post wound closure, hyaluronidase electrophoresis alternated with hydrocortisone, can withstand vigorous prospectively randomized clinical trials, it would be a real advance. The children described here were not treated with compression therapy, yet many had more acceptable scarring than is routinely seen in American burn centers.—M.C. Robson, M.D.

Long-Term Assessment of the Effects of Circumferential Truncal Burns in Pediatric Patients on Subsequent Pregnancies

McCauley RL, Stenberg BA, Phillipps LG, Blackwell SJ, Robson MC (Shriners Burns Inst, Galveston)
J Burn Care Rehabil 12:51–53, 1991   7–9

Introduction.—Documentation of the incidence and long-term follow-up of circumferential truncal burns is scarce. The impact of the childhood trauma of circumferential burns and split-thickness skin grafts on subsequent pregnancy were studied longitudinally in 22 women, all of whom had been available for long-term follow-up into early adulthood.

Long-Term Follow-Up of Patients With Circumferential Truncal Burns Who Later Became Pregnant

	First pregnancy (*n* = 7)	Second pregnancy (*n* = 4)	Third pregnancy (*n* = 3)
Age (yr)*	19.83 ± 1.77	22.00 ± 0.58	23.41 ± 0.88
Time from burn injury to delivery (yr)*	12.19 ± 2.97	14.25 ± 2.64	14.39 ± 1.06
Prenatal complications	1	0	0
Labor and delivery complications	0	0	0

* Mean ± SD.
(Courtesy of McCauley RL, Stenberg BA, Phillips LG, et al: *J Burn Care Rehabil* 12:51–53, 1991.)

Findings.—Seven of the 22 patients conceived. All 7 had sustained flame-burn injuries that were treated with excision and split-thickness skin grafting during their initial hospitalization. The mean total body surface area of burns was 63.21% ± 16.69% with 44.21% ± 17.54% of the injuries full thickness.

Outcome.—During a follow-up period of 12.19 ± 2.97 years, the 7 patients had a total of 14 full-term pregnancies. Four patients had second pregnancies and 3 had third pregnancies (table). There were no labor and delivery complications in 13 vaginal deliveries and 1 elective cesarean section. In 1 case, a patient had breakdown of abdominal scar tissue during the third trimester of pregnancy. The burn treatment of maximal tissue preservation appears to have resulted in strong and flexible mature burn scars.

Conclusion.—In 7 pediatric circumferential truncal burn patients followed into early adulthood, there were 14 full-term pregnancies. The strong and flexible mature burn scars created no significant prenatal complications or labor and delivery complications.

▶ Burn surgeons are constantly asked by patients, parents, insurance carriers, and lawyers about the effects of deep truncal burns on future pregnancies. This is the first series reporting the longitudinal follow-up into adulthood of patients who sustained burn injuries as children. Seven of these women became pregnant. Surprisingly, there were few problems, these patients having normal pregnancies and uncomplicated vaginal deliveries. The paper should be of use for counseling purposes.—M.C. Robson, M.D.

Electrical Injury of Wrist: Classification and Treatment—Clinical Analysis of 90 Cases

Shen Z-Y, Chang Z-D, Wang N-Z (Ji Shui Tan Hosp, Beijing, China)
Burns 16:449–456, 1990   7–10

Objective.—Electrical injuries of the wrist are likely to produce full-thickness necrosis of the skin and damage to deep structures beneath the eschar. In a prospective study conducted from 1980 to 1989, 90 consecutive patients with 114 upper limbs with typical electrical injury of the wrist were treated.

Management.—Based on extensive clinical investigation of arterial injury and its adverse effects on hand circulation, a grading system was developed for electrically injured wrists based not only on the extent and severity of the devitalized tissues, but more importantly, on the degree of damage of the radial and/or ulnar arteries.

Results.—The overall amputation rate was 39.4%. However, amputation was necessary only in patients with circumferential injuries—type III and type IV—with rates of 80% and 100%, respectively. Most patients with type II injuries required late reconstruction. Type III injuries, i.e., circumferential deep burns of the wrist with extensive necrosis and inflammation, necessitated amputation in 8 of 10 hands. However, a pedicle greater omentum transfer with an arterial bypass between the gastroepiploic artery and palmar arch artery and a vein graft bridge between the hand and forearm, then covered with split-thickness skin grafts and an abdominal flap, was successfully used in 1 patient with type III injury.

Conclusion.—Amputation rates associated with electrically injured upper extremities are high. The grading system proposed for electrical injuries of the wrist is relevant for both prognosis and better treatment. The new method designed to repair circumferential wounds of the electrically injured wrist overcomes 3 difficulties, including too-long segmental necrosis of the radial and ulnar arteries to permit reconstruction, resurfacing an extensive circumferential wound at the wrist and forearm without infection, and avoiding adhesions between tendons and their surrounding tissues.

▶ A carefully studied series of 114 electrical injuries of the wrist has allowed a useful classification to be developed. These authors demonstrate that, unless the injury involves skin circumferentially, amputation can be avoided. Any classification system becomes useful only after being verified by other groups. This one may well withstand the test. The authors' use of an omental flap in these devastating injuries deserves attention. The arcade of vessels allows revascularization of multiple digits and gliding function of the tendons.—M.C. Robson, M.D.

8 Transplantation

Pretransplantation Blood Transfusion Revisited
van Twuyver E, Mooijaart RJD, ten Berge IJM, van der Horst AR, Wilmink JM, Kast WM, Melief CJM, de Waal LP (Univ of Amsterdam; Univ Hosp Leiden, The Netherlands)
N Engl J Med 325:1210–1213, 1991   8–1

Background.—By an unknown mechanism, blood transfusion before organ transplantation improves allograft survival. Studies in mice have shown that the presence of common histocompatibility antigens in the donor and recipient favors induction of allograft tolerance. Twenty-three patients awaiting a first renal transplant were studied to evaluate the impact of HLA compatibility between blood donor and recipient on induction of allograft tolerance.

Methods.—The 23 subjects were given transfusions with HLA-typed buffy coat-depleted packed cells. The average leukocyte content of the transfusions was $7.7 \pm 3.5 \times 10^8$, and each transfusion was given within 36 hours of donation. Limiting dilution cultures were used to determine the relative frequency of cytotoxic T lymphocyte precursors before transfusion and several times thereafter.

Results.—In 10 patients T cell nonresponsiveness against the donor cells developed. Tolerance developed in 9 of those patients, all of whom had 1 HLA haplotype or at least 1 HLA-B and 1 HLA-DR antigen in common with the donor (Fig 8-1). It took 1 to 2 months for tolerance to develop, and it could still be measured 1 year after transfusion in 2 patients. Of the 13 patients who received transfusions from donors without HLA-antigen compatibility, no decline in T cell response against donor alloantigens occurred in any.

Conclusions.—Tolerance to donor antigens is induced by blood transfusion in which there is a common HLA haplotype or shared HLA-B and HLA-DR antigens. New strategies can now be developed to induce tolerance for transplantation, possibly by selecting donors on the basis of acceptable HLA-antigen mismatches associated with T cell nonresponsiveness.

▶ Although pretransplant blood transfusions are required less frequently than in years before recombinant erythropoietin was available for patients with chronic renal failure, donor-specific transfusions may still have an important role. In this series and in other reports, haploidentical blood donations have induced a state of tolerance in some patients, at least as measured by

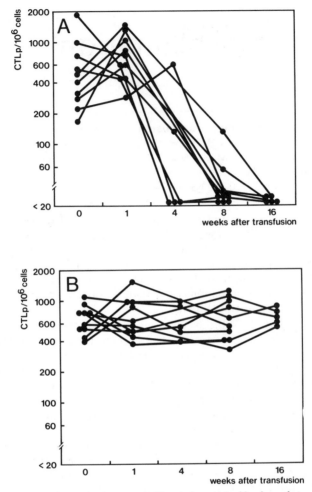

Fig 8–1.—Estimates of precursor frequency in 10 patients receiving blood transfusions from donors with whom they had HLA antigens in common. **A,** frequencies determined after incubation with donor cells. Four, 8, and 16 weeks after transfusion, the frequencies of precursors against donor cells showed a marked and statistically significant decrease in all recipients (P < .005). **B,** no significant variations in the frequencies of precursors against cells of third-party blood donors were observed in the recipients 1, 4, 8, and 16 weeks after transfusion (P > .05). (Courtesy of van Twuyver E, Mooijaart RJD, ten Berge IJM, et al: N Engl J Med 325:1210–1213, 1991.)

the absence of donor-specific cytotoxic T cells. Whether this state is related to compatibility or incompatibility of the mismatched haplotype is arguable, but the beneficial effect on transplantation is clear.—O. Jonasson, M.D.

Downregulation of Antidonor Cytotoxic Lymphocyte Responses in Recipients of Donor-Specific Transfusions

Hadley GA, Kenyon N, Anderson CB, Mohanakumar T (Washington Univ; Diabetes Research Inst, Miami)
Transplantation 50:1064–1066, 1990   8–2

Background.—Research results have demonstrated that donor-specific blood transfusions (DSTs) lengthen the survival of HLA-disparate allografts to that achieved with HLA-identical transplants. The types of changes in cellular immunity that occur in human DST recipients were investigated, using a limiting dilution assay for cytotoxic T lymphocyte precursors (CTLp) in 7 patients before and after they underwent DST conditioning.

Methods.—The patients had 3 transfusions of 200 mL of donor blood spaced 2 weeks apart while taking azathioprine continuously for immunosuppression. Pre-DST blood samples were taken 1–2 weeks before the initial transfusion and post-DST samples were taken 2 weeks after the final infusion. Limiting dilution analysis was used to evaluate antidonor CTL responses.

Findings.—After the DST procedures, 2 different kinds of antidonor limiting dilution analysis plots were seen. One group (4 patients) had post-DST antidonor plots with single-hit kinetics, whereas the other group (3 patients) had biphasic post-DST plots to donor antigens. Six of the 7 patients receiving transfusions had no significant change in reactivity to any third-party antigens after DST. One patient had a significant increase in the third-party reactivity after DST, and another patient had a significant decrease.

Comment.—The findings are consistent with the hypothesis that the DST-conditioning procedure increases an immunoregulatory cell population responsible for the downregulation of production of antidonor CTL responses in a subset of DST recipients. This type of mechanism could partially explain the beneficial effects of DST conditioning on renal allograft survival.

▶ These investigators, using limiting dilution techniques similar to those of van Twuyver et al. (Abstract 8–1), found that a suppressor cell population had likely been generated in some patients and suggest that donors whose incompatibility was the noninherited maternal haplotype were associated with this event. All together, regardless of mechanism—suppressor cells, anti-idiotypic antibody, CTL elimination or inactivation—blood transfusions in these recipients have had a predictable beneficial effect and probably should still be administered.—O. Jonasson, M.D.

Comparison of RFLP-DR Beta and Serological HLA-DR Typing in 1500 Individuals

Mytilineos J, Scherer S, Opelz G (Univ of Heidelberg, Germany)
Transplantation 50:870–873, 1990   8–3

Background.—For technical reasons, serologic typing of HLA-DR antigens is often problematic. However, HLA-DR typing by analysis of DNA restriction fragment-length polymorphisms (RFLP), introduced recently, permits an exact definition of HLA-DR alleles. The reliability of RFLP typing was tested in a clinical laboratory setting.

Methods and Findings.—The standard serologic technique and the RFLP method were both used to type 1,522 persons. Although 11% of the serologic typings were unsuccessful or doubtful technically, all RFLP typings were successful (table). An error rate of 25% was noted in the results of the remaining 1,358 typings. In 16%, a serologic "blank" was a definable allele by RFLP. In 9%, an allele was incorrectly interpreted serologically. Eleven percent of individuals tested were HLA-DR homozygous by RFLP.

Conclusions.—Although the RFLP method for HLA-DR typing is time consuming and involves the use of radioactivity, it has an impressive qualitative advantage over serology. All serologic typing failures in this study could be typed successfully by RFLP. Nearly all "blanks" were resolved. Another important advantage of this method is that it can recognize homozygous individuals without family typing. The RFLP typing is especially useful for typing bone marrow transplant recipients in whom serology often fails and for kidney transplant candidates with "blanks."

▶ Poor cell preparations often make HLA typing of sick patients quite difficult. Although the molecular techniques presently available are expensive and time consuming, the HLA phenotype can be precisely defined—a real advantage for bone marrow recipients, especially of unrelated donor marrow, or for difficult renal transplant recipients. Another study (Abstract 8–28) used a newer method, polymerase chain reaction fingerprinting, which adds information about compatibility.—O. Jonasson, M.D.

Serologic Blanks Clarified by RFLP-DRβ Typing

	All individuals (n = 1358)	Kidney recipients (n = 236)	Organ donors (n = 55)	Leukemia patients (n = 93)	Healthy individuals (n = 908)
DR "blank" by serology	28.0%	36.4%	21.8%	24.7%	26.8%
RFLP homozygous	11.4%	16.1%	9.1%	8.6%	10.7%
Second antigen determined by RFLP	15.6%	19.9%	10.9%	14.0%	15.4%
DR-Br	0.7%	0.0%	0.0%	0.0%	0.7%
DR "blank" by RFLP	0.3%	0.4%	1.8%	2.2%	0.0%

(Courtesy of Mytilineos J, Scherer S, Opelz G: *Transplantation* 50:870–873, 1990.)

The Immunosuppressive Properties of New Oral Prostaglandin E₁ Analogs

Pollak R, Dumble LJ, Wiederkehr JC, Maddux MS, Moran M (Univ of Illinois, Chicago; Univ of Melbourne, Australia; G D Searle & Co, Skokie, Ill)
Transplantation 50:834–838, 1990
8–4

Objective and Methods.—Both endogenous and synthetic prostaglandins, particularly the E series, have marked effects on immune responses. The immunosuppressive actions of a new synthetic oral PGE₁ analogue were examined by evaluating misoprostol, its active acid metabolite MPA, and enisoprost in an in vitro mixed lymphocyte reaction (MLR) immunosuppressive assay. A lymphoblastoid B cell line derived from Epstein-Barr virus transformation of a human B cell served as a source of stimulator cells in 1-way allogeneic MLR.

Observations.—The PGE₁ analogs suppressed lymphocyte proliferative responses in the MLR in a dose-dependent manner. The active analog MPA enhanced the inhibitory effect of cyclosporine in the immunosuppressive assay. By themselves, the PGE₁ analogs failed to alter phytohemagglutinin-stimulated lymphocyte mitogenesis at concentrations that were effective in the MLR. Adding recombinant interleukin-2 to PGE₁ analogs in the MLR restored lymphocyte responsiveness in a dose-dependent manner. The prostaglandins had the effect of downregulating HLA-DR expression as well as expression of the interleukin-2 receptors.

Conclusions.—The new synthetic PGE₁ analogs, which are bioavailable orally, warrant further consideration for use in clinical transplantation, as well as in treating various immunologically mediated disorders.

▶ In these in vitro experiments, a PGE₁ analog was impressive in suppression of MLRs, apparently through inhibition of interleukin-2-related events. Because immunosuppression by cyclosporine seemed to be enhanced by the addition of PGE₁, the pathways of suppression, although each related to interleukin-2, should be different. The prostaglandins cause diarrhea, but they are well tolerated in appropriate doses and may be important adjuncts to immunosuppression.—O. Jonasson, M.D.

Evidence That Glucocorticosteroid-Mediated Immunosuppressive Effects Do Not Involve Altering Second Messenger Function

Almawi WY, Hadro ET, Strom TB (Harvard Med School; Beth Israel Hosp, Boston)
Transplantation 52:133–140, 1991
8–5

Background.—Several immune disorders have been treated with glucocorticosteroids (GCS) as immunosuppressive agents, although the exact mechanism of GCS action remains unknown. Glucocorticosteroids block transcription of interleukin (IL)-1 and IL-6 genes in a concentration-dependent manner. How GCS suppress proliferation of human peripheral blood mononuclear leukocytes (PBML) was investigated. Proliferative responses to immobilized anti-CD3 mAb or mitogens were studied.

Results.—Dexamethasone and 6-α-methylprednisolone inhibited PBML in a concentration-dependent manner. Dexamethasone did not block the entry of Ca^{2+} into cells stimulated by anti-CD3 plus phorbal-12-β-myristate-13-α-acetate, and dexamethasone-mediated suppression was not circumvented by Ca^{2+} ionophores. Thus the GCS mechanism did not involve interference with Ca^{2+} fluxes. Protein kinase C inhibitors and stimulators did not prevent dexamethasone-mediated suppression. Nor did dexamethasone affect upregulation of CD4 and CD8 expression, which is an indirect index of protein kinase C activity, or change the translocation of protein kinase C from cytosolic to membrane-bound compartments. Thus dexamethasone had no effect on PKC activity.

Conclusions.—Given that GCS inhibit cytokine gene transcription, and that rIL-1 plus rIL-6 plus rIFN-γ completely abrogates the suppressive effects of GCS, the findings suggest that the immunosuppressive effects of GCS result from inhibition of cytokine gene expression. Glucocorticosteroids may enter the cytoplasm of T cells and accessory cells and bind to the GCS receptor, which becomes a DNA-binding protein.

▶ Clarification of the mechanism of action of steroids in immunosuppression may be useful in isolating the desired immunosuppressive effects from those causing undesirable side effects, although the hypothesis that the steroid-receptor complex becomes a DNA-binding protein may make this unlikely. The action causing IL-1 transcription to fail may similarly cause widespread effects.—O. Jonasson, M.D.

Cyclosporine-Induced Enhancement of Interleukin 1 Receptor Expression by PHA-Stimulated Lymphocytes
Degiannis D, Stein S, Czarnecki M, Raskova J, Raska K Jr (Univ of Medicine and Dentistry of New Jersey, Piscataway and Newark)
Transplantation 50:1074–1076, 1990   8–6

Introduction.—Cyclosporine (CsA) exerts an immunosuppressive action by inhibiting the transcription of the interleukin-2 (IL-2) mRNA and DNA synthesis in mitogen-induced peripheral blood mononuclear cells. The effect of CsA on expression of the IL-1 receptor on the surface of phytohemagglutinin (PHA)-stimulated lymphocytes and on the secretion of IL-1 β in the culture supernatant was examined.

Findings.—The presence of PHA increased the proportion of lymphocytes binding IL-1. Adding CsA further increased the expression of IL-1 receptor, but prednisolone had no such effect. Also, PHA induced the secretion of IL-1 β in mononuclear cell culture supernatants, and this effect was inhibited by prednisolone. Cyclosporine only slightly increased the secretion of IL-1 β.

Interpretation.—These findings are consistent with induction of cytokine bioactivity by CsA, constituting a link between CsA and polyclonal lymphoproliferation. The similarities in function between IL-1 and IL-6 suggest that CsA-induced enhancement of the accessory signals provided by these agents may help to explain the association between CsA treatment and lymphoproliferative disorders.

▶ Although CSA inhibits IL-2 synthesis, it appears to enhance IL-1 production and subsequent B cell activation. Steroids inhibit IL-1 production, as discussed in the previous paper, making sense of using the 2 drugs in combination. Whether the increased IL-1 receptor expression and IL-1 secretion facilitates the development of Epstein-Barr virus lymphomas is an interesting speculation.—O. Jonasson, M.D.

OKT3 F(AB')₂ Fragments—Retention of the Immunosuppressive Properties of Whole Antibody With Marked Reduction in T Cell Activation and Lymphokine Release

Woodle ES, Thistlethwaite JR, Ghobrial IA, Jolliffe LK, Stuart FP, Bluestone JA (Univ of Chicago; Ortho Pharmaceutical Corp, Raritan, NJ)
Transplantation 52:354–360, 1991   8–7

Objective.—Previous in vivo studies with whole and F(ab')₂ fragments of an antimurine CD3 monoclonal antibody (mAb) suggested that, although the fragments produce minimal T cell activation, they retain significant immunosuppressive effects. An attempt was made to examine the immune activating and suppressing properties of pepsin-derived OKT3 F(ab')₂ digest fragment preparations of OKT3 on human peripheral-blood mononuclear cells.

Methods.—Immunosuppressive effects were assessed by quantifying T cell receptor modulation and coating, and also by examining inhibition of cytotoxic T lymphocyte activity.

Observations.—Whole mAb modulated the T cell receptor complex more efficiently than did F(ab')₂ fragments. Whole OKT3 and fragments were equally effective in suppressing cytotoxic T lymphocyte activity. Purified F(ab')₂ preparations exhibited minimal T cell activating ability, as gauged by proliferation, the expression of interleukin-2R and Leu-23, and lymphokine release. In contrast, whole OKT3 mAb induced the expression of IL-2R and Leu-23 and induced the release of tumor necrosis factor and interferon in low concentrations. Progressive contamination of fragments with whole antibody led to the increasing mitogenic potency of the F(ab')₂ preparation.

Conclusions.—These findings indicate that OKT3 F(ab')$_2$ digest fragments are much less potent than whole mAb in activating T cells, but retain significant immunosuppressive activity. The role of nonactivating forms of OKT3 in clinical immunosuppression will rely on reducing or eliminating T cell-activating properties while retaining adequate selective immunosuppressive effects.

▶ The non–complement-fixing F(ab')$_2$ fragments of OKT3 appear to have at least immediate immunosuppressive effects without the adverse accompanying side effects of cytokine liberation from T cell activation. The authors speculate that T cell activation, however, may be necessary for long-term immunosuppression. Striking the right balance between activation and suppression will be required.—O. Jonasson, M.D.

Activation-Independent Binding of Human Memory T Cells to Adhesion Molecule ELAM-1

Shimizu Y, Shaw S, Graber N, Gopal TV, Horgan KJ, Van Seventer GA, Newman W (Natl Cancer Inst, Bethesda, Md; Otsuka America Pharmaceutical Inc, Rockville, Md)
Nature 349:799–802, 1991   8–8

Background.—It is likely that the induction of adhesion molecules on endothelial cells by inflammatory cytokines is a critical step in the differential migration of T lymphocyte subsets into sites of inflammation. Molecular pathways involving the integrins VLA-4 and LFA-1 mediate the adhesion of T cells to activated endothelium. A third pathway, involving the rapidly inducible endothelial cell surface adhesion molecule ELAM-1, contributes to the binding of resting CD4+ T cells to human endothelial cells induced by interleukin-1.

Observations.—The ability of ELAM-1 to mediate CD4+ T cell adhesion was confirmed by cell adhesion assays that demonstrated specific binding of T cells to purified ELAM-1 immobilized on plastic. Purified resting memory CD4+ T cells bound much more strongly than naive cells to human umbilical vein endothelial cells. Studies with purified ELAM-1 demonstrated greater binding of memory CD4+ T cells to ELAM-1 than to integrin ligands such as fibronectin. Also, ELAM-1 mediates the adhesion of granulocytes and monocytes to induced human umbilical vein endothelial cells.

Implications.—The induction of adhesion molecules such as ELAM-1 by inflammatory cytokines provides a means by which lymphocytes can selectively attach to endothelium and then migrate into a site of tissue injury. The ELAM-1 pathway may be critical for the initial attachment of T cells to inflamed endothelium in vivo. The finding that memory, but not naive, T cells bind to ELAM-1 suggests that this pathway may contribute to the different recirculation patterns of these T cell types.

▶ Rejection is an inflammatory event, and the mechanisms for T cell invasion of the inflamed endothelium are just being uncovered. As these authors put it, there is an "ensemble" of adhesion molecules related to the differential migration of cells. In these studies, presensitized (memory) T cells are specifically attracted by the ELAM-1 molecule.—O. Jonasson, M.D.

Prevention of Xenograft Rejection by Masking Donor HLA Class I Antigens

Faustman D, Coe C (Massachusetts Gen Hosp, Boston)
Science 252:1700–1702, 1991   8–9

Background.—Activation of cytotoxic T cells (CTLs) underlies the xenogeneic response leading to the rejection of transplants and, presumably, to the autoimmune rejection of tissues. Many methods of interfering with T cell-target cell adhesion have produced recipient immune responses that interfere with treatment. An alternative approach is to treat the target cell to avoid T cell adhesion and activation, thereby precluding the need to treat the host.

Treatment of Human Donor Islets With
Polyclonal Mouse Antibodies to Human Islets
Before Transplanation

Islet treatment	C (ng/ml)	Histology
Polyclonal mouse antibodies to human islets	<2	No islets visible at 30, 60, 90, and 120 days after transplantation
Polyclonal mouse F(ab')$_2$ to human islets	>2.8	Well-granulated islets visible at 30, 60, 90, and 120 days after transplantation
Polyclonal mouse F(ab')$_2$ to human islets depleted of antibodies to HLA class I	<2	No islets visible at 30 days after transplantation
Untransplanted mice	<2	

Polyclonal mouse antibodies to human islets were produced by 7 intraperitoneal immunizations of mice at weekly intervals with human islets. The antibody preparation was depleted of antibodies to HLA class I or CD 29.
There were 4 mouse recipients in each group.
The human C peptide concentration was measured at day 30.
(Courtesy of Faustman D, Coe C: *Science* 252:1700–1702, 1991.)

Methods.—This approach was used to conceal the HLA class I antigens on pancreatic islets before their transplantation. Human islets lack large amounts of 2 adhesion epitopes, and for this reason there is a lesser need to conceal them from the CTLs. Therefore, the HLA class I antigens become the chief candidates for masking. Mice were given transplants of human islets treated with an antibody to HLA class I, polyclonal antibodies to islet cells, or antibody to CD29.

Results.—Treatment of donor xenogeneic islets with antibody to HLA class I led to total survival of the islets. The large islet clusters were well granulated. Untreated islets were rejected within 1 week. It appeared necessary to remove the fragment (Fc) domain from the antibody to circumvent complement lysis. Those mice given islets coated with HLA class I antibody had increased C peptide levels. In addition, immunofluorescence studies confirmed that prolonged islet survival resulted from antigen masking by F(ab')$_2$ antigen-binding fragments of the antibody (table).

Discussion.—Concealing foreign HLA class I determinants permits the prolonged survival of islet xenografts without the need for treatment of the recipient. Also, an intact immune system is preserved.

▶ These are elegantly simple experiments; the F(ab')$_2$ antibody fragments lack complement fixation ability but effectively masked the key antigenic structure on the surfaces of islet cells, the major histocompatibility complex class I antigens. Without this antigenic expression, cytotoxic T cells failed to adhere and effect cell killing, even in a xenograft model. Availability of large quantities of islets from xenograft sources would make it feasible to entertain the possibility of therapeutic application of islet transplantation, and the major differences in the xenografted islet cells would lessen the likelihood of autoimmune destruction from the primary diabetes.—O. Jonasson, M.D.

Use of Yttrium-90-Labeled Anti-Tac Antibody in Primate Xenograft Transplantation
Cooper MM, Robbins RC, Goldman CK, Mirzadeh S, Brechbiel MW, Stone CD, Gansow OA, Clark RE, Waldmann TA (Natl Heart, Lung, and Blood Inst; Natl Cancer Inst, Bethesda, Md)
Transplantation 50:760–765, 1990   8–10

Background.—T cells express interleukin-2 receptor (IL-2R) in the presence of foreign histocompatibility antigens but not normal resting cells. Selective immunosuppression might therefore be achieved if the interaction of interleukin-2 (IL-2) and IL-2R could be blocked. Anti-Tac, IgG$_{2a}$, a monoclonal antibody that is specific to IL-2R, was used with or without yttrium-90 to inhibit rejection in a primate xenograft model.

Methods.—Cardiac xenografts from cynomolgus monkey donors were transplanted to the cervical or abdominal region of rhesus monkey recipients. Group I included 3 animals that received no immunosuppression; group II, 5 animals that received 2 mg of unmodified anti-Tac per kg every other day; group III, 5 animals that received 16 mCi of 90Y-anti-Tac. Four animals, comprising group IV, received the same dose of 90Y bound to UPC-10, another murine monoclonal antibody that does not recognize activated immunoresponsive cells specifically. Immunosuppressive regimens were given in divided doses during the first 2 weeks after transplantation.

Results.—The mean rejection time in group I was 6.7 days, with an increase in soluble IL-2R levels at the time of rejection; this indicated the generation of Tac-releasing and -expressing cells. The mean survival was 6.2 days in group II, whereas that in group III was 38.4 days. Although the mean survival was 21.3 days in group IV, this was significantly less than in group III, in which half of the radioactive dosage was given in specific fashion via anti-Tac. In group IV the animals had reversible bone marrow suppression without associated toxicity to the kidney or liver; antibodies to the murine monoclonal developed in almost all the animals.

Conclusions.—It appears that 90Y-anti-Tac therapy directed at IL-2R might have uses in organ transplantation and in the treatment of neoplastic diseases that express Tac. The inhibitory effect of T suppressor lymphocytes that are active during acute rejection appears to be exceeded by the helper-cytotoxic response driven by IL-2. Prolongation of graft survival depends on deleting or killing the activated T cell clones generated, rather than just blocking IL-2R.

▶ In this xenograft model using concordant (closely related) species, a cytotoxic combination of antibody blocking the T cell receptor with a therapeutic isotope prolonged organ survival substantially. Discordant xenografts will undoubtedly require additional measures to mitigate antibody-related events.—O. Jonasson, M.D.

Inhibition of Complement-Mediated Endothelial Cell Cytotoxicity by Decay-Accelerating Factor: Potential for Prevention of Xenograft Hyperacute Rejection

Dalmasso AP, Vercellotti GM, Platt JL, Bach FH (Univ of Minnesota)
Transplantation 52:530–533, 1991   8–11

Background.—Hyperacute rejection, initiated by host antibody binding to endothelial cells of the donor organ, remains the chief obstacle to the xenotransplantation of vascularized organs. Complement may participate in the rejection process by mediating endothelial cell activation and by the adhesion of leukocytes to endothelium, which events are followed by thrombosis and tissue necrosis.

Objective.—The potential value of decay accelerating factor (DAF), a membrane-associated complement inhibitor, in preventing complement-mediated tissue injury was examined. An in vitro model of xenotransplantation was used consisting of porcine aortic endothelial cells incubated with human serum (as a source of xenogeneic natural antibodies) and complement.

Findings.—Purified labeled human DAF, incorporated into the porcine aortic endothelial cells in a dose-dependent manner, protected them against the cytotoxic effects of human complement.

Implications.—This is the first study of the feasibility of using complement inhibition in xenotransplantation. The long-term goal is to engineer a transgenic donor animal with human membrane-associated complement inhibitor genes to achieve high-level expression of the corresponding proteins in xenograft endothelial cells. In this way, the role of complement in hyperacute rejection might be largely eliminated when transplanting such an organ into a human recipient.

▶ The ultimate plan suggested by these authors is to genetically engineer a large animal species, such as the pig, so that endothelial cells express those human factors (e.g., DAF) that prevent human complement activation. The experiments reported here demonstrate that human DAF, when incorporated into porcine endothelial cells, is effective in preventing cell lysis by human complement in vitro—an important first step.—O. Jonasson, M.D.

Kidney Graft Survival in Rats Without Immunosuppressants After Intrathymic Glomerular Transplantation
Remuzzi G, Rossini M, Imberti O, Perico N (Mario Negri Inst for Pharmacological Research, Bergamo, Italy; Ospedali Riuniti, Bergamo, Italy)
Lancet 337:750–752, 1991   8–12

Background.—The life-long immunosuppression usually required by renal allograft recipients may produce life-threatening complications and not infrequently compromises the quality of the patient's life. Complications could be avoided if it were possible to achieve a state of antigen-specific unresponsiveness approximating true tolerance. This probably would entail altering initial host contact with the graft.

Objective and Methods.—An attempt was made to induce tolerance in 6 rats by the intrathymic placement of renal glomeruli before transplanting the contralateral kidney in genetically unrelated animals. Isolated glomeruli were inoculated into the thymus of rats pretreated orally for 2 days with cyclosporine, 40 mg/kg daily. A dose of dexamethasone, 2.5 mg/kg, was given subcutaneously at the time of inoculation. Orthotopic renal transplantation was carried out 10 days later.

Results.—Control rats injected intrathymically with medium alone rejected their allografts within 7–9 days. In contrast, induction of donor-specific unresponsiveness permitted indefinite survival of allografts without further immunosuppressive measures. All of the experimental animals were in good health at the end of the study.

Conclusion.—Intrathymic instillation of allogeneic glomeruli can induce a state of natural donor-specific immune tolerance in major histocompatibility complex-incompatible rats, allowing the indefinite survival of a subsequent renal allograft without immunosuppressive treatment.

▶ This group has taken intrathymic inoculation of allogeneic tissue one step further by inoculating glomeruli and subsequently transplanting a whole kidney allograft from the glomeruli donor. The ultimate test of this experiment in a large animal species and then in man is eagerly anticipated.—O. Jonasson, M.D.

Minimal Sensitization and Excellent Renal Allograft Outcome Following Donor-Specific Blood Transfusion With a Short Course of Cyclosporine
Cheigh JS, Suthanthiran M, Fotino M, Riggio RR, Schechter N, Stubenbord WT, Stenzel KH, Rubin AL (The Rogosin Inst, New York; New York Hosp/Cornell Univ Med Ctr)
Transplantation 51:378–381, 1991   8–13

Introduction.—Donor-specific transfusion (DST) has significantly improved graft survival rates in recipients of living-related kidney transplants. It is associated, however, with a high rate of sensitization, which precluded many patients from receiving kidneys from their blood donors. A new protocol of DST under cyclosporine A (CsA) coverage was developed and its immunologic consequences and clinical efficacy examined.

Patients.—Between 1985 and 1989, 65 prospective kidney transplant recipients received DST from a 1-haplotype-matched living-related prospective kidney donor; 10 other prospective recipients received DST from a zero-haplotype-matched living donor. Recipients were transfused with 100 mL of stored whole blood 1, 8, and 15 days after storage. All recipients were given CsA, 6 mg/kg/day, starting the day before DST and finishing 1 week after DST, for a total of 23 days. Recipients were monitored by donor-specific mixed lymphocyte culture before and after DST and serially for antibodies by standard complement-dependent lymphocytotoxicity assay.

Results.—Only 3 of the 65 recipients (4.6%) who received blood from a 1-haplotype-matched donor had donor-specific lymphocytotoxic antibodies. One sensitized patient's serum became free of donor-specific antibodies after 2 additional blood transfusions from her original blood donor, and she received a successful transplant shortly thereafter from the same donor. Thus only 2 of the 65 recipients were prevented from receiving a transplant from their blood donors. None of the 10 patients who received DST from zero-haplotype-matched donors had sensitization after DST, and all received kidney transplants from their respective donors. Graft survivals were 96% at 1 year and 92% at 2 years for the 57 patients who received a kidney transplant from a 1-haplotype-matched donor. The rates were 90% at both 1 year and 2 years for the 10 patients who received a kidney transplant from a zero-haplotype-matched donor.

Conclusion.—Donor-specific transfusion with a short course of CsA produced a remarkably low incidence of sensitization and excellent graft outcome.

▶ In the previous study, a state of chimerism was postulated to account for the immunologic tolerance achieved by transfusion of haplo-identical blood. In this series, in which both haplo-identical and zero-matched donors were used, the blood transfusions were small (100 mL) and 2 of the 3 transfusions were more than a week old. It is unlikely that viable leukocytes were present in large numbers, and the hypothesis that chimerism was induced is even less likely. Immunosuppression given concomitantly with the transfusion may change the type of response—no detailed studies of tolerance or the absence of precursor cytotoxic cells were conducted—but the outcome of renal transplantation was excellent. An anti-idiotypic immune response also has been suggested as a plausible mechanism for this effect.—O. Jonasson, M.D.

Donor-Specific Cytotoxic T Lymphocyte Hyporesponsiveness Following Renal Transplantation in Patients Pretreated With Donor-Specific Transfusion

Grailer AP, Sollinger HW, Kawamura T, Burlingham WJ (Univ of Wisconsin)
Transplantation 51:320–324, 1991   8–14

Background.—Research on donor-specific transfusion (DST) has shown numerous effects on donor-specific T lymphocyte responses. Although the effects of DST on the mixed leukocyte culture response are generally suppressive, the effects on cytotoxic T lymphocyte (CTL) responses vary. Posttransplant CTL hyporesponsiveness to donor alloantigens has been described in prednisone/azathioprine-immunosuppressed renal transplant recipients with cadaveric organs. Whether the development of antidonor CTL hyporesponsiveness correlates with a decreased incidence of rejection in DST-treated patients in the first year after transplantation was investigated.

Methods and Findings.—Donor-specific CTL hyporesponsiveness developed in peripheral blood lymphocytes up to 2 years after transplantation in patients preconditioned with 3 DSTs plus azathioprine. In 12 patients, the hyporesponsiveness developed gradually. It became detectable in some patients as soon as 1 month after transplantation. It was statistically significant for the whole group at 9–12 months after the transplant. Some patients had a complete specificity for donor alloantigens, and others had partial suppression of the response to a third-party HLA-mismatched control. In 1 patient, the mechanism of donor-specific CTL hyporesponsiveness was explored 2 years after transplantation. The patient had received a 2-HLA haplotype-mismatched kidney transplant from her husband. Bulk culture CTL analysis demonstrated specific nonresponsiveness to donor stimulators. However, the antidonor response was restored to pretransplant peripheral blood lymphocyte levels in the presence of exogenous recombinant interleukin-2. Limiting dilution analysis showed equivalent precursor frequency of antidonor CTL in pretransplant and posttransplant peripheral blood lymphocytes.

Conclusions.—The findings suggest that posttransplant CTL hyporesponsiveness to donor develops gradually in the peripheral blood of kidney transplant recipients after DST. Although clonal deletion of antidonor CTL precursors may contribute to the protective DST effect in some cases, defective lymphokine production may be a more important mechanism in others.

▶ Yet another hypothesis for the beneficial effect of donor-specific blood transfusion is raised in this paper. Here, there clearly was no chimerism or a state of tolerance, because CTL precursors were present, merely not activated.—O. Jonasson, M.D.

National Allocation of Cadaveric Kidneys by HLA Matching: Projected Effect on Outcome and Costs
Gjertson DW, Terasaki PI, Takemoto S, Mickey MR (Univ of California, Los Angeles, Tissue Typing Lab)
N Engl J Med 324:1032–1036, 1991   8–15

Objective.—Transplantation of a cadaveric kidney matched at the HLA-A, -B, and -DR loci enhances graft survival in cyclosporine-treated patients. The value of a national system of kidney allocation based on HLA matching, however, is still debated. Some fear that the costs of such a system are unjustified. The effect of HLA matching on graft survival for all allocations of cadaveric kidneys in the United States was estimated.

Methods.—Data on 22,190 first-time cadaveric kidney recipients were partitioned to estimate the graft survival rates in 5 mutually exclusive groups of transplants with increasing numbers of HLA mismatches (Fig 8–2). Overall graft survival was projected as a weighted average, using percentages of transplants in the hierarchical groups in recipient waiting pools of various sizes. The costs and benefits of HLA matching in a national system were compared with those of cyclosporine introduction, which was estimated to enhance graft survival by 7% at 10 years.

Outcome.—Sharing kidneys nationally on the basis of hierarchical HLA matching would enhance graft survival by an estimated 5% at 10

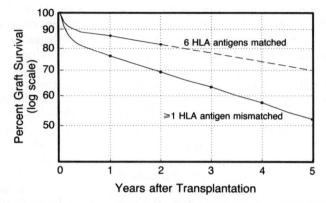

Fig 8–2.—Actuarial 5-year graft-survival curves (*solid line*) and projections (*dashed line*) for 365 first-time recipients of cadaver kidneys matched for 6 HLA antigens and 21,621 recipients of transplants with at least 1 HLA-antigen mismatch. The differences between groups after 3, 6, 12, and 24 months were all significant (P < .0001). (Courtesy of Gjertson DW, Terasaki PI, Takemoto S, et al: N *Engl J Med* 324:1032–1036, 1991.)

years. The anticipated 5-year cost of this national system for 7,000 recipients would be $6.5 million less than the cost of using cyclosporine alone. That estimated cost includes costs of graft removal and dialysis after transplant rejection (table).

Conclusion.—A national HLA allocation system will not add to the cost of renal transplantation. It will improve the long-term results by 5%, similar to the effect of cyclosporine. A national kidney-sharing system based on hierarchical levels of HLA matches should be established.

▶ The debate over the benefits of HLA matching of donor and recipient in kidney transplantation should have long since been over. Although, as is

Present-Value Costs for the First 5 Years After Transplantation for 7,000 First-Time Recipients of Cadaver Kidneys

Inflation Factor	No Cyclosporine, Random Matching	Differential	Cyclosporine, Random Matching	Differential	Cyclosporine, Hierarchical HLA Matching, 20,000-Patient Pool
%			*millions of dollars*		
0	601.0	52.4	653.4	−6.5	646.9
2.5	615.4	54.4	669.8	−7.1	662.7
5.0	630.6	56.4	687.0	−7.8	679.2
10.0	663.2	60.7	723.9	−9.2	714.7

Note: The discount rate was assumed to be 8%. Costs were based on the following charges per patient per year: transplantation (includes hospitalization, workup, and procurement), $35,0000; first year after transplantation (clinic visits and medications), $20,000 with cyclosporine and $15,000 without cyclosporine; subsequent years after transplantation, $8,000 with cyclosporine and $3,000 without cyclosporine; graft removal, $10,000; dialysis, $17,000; and additional charges for kidney sharing, $1,000.

(Courtesy of Gjertson DW, Terasaki PI, Takemoto S, et al: N *Engl J Med* 324:1032–1036, 1991.)

clear from the 2 preceding papers (Abstracts 8–14 and 8–15), serologic typing for HLA is imperfect—perhaps accounting for the numbers of failures even in 6-antigen "matches"—the evidence that 6 antigen-matched recipients have a far better long-term graft survival is incontrovertible. Resistance to sharing of kidneys is widespread, and it will be difficult to overcome the strong motivation of the organ-procuring center to use its organs in local patients, even in the face of such powerful evidence. It may take cost-based rules to finally see effective organ sharing.—O. Jonasson, M.D.

Renal Transplantation Despite a Positive Antiglobulin Crossmatch With and Without Prophylactic OKT3
Dafoe DC, Bromberg JS, Grossman RA, Tomaszewski JE, Zmijewski SM, Perloff LJ, Naji A, Asplund MW, Alfrey EJ, Sack M, Zellers L, Kearns J, Barker CF (Hosp of the Univ of Pennsylvania)
Transplantation 51:762–768, 1991   8–16

Background.—Many transplant centers use the antiglobulin crossmatch (AGXM) to enhance detection of preformed antibody to donor antigens that may cause hyperacute rejection. However, positive AGXM sometimes detects irrelevant or very low titers of anti-HLA antibody, which precludes transplantation in suitable recipients. The significance of a positive AGXM was determined.

Results.—Cadaveric renal transplantation was done in 48 patients despite a weakly positive AGXM, which is defined as cell killing above background but no greater than 20%. In an initial group of 10 patients who received cyclosporine, azathioprine, and prednisone, accelerated rejection occurred in 4 patients and graft loss in 3. A subsequent group of 38 patients received a prophylactic course of OKT3 and then triple therapy. There were no episodes of accelerated acute rejection in this group, although clinical hyperacute rejection occurred in 1 patient. Also, the incidence of delayed graft function was high—75%. Patients treated prophylactically with OKT3 had a decreased incidence of acute rejection per recipient and a delayed onset of first episodes. The 1-year actuarial primary graft survival rate was 88% in the group treated with OKT3 and 50% in the initial group. Overall, the outcome in patients with a weakly positive AGXM was similar to that in a comparison group of 32 patients with a negative AGXM and immediate graft function. However, a subset of positive AGXM regraft recipients treated prophylactically with OKT3 did not do well, with a 36% incidence of primary nonfunction.

Conclusion.—A positive AGXM, as defined in this study, is not a contraindication to primary renal transplantation. The use of the AGXM can identify transplant recipients who would benefit from prophylaxis with OKT3.

▶ Although the authors conclude that a current positive antiglobulin cross-match test was not necessarily a contraindication to renal transplantation if OKT3 was used prophylactically, their data suggest otherwise. Few patients died, but early nonfunction was common and primary nonfunction occurred frequently in OKT3 recipients with a positive cross-match. These events have long been known to be associated with an eventual poor transplant outcome. Treatment with OKT3 is not without a price—it caused severe reactions in 10% of the prophylactically treated group; the rate of infections and other complications was not reported. Even in these high-risk patients, HLA matching was poor. Perhaps an improved strategy would be to match better with organ-sharing protocols and avoid transplantation when the cross-match is positive.—O. Jonasson, M.D.

Cytokine Regulation of ICAM-1 Expression on Human Renal Tubular Epithelial Cells In Vitro
Ishikura H, Takahashi C, Kanagawa K, Hirata H, Imai K, Yoshiki T (Hokkaido Univ, Sapporo, Japan; Sapporo Med College)
Transplantation 51:1272–1275, 1991   8–17

Background.—The intercellular adhesion molecule-1 (ICAM-1) has an important role in adhesion of lymphocytes to nonlymphocytes. An example is the adhesion of lymphocytes to renal tubular epithelial cells, which appears to be a critical event in renal allograft rejection. The expression of ICAM-1 on several cell types is upregulated by cytokines such as interleukin-1 (IL-1), interferon-gamma (IFN-γ), and tumor necrosis factor (TNF-α). The regulation of ICAM-1 expression on human renal tubular epithelial cells in culture was examined.

Findings.—Many tubular epithelial cells from primary cultures expressed the ICAM-1 antigen. Supernates of mixed lymphocyte reactions (MLRs) from both specific and third-party combinations augmented the expression of ICAM-1 in a dose-dependent manner. Recombinant human cytokines that augmented the expression of ICAM-1 included IFN-γ, TNF-α, IL-1, and IL-4. The MLR supernatants contained IFN-γ and TNF-α, and their activity was partly inhibited by neutralizing antibody against IFN-γ.

Implications.—These findings indicate that cytokines released by T cells and antigen-presenting cells upregulate the expression of ICAM-1 on renal tubular epithelial cells. This may lead to increased attachment of graft-infiltrating T cells to the renal tubular cells preceding allograft rejection.

▶ In contrast to pancreatic islet cells that do not regularly express ICAM-1 but bind cytotoxic T lymphocytes to class I major histocompatibility complex molecules, these investigators have shown that ICAM-1 is expressed prominently by renal cells and may be important in the cell-cell interaction of renal cells and T cells during rejection. In Faustman and Col's work (Abstract 8–9), antibody blockade of the class I antigens prevented T cell adherence to islet cells; Ishikura et al.'s study here may suggest that ICAM-1 could be the most important adhesion factor in renal cell rejection.—O. Jonasson, M.D.

The Effects of Tissue-Associated and MHC Class II Antigen Presentation on In Vitro Lymphoproliferative Responses Against Canine Liver and Kidney Cell Subpopulations

Ranjan D, Roth D, Esquenazi V, Carreno M, Fuller L, Leif RC, Burke G, Miller J (Miami VA Hosp; Univ of Miami)
Transplantation 51:475–480, 1991   8–18

Background.—After allografting there is an increased expression of class II antigens in the grafted organ tissue. Because transplanted organs differ in their sensitivity to rejection, it has been thought that this difference in immunogenicity may be caused by differential expression of class II antigens. The apparent difference in the immunogenicity of canine liver and kidney cells in vitro was examined as it relates to the expression of class II and nominal antigens.

Methods.—Purified hepatocytes (LH), Kupffer cells (LKu), interhepatic biliary duct cells (LD), and kidney tubular cells were isolated. These cells were then incubated for 48 hours in a 2-compartment diffusion chamber with either 2-way mixed lymphocyte cultures or canine interferon-γ. Class II expression was detected by a monoclonal antibody in a cell analyzer.

Results.—Incubation of LH, LKu, and LD with either lymphocyte cultures or interferon resulted in significantly increased class II expression. Interferon-γ preinduction of canine class II expression by LKu and LD cells amplified the allogeneic mixed lymphocyte liver cultures by twofold. However, there was no autologous response. There was both an allogeneic and an autogenous response against kidney tubular cells, which was further stimulated by interferon-γ. Antibody to class II antigens blocked the uptake of labeled thymidine, indicating dependence of amplification in all cases on class II antigen gene expression. An antibody against tubular cells had no effect.

Conclusion.—Normal canine liver cells are significantly different in immunogenicity from normal canine kidney tubular cells. Cells of the normal canine liver do not readily stimulate a primary lymphoproliferative autoimmune reaction in vitro despite class II amplification. Therefore, autoreactivity is less important in the immune recognition of purified cellular components of liver tissue than of kidney tissue.

▶ In these complex experiments, tissue-associated antigens clearly participated in immune stimulation by kidney, but not liver, cells. Induction of the allogeneic or even the autologous immune response is a series of events involving class II antigens, cytokines, adhesion molecules, and tissue antigens, which seems to vary from organ to organ.—O. Jonasson, M.D.

Immunomodulation of Kidney and Heart Transplants by Anti-Idiotypic Antibodies

Hardy MA, Suciu-Foca N, Reed E, Benvenisty AI, Smith C, Rose E, Reemtsma K (Columbia Univ)
Ann Surg 214:522–530, 1991   8–19

Introduction.—Apart from donor availability, inability to manipulate the immune response remains a major obstacle to successful kidney and heart transplantation. Whether long-term allograft survival is influenced by circulating HLAs from the graft and by anti-anti-HLA (anti-idiotypic) antibodies was investigated.

Methods.—Studies were done in 330 recipients of renal allografts and 174 patients given cardiac allografts. All patients received cyclosporine-based triple immunosuppressive therapy. Rejection was treated with either an increased steroid dose or OKT3 antibody. Anti-donor HLA antibodies were uncovered by dissociation of immune complexes and depletion of soluble antigens using magnetic beads coated with monoclonal antibody.

Findings.—The presence of anti-donor-HLA antibodies (Ab1) before or after transplantation was associated with graft failure. Other anti-HLA antibodies failed to influence graft survival rates. Patients with cyclic variations of Ab1 in association with anti-Ab1 antibodies (Ab2) all had surviving grafts. Those with cyclically varying Ab1 but no anti-Ab1 antibodies had much lower 2-year graft survival rates. The continuous presence of Ab1 also compromised allograft survival.

Conclusions.—Serial estimates of anti-HLA antibodies after organ transplantation are a useful means of predicting long-term graft survival. All recipients exhibit an active immune response to mismatched graft HLA antigens. Graft survival depends in part on whether suppressive anti-idiotypic antibodies can develop.

▶ The concept of anti-idiotypic antibodies is also discussed in a number of papers selected for review in the chapter on Tumor Immunology. In this concept, antigen [in this case, major histocompatibility complex (MHC) antigens represented on endothelial cells of the donor organ] elicits antibody (Ab1-anti-MHC or HLA antibody). The antigen-binding site of Ab1 elicits a new antibody, Ab2, the anti-idiotypic antibody, actually a mirror image of the original antigen. As a mirror image, Ab2 serves to block the binding sites of Ab1. In these detailed and comprehensive serologic studies, the authors have shown a strong correlation with the success and development of blocking anti-idiotypic antibodies.—O. Jonasson, M.D.

Detection of Allograft Endothelial Cells of Recipient Origin Following ABO-Compatible, Nonidentical Cardiac Transplantation
O'Connell JB, Renlund DG, Bristow MR, Hammond EH (Univ of Utah)
Transplantation 51:438–442, 1991   8–20

Introduction.—Endothelial cells play an important role in augmenting immune responses by promoting the expression of major histocompatibility complex (MHC) class II antigens. After an immune-mediated vascular injury associated with rejection, reendothelialization is necessary to restore vascular integrity. The origin of the replacement endothelial cells can be determined if the ABO antigens expressed on the cells differ in the donor and recipient.

Objective and Methods.—The significance of reendothelialization by recipient endothelial cells was determined by staining serial endomyocardial biopsy specimens for ABO antigens; the specimens were obtained from 34 compatible, nonidentical cardiac allograft recipients. They represented 13% of 268 heart transplant procedures carried out from 1985 to 1990. Immunoperoxidase staining was carried out.

Findings.—In 10 instances (30%) the allograft endothelial cells expressed recipient characteristics, 5 of them completely, within a mean of 7.5 months after transplantation. Follow-up for 26 months on average failed to reveal significant differences in pretransplant features, graft survival, morbidity, or long-term allograft function between recipients whose endothelial cells expressed recipient blood group antigens and the others. The prevalence of chronic rejection also did not differ significantly in these groups.

Summary.—Endothelial cells expressing recipient ABO blood group antigens are found in nearly one third of cardiac allograft recipients.

▶ It has long been postulated that the endothelial cells of an allograft will, in time, be replaced by migrating monocytic cells of the recipient to form a new, host-derived endothelium. That this was documented only in 10% of successful cardiac allografts is surprising, because it would be logical to suppose that a nonrejecting graft would be repopulated routinely. However, as these authors and others have suggested, the repopulation may occur only on endothelium that has been injured, and the prognostic implications of this finding might be adverse.—O. Jonasson, M.D.

Intragraft Delivery of 16,16-Dimethyl PGE_2 Induces Donor-Specific Tolerance in Rat Cardiac Allograft Recipients
Kamei T, Callery MP, Flye MW (Washington Univ)
Transplantation 51:242–246, 1991   8–21

Rationale.—The E prostaglandins (PGEs) reportedly downregulate immune responses. If, as appears likely, T cell precursors can mature within an allograft before mediating graft rejection, direct local treatment of an allograft with an effective immunosuppressant could modify rejection while minimizing systemic side effects.

Methods.—The stable PGE_2 analogue 16,16-dimethyl PGE_2 (di-M-PGE_2) was infused by osmotic pump into rats bearing heterotopic cardiac allografts. The analogue was delivered intravenously via a lumbar vein, intraperitoneally, or directly into the graft via the innominate artery.

Results.—Delivery of di-M-PGE_2 directly into the allograft, in a daily dose of 20 µg/kg for 2 weeks, totally prevented graft rejection for longer than 150 days (Fig 8–3). No drug toxicity was evident. Allografts were rejected within 8 days in untreated recipients. Treatment for 1 week only had a partial effect. The intravenous administration of di-M-PGE_2 failed to prolong graft survival. Long-term recipients accepted skin grafts from donor-strain rats for longer than 35 days but rejected third-party skin grafts in a normal manner. When long-surviving allografts were retransplanted into naive recipients they were rejected within a week.

Conclusions.—A 2-week infusion of di-M-PGE_2 directly into a strongly mismatched cardiac allograft permits long-term engraftment and the development of donor-specific tolerance in the recipient. No other treatment is needed to prevent subsequent rejection after withdrawal of di-M-PGE_2. This approach warrants consideration for use in clinical transplantation.

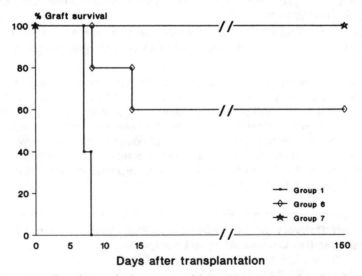

Fig 8–3.—The effect of intragraft administration of di-M-PGE_2 on Lewis cardiac allograft survival in Buffalo recipients. A daily dose of 20 µg of di-M-PGE_2 per kg was administered directly into the graft for either 1 (group 6) or 2 weeks (group 7) after transplantation. The control group received no treatment (group 1). (Courtesy of Kamei T, Callery MP, Flye MW: *Transplantation* 51:242–246, 1991.)

▶ Although the donor and recipient combination used in these experiments was not stringent, the results of intragraft administration of a PGE_2 analog were most impressive, especially tolerance to a subsequent skin graft. As also indicated in the experiments with intrathymic inoculation, the first encounter of host with donor may program the immune response that follows. In these experiments, that first encounter took place in an environment modified by PGE_2, and lymphocyte activation to those antigens was permanently altered.—O. Jonasson, M.D.

Induced Expression of Endothelial-Leukocyte Adhesion Molecules in Human Cardiac Allografts
Briscoe DM, Schoen FJ, Rice GE, Bevilacqua MP, Ganz P, Pober JS (Children's Hosp; Brigham and Women's Hosp, Boston)
Transplantation 51:537–539, 1991   8–22

Introduction.—Adhesion of leukocytes to postcapillary venules is an important step in the development of an inflammatory response. The venular endothelial cells express several inducible cell surface molecules that bind leukocyte populations.

Objective.—The expression of endothelial leukocyte adhesion molecule-1 (ELAM-1), inducible cell adhesion molecule-110 (INCAM-110), and intercellular adhesion molecule-1 (ICAM-1) by microvascular endothelial cells was examined in endomyocardial biopsy specimens obtained from heart transplants. Whereas ELAM-1 is a ligand for neutrophils, IN-CAM-110 is a ligand for monocytes and lymphocytes, and ICAM-1 is a ligand involved in the adhesion and transmigration of all leukocytes. The study included 5 specimens with minimal infiltration, 5 with focal infiltrates, and 5 with multifocal and diffuse infiltration.

Observations.—Scores for ICAM-1 increased substantially in the presence of CD3+ T-cell infiltrates. Scores for INCAM-110 induction more than tripled under the same conditions. In contrast, ELAM-1 was not detected in any of the specimens. In specimens containing infiltrates of CD3+ cells, ICAM-1 was diffusely increased in both capillaries and venules, whereas INCAM-110 was largely limited to venules. Expression of both ligands was increased in acute rejection.

Conclusion.—These preliminary findings suggest that ICAM-1 and INCAM-110, but not ELAM-1, are increased on postcapillary venular endothelial cells in posttransplant myocardial biopsy specimens exhibiting CD3+ T cell infiltration.

▶ Endothelial cells in cardiac allografts express the adhesion molecules, ICAM-1 and INCAM-110. The level of expression of these molecules on endothelial cells of capillaries and venules correlates with rejection activity and may be responsible for the adherence and invasion of the cytotoxic T effector cells into the parenchyma during rejection. In these studies, INCAM-110 seemed to be the most relevant molecule. Class I antigens were not studied in this context, but the expression of 1 or more of these key adhesion elements on the endothelium and parenchyma of the allograft may be essential for the rejection reaction to begin.—O. Jonasson, M.D.

Intrathymic Islet Transplantation in the Spontaneously Diabetic BB Rat

Posselt AM, Naji A, Roark JH, Markmann JF, Barker CF (Hosp of Univ of Pennsylvania)
Ann Surg 214:363–371, 1991   8–23

Background.—Current immunosuppressive regimens have failed to prolong the survival of pancreatic islet allografts. It has been shown that islet allografts placed in the thymus of chemically diabetic rats are not rejected, and that animals bearing such grafts are specifically unresponsive to donor alloantigens.

Study Design.—The mechanisms underlying the prolonged survival of intrathymic grafts were examined in spontaneously diabetic BB rats, in which both autoimmunity and rejection can destroy islet tissue. Also, WF rats made by hyperglycemic by streptozotocin injection were studied. Pancreatic islets isolated from Lewis donors were transplanted by portal venous inoculation into the renal subcapsular position and intrathymically.

Observations.—Islets given intraportally to spontaneously diabetic rats were consistently destroyed, and islet failure also was frequent in recipients of renal subcapsular grafts. In contrast, intrathymically placed islets lived and maintained a normal serum glucose for longer than 4 months (table). The intrathymic islets appeared normal histologically; the liver of animals that remained normoglycemic also contained well-granulated

The Survival of MHC-Compatible and MHC-Incompatible Islet Allografts in BB Rats

Transplant Site	Donor Strain (MHC)	Days of Allograft Survival (MST)*
Liver (intraportal)	Lewis (RT1^l)	8, 9, 9, 19, 24, (9)*
Renal subcapsule	Lewis (RT1^l)	41, 47, 59, >70† >120 × 2 (>64.5)
	WF (RT1^u)	23, 64, >120 (64)
Thymus	Lewis (RT1^l)	>50 × 5, >120 × 6 (>120)‡
	WF (RT1^u)	>120 × 5 (>120)

* MST, median survival time.
(Courtesy of Posselt AM, Naji A, Roark JH, et al: *Ann Surg* 214:363–371, 1991.)

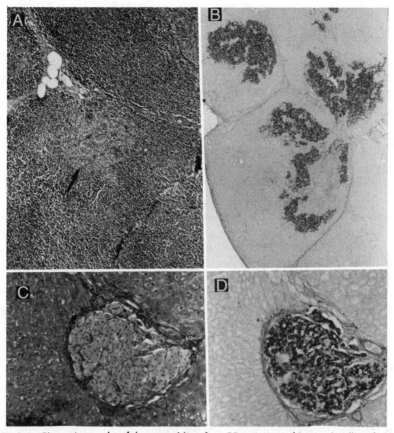

Fig 8–4.—Photomicrographs of thymus and liver from BB recipients of Lewis islet allografts. **A**, a section of a thymus removed 180 days after implantation of Lewis islets. The islets *(arrow)* appear healthy and there is no mononuclear infiltration (hematoxylin-eosin; original magnification, ×80). **B**, an aldehyde-fuchsin-stained section from the same specimen demonstrating abundant insulin granules (original magnification, ×20). **C**, a section of liver from a rat that was transplanted with intraportal Lewis islets 120 days after intrathymic islet transplantation. The removal of the liver was peformed 110 days after intraportal islet transplantion (hematoxylin-eosin; original magnification, ×160). **D**, the presence of beta cells in the same section is indicated by insulin-specific staining (aldehyde-fuchsin; magnification, ×16C). (Courtesy of Posselt AM, Naji A, Roark JH, et al: *Ann Surg* 214:363–371, 1991.)

islets (Fig 8–4). Thymic placement did not prevent allograft rejection in WF rats sensitized with donor-strain skin. Adoptive transfer of spleen cells from WF rats bearing intrathymic Lewis islets failed to prolong islet survival in secondary hosts.

Implications.—The success of intrathymic islet allograft placement appears to depend on both the immunologically privileged state of the thymus and systemic changes in the immune system. Intrathymic islet transplantation can restore permanent euglycemia in spontaneously diabetic rats. Whether this approach is practical for treating insulin-dependent diabetes remains to be determined.

▶ A year ago these investigators reported that pancreatic islet allografts survived when inoculated into the thymus, a privileged site. These experiments are an important addition to this information, in that compatible islet grafts from major histocompatibility complex-identical donors survived and functioned in spontaneously diabetic BB rats. The BB rat becomes diabetic from autoimmune destruction of pancreatic islets akin to the disease in humans resulting in type I (insulin-deficient) diabetes. Thus animals already sensitized to islets failed to destroy the thymic transplants. Moreover, subsequent islet grafts inoculated into the portal circulation survived and functioned, whereas compatible islet grafts inoculated primarily into the liver were always promptly destroyed by an autoimmune process. The mechanisms by which this is accomplished are unknown, but the implications are very exciting.—O. Jonasson, M.D.

Angiogenic Peptides in Pancreatic Islet Transplantation to Diabetic Rats
Hayek A, Lopez AD, Beattie GM (Whittier Inst for Diabetes and Endocrinology, La Jolla, Calif)
Transplantation 50:931–933, 1990   8–24

Background.—It is not clear whether the newly characterized angiogenic peptides enhance pancreatic islet transplantation when given exogenously. It is possible that hyperglycemia counters initial islet engraftment, possibly by interfering with angiogenic processes that produce fully revascularized islets.

Methods.—The effects of basic fibroblast growth factor (FGF), an angiogenic peptide, were studied in rats with severe diabetes that had syngeneic neonatal rat islets placed intrasplenically. Basic FGF or diluent was delivered by a minipump secured to the spleen. Functional in vitro studies of hormone release and mitogenesis were carried out to exclude a direct peptide effect on the islets.

Findings.—Significantly more animals given islets plus FGF than control animals were cured (70% vs 20%). Control rats that were cured had relatively low glucose concentrations. The difference could not be ascribed to either increased islet cell replication or a direct effect of the peptide on islet function.

Implications.—The cure rate of diabetes is significantly improved when basic FGF is delivered to the site of islet transplantation in the diabetic rat. Angiogenic factors might have general application in improving the results of transplanting avascular cell systems.

▶ Although it would seem logical that hyperglycemia would stimulate the proliferation of islet cells after implantation in diabetic animals, it has long been recognized that hyperglycemia causes failure of the islet grafts unless a large excess of islet cells is administered. These investigators have shown that only 1,000 islets, a number that is routinely insufficient to reverse diabetes in mice, produces lasting euglycemia if an angiogenesis-promoting factor, FGF, is continuously pumped into the implantation environment. Unfortunately, histologic studies were not reported to verify that the islets had developed a rich blood supply in their implantation site in the spleen, but if this is the case, one of the most frustrating dilemmas of islet transplantation may have been resolved.—O. Jonasson, M.D.

Selective Enhancement of β Cell Activity by Preparation of Fetal Pancreatic Proislets and Culture With Insulin Growth Factor 1
Eckhoff DE, Sollinger HW, Hullett DA (Univ of Wisconsin)
Transplantation 51:1161–1165, 1991   8–25

Introduction.—Human fetal pancreas (HFP) has several advantages over whole organ and islet transplantation. It is more widely available and is readily transplanted without the technical difficulties attending islet isolation. Transplantation of HFP has not, however, reversed diabetes secondary to decreased insulin production and graft rejection.

Objective and Methods.—An attempt was made to improve function using proislets obtained by limited collagenase digestion of HFP and culture with insulin-like growth factor 1 (IGF-1). The digestion time, collagenase concentration, and culture conditions were optimized by estimating insulin release in response to low and high glucose concentrations and a high glucose level plus theophylline.

Observations.—The presence of IGF-1 enriched β cell viability, as was evident from insulin-specific immunoperoxidase staining and insulin release in response to high glucose plus theophylline. Staining of proislets suggested selective enrichment of β cells. Streptozocin-diabetic mice that received renal capsular transplants of proislets cultured with IGF-1 regained normoglycemia much sooner than control animals. Their serum glucose control on tolerance testing was equivalent to that seen in nondiabetic mice.

Conclusion.—The use of HFP proislets cultured with endocrine growth factors such as IGF-1 may provide enriched β cells that are less immunogenic than previous preparations and therefore more suitable for clinical use.

▶ Fetal islet tissue is theoretically advantageous as the islet transplant material, because it is rich in β cells and islets are relatively easy to isolate. In this paper, IGF-1 was used in the process of isolation and culture of fetal tissue to enhance β cell differentiation and function, with good effect. Perhaps in combination with an angiogenic factor, as described in Abstract 8–24, more efficient "take" of fetal islet tissue transplants can be obtained.—O. Jonasson, M.D.

Biohybrid Artificial Pancreas: Long-Term Implantation Studies in Diabetic, Pancreatectomized Dogs

Sullivan SJ, Maki T, Borland KM, Mahoney MD, Solomon BA, Muller TE, Monaco AP, Chick WL (BioHybrid Technologies Inc, Shrewsbury, Mass; New England Deaconess Hosp, Brookline, Mass; Grace & Co–Conn, Lexington, Mass)
Science 252:718–721, 1991   8–26

Background.—Although pancreatic transplantation can produce normoglycemia, many problems attend the use of whole or segmental pancreatic transplants, including the limited availability of donor organs. The biohybrid artificial implantable pancreas uses a selectively permeable membrane that is coiled inside a housing for the islet cells (Fig 8–5) and connected to a polytetrafluoroethylene graft that joins the implant to the vascular system as an arteriovenous shunt.

Methods.—Islets from either adult mongrel dogs or bovine calves were seeded into devices both for implantation in vivo in dogs and for in vitro perfusion culture. Long-term insulin secretion was examined in vitro for up to 9 months. In vivo function was assessed in pancreatectomized dogs.

Observations.—In vitro insulin secretion peaked within 2 months of culture and then decreased slowly. Insulin secretion responded to shifts in the glucose concentration. The dogs exhibited significantly altered needs for exogenous insulin after implantation (Fig 8–6). The implantation of 2 devices into each animal totally eliminated the need for exogenous insulin therapy in most instances. Nevertheless, the response to intravenous glucose remained abnormal.

Conclusions.—The biohybrid artificial pancreas holds promise as a treatment for diabetes. Improvements in design may allow the device to

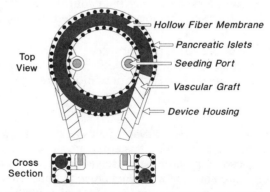

Fig 8–5.—Schematic diagram of the biohybrid pancreas device. The biohybrid pancreas device consists of an annular-shaped acrylic housing containing 30–35 cm of coiled, tubular membrane with an inner diameter of 5–6 mm and a wall thickness of 120–140 μm. This provides approximately 60 cm² of membrane surface area and a cell compartment volume around the membrane of 5–6 mL. (Courtesy of Sullivan SJ, Maki T, Borland KM, et al: *Science* 252:718–721, 1991.)

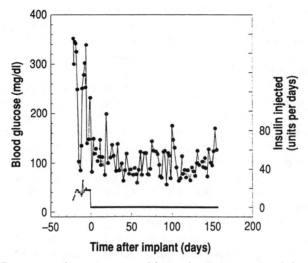

Time after implant (days)

Fig 8–6.—Exogenous insulin requirements and fasting glucose concentrations before and after device implantation. These data were obtained for an animal PS22 that received 2 devices containing a total of 4×10^5 islets. This pancreatectomized dog had required 18 units of insulin per day to maintain an average fasting glucose of 246 mL/dL. After implantation of the device, the fasting glucose levels averaged 107 mg/dL in the absence of any endogenous solution. *Small dots* indicate insulin; *large filled circles*, glucose (Courtesy of Sullivan SJ, Maki T, Borland KM, et al: *Science* 252:718-721, 1991.)

provide glycemic regulation resembling that normally provided by the pancreatic islets.

▶ An artificial pancreas has been the goal of these investigators for many years. Technological developments have permitted the successful application of an isolated islet cell mass that is protected by semipermeable membranes from immunologic destruction for as long as 5 months, a remarkable achievement that makes possible the application of xenografted islets, e.g., from bovine or porcine sources.—O. Jonasson, M.D.

Replacement of Donor Lymphoid Tissue in Small-Bowel Transplants
Iwaki Y, Starzl TE, Yagihashi A, Taniwaki S, Abu-Elmagd K, Tzakis A, Fung J, Todo S (Univ of Pittsburgh)
Lancet 337:818–819, 1991   8–27

Introduction.—Little is known about the fate of lymphocytes in intestinal grafts, in part because long-term survival has been infrequent. The first patients successfully having complete small bowel transplantation with cyclosporine infusion briefly had donor lymphocytes in the peripheral blood and had symptoms of graft-vs.-host disease at the same time.

Cases.—The fate of host and donor lymphocytes was followed in 3 patients who received FK506 for immunosuppression, 1 after complete small bowel transplantation and 2 after transplantation of both the entire small bowel and liver from the same donor. One of the patients had lost the entire small bowel from a gunshot wound, and 2 had total small bowel resection for necrotizing enterocolitis and superior mesenteric thrombosis, respectively.

Observations.—From 5% to 11% of lymphocytes in the recipients' peripheral blood were of donor origin in the early postoperative phase. Clinical signs of graft-vs.-host disease were absent at this time. Donor cells became undetectable within 12–54 days after surgery. Serial biopsy specimens of the grafted bowel showed progressive replacement of lymphocytes in the lamina propria by cells bearing the recipient's HLA phenotype. This repopulating process was complete after 10–12 weeks, while donor intestinal epithelial cells persisted. All 3 patients had histologically normal, or nearly normal, bowel within 5–8 months postoperatively when receiving enteral alimentation.

Implications.—These findings and those from animal studies indicate that the presence of recipient lymphocytes in the transplanted small bowel does not necessarily imply rejection. Lymphoreticular repopulation is probably a part of the successful transplantation of any graft containing lymphoid tissue. It is not clear whether this contributes to acceptance of the graft.

▶ In these interesting observations, donor lymphocytes were found to circulate in recipients of small bowel transplants and were replaced by recipient lymphocytes in the transplanted small bowel within 10–12 weeks. The authors suggest that the circulating donor cells may have survived and become established in the recipient's tissues, thus serving as a potential source for graft-vs.-host disease, and that recipient repopulation of transplanted tissues is a routine event, even in the absence of rejection. Without phenotyping and functional analysis of the lymphocyte infiltrate in an organ allograft, the significance of the presence of the cells is not clear and may not indicate a rejection reaction.—O. Jonasson, M.D.

PCR-Fingerprinting for Selection of HLA Matched Unrelated Marrow Donors

Clay TM, Bidwell JL, Howard MR, Bradley BA for the Collaborating Centres in the IMUST Study (UK Transplant Service, Bristol, England)
Lancet 337:1049–1052, 1991   8–28

Introduction.—The average time it takes to find an HLA-matched unrelated bone marrow donor for a patient with leukemia or marrow failure is 6 months. The long delay is attributable, in part, to the time it takes to establish HLA-DR identity between patient and donor. A novel DNA matching technique for testing the DR match between patients and unrelated marrow donors was evaluated.

Methods.—During the final annealing stage of the polymerase chain reaction (PCR), heteroduplexes are formed between heterologous amplified coding and noncoding DNA sequences; different HLA-DR/Dw types given unique banding patterns, termed "PCR fingerprints," after electrophoresis on nondenaturing polyacrylamide gels. Matching is done by visual comparison of patients' and donors' fingerprints. Identity can be confirmed by mixing donor and recipient DNA before the final stage of the PCR as a "DNA cross-match." The DNA matching technique was evaluated in 53 unrelated HLA-A and HLA-B matched patient-donor pairs. The results were compared with HLA-DR matching by DNA-restriction fragment-length polymorphism (RFLP), supplemented by PCR typing with selected sequence-specific oligonucleotides (SSO) for DR4 subtypes.

Results.—Forty-two of the 53 pairs gave the same results with PCR fingerprinting and with DNA-RFLP analysis. In the remaining 11 pairs, DR/Dw mismatches were detected by PCR fingerprinting but not by the standard DNA-RFLP method. Probing with PCR-SSO confirmed that mismatches represented different subtypes of DR4.

Conclusions.—Polymerase chain reaction fingerprinting is a rapid technique. Results are available less than 8 hours after DNA isolation, compared with the 2 weeks required for DNA-RFLP. Moreover, PCR fingerprinting requires less equipment and less technical skill than conventional HLA-DR typing. Probably, PCR fingerprinting will improve the efficiency of donor searches for unrelated HLA-matched marrow donors.

▶ Using PCR amplification of minute quantities of DNA, these investigators demonstrated that 2 unrelated individuals who are "identical" by conventional HLA serotyping, and even by sophisticated RFLP molecular techniques, may actually have different HLA antigens. Bone marrow transplantation between unrelated persons is the crucible for donor-recipient matching, and the novel "DNA cross-match" proposed in this paper will visibly display nonidentity in a relatively inexpensive and rapid test.—O. Jonasson, M.D.

Anti-B-Cell Monoclonal Antibodies in the Treatment of Severe B-Cell Lymphoproliferative Syndrome Following Bone Marrow and Organ Transplantation

Fischer A, Blanche S, Le Bidois J, Bordigoni P, Garnier JL, Niaudet P, Morinet F, Le Deist F, Fischer A-M, Griscelli C, Hirn M (Hôpital des Enfants-Malades, Paris; Centre Hospitalier Régional, Nancy; Hôpital E Herriot, Lyons; Hôpital Saint-Louis, Paris; et al)
N Engl J Med 324:1451–1456, 1991   8–29

Introduction.—The B cell lymphoproliferative syndrome, which results from immunosuppression, can cause life-threatening complications in patients undergoing marrow or organ transplantation. In an open, multicenter, prospective trial, the effects of CD12 and CD24 monoclonal antibodies were assessed in the treatment of 26 patients in whom the syndrome developed after organ or marrow transplantation.

Methods.—The B-cell-specific antibodies, including those with anti-immunoglobulin heavy chain and light chain isotype antibodies, were used to characterize B cells in the blood and biopsy samples of tissue from 26 patients with B cell lymphoproliferative syndrome. All patients had required aggressive immunosuppression. The monoclonal antibodies used included the ALB9, a mouse IgG1 specific for CD24 that was infused for 4–6 hours every day for 10 days (dose, .2 mg/kg).

Findings.—Three patients experienced grade 2 fever, whereas 2 had pain and 1 had vomiting, diarrhea, and thrombocytopenia. No patient produced antibodies against the mouse immunoglobulins during the study period. No B cells were detected in the serum of the 18 patients who were analyzed. Some patients had received antiviral drugs during the study. The anti-B-cell antibodies produced complete remission in 16 of the 26 patients who received treatment within 15–45 days (median, 21 days). Complete remission occurred only in those individuals with oligoclonal B cell lymphoproliferative syndrome. All patients with the monoclonal B cell lymphoproliferative syndrome died within 38 days of beginning therapy. Of the 15 patients in complete remission who could be evaluated, CD21 and CD24 expression occurred on the proliferative B cells in 10 and CD21 or CD24 expression occurred in 5. Of the 16 patients in complete remission, 2 marrow-transplant recipients had a relapse. Figure 8–7 shows the outcomes of all 18 patients.

Conclusions.—The intravenous infusion of the anti-B-cell antibodies may be able to control the oligoclonal B cell proliferation of cells as long as the CNS is not involved. A randomized, controlled trial is recom-

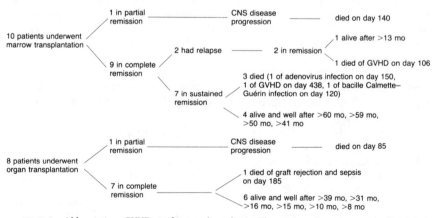

Fig 8–7.—*Abbreviation:* GVHD, graft versus host disase. The outcome in patients with oligoclonal B-cell lymphoproliferative syndrome who were treated with anti-B-cell antibodies. (Courtesy of Fischer A, Blanche S, Le Bidois J, et al: *N Engl J Med* 324:1451–1456, 1991.)

mended to further test this monoclonal antibody as treatment for the B cell lymphoproliferative syndrome.

▶ Remarkable results were achieved in this selected group of patients with aggressive B cell lymphomas after bone marrow or organ transplantation. The results in organ recipients were especially good, even those in whom reduction of immunosuppressive drugs had failed to reverse the disease. The authors suggest that organ recipients in whom nonmonoclonal lymphoma develops might be treated primarily with anti-B-cell antibodies and be able to retain their organ grafts.—O. Jonasson, M.D.

9 Oncology and Tumor Immunology

Effect of Prior Cancer Chemotherapy on Human Tumor-Specific Cytotoxicity In Vitro in Response to Immunopotentiating Biologic Response Modifiers
Weisenthal LM, Dill PL, Pearson FC (Oncotech Inc, Irvine, Calif; Cell Technology Inc, Boulder, Colo)
J Natl Cancer Inst 83:37–42, 1991   9–1

Background.—Many attempts have been made to treat cancer with bacterial products that produce "nonspecific" stimulation of the immune system. The clinical benefit has been inconsistent at best and, apart from bacille Calmette-Guérin, the use of biological response modifiers (BRMs) has not found a routine place in management.

Objective and Methods.—Tumor-specific cytotoxicity was quantified in fresh biopsy specimens of human tumors by a modified form of the differential staining cytotoxicity assay. The suspension cultures of freshly dissociated tumors were incubated with and without drugs for several days before evidence of membrane damage was sought. The test agents included interleukin-2, interferons α and γ, tumor necrosis factor, and ImuVert, a suspension of ribosomes and membrane vesicles from *Serratia marcescens*.

Observations.—ImuVert was much more effective against tumors from chemotherapy-response patients (including those with breast and ovarian adenocarcinomas) than against tumors from either untreated or treatment-resistant patients. The refractory tumors included adenocarcinomas of the lung, colon, pancreas, stomach, gallbladder, uterus, and prostate. Similar findings were obtained for tumor necrosis factor and interferon-γ, but not for interferon-α or interleukin-2. The findings could not be ascribed to a larger number of effector cells in tumors from previously treated patients.

Conclusions.—Macrophage-activating BRMs may prove most helpful in treating patients whose tumors have responded to chemotherapy. Such agents warrant further trial as adjuncts to chemotherapy in patients with responsive adenocarcinomas.

▶ The systemic release of antigenic material from tumor cells undergoing necrosis during chemotherapy may specifically sensitize cytotoxic cells, which are then more likely to respond to activation by cytokines. This explanation of an effect of biological response modifiers, inducing the release of cytokines, is supported by these interesting data.—O. Jonasson, M.D.

Increased Serum Levels of Soluble Receptors for Tumor Necrosis Factor in Cancer Patients
Aderka D, Engelmann H, Hornik V, Skornick Y, Levo Y, Wallach D, Kushtai G (Tel Aviv Univ; Weizmann Inst of Science, Rehovot, Israel)
Cancer Res 51:5602–5607, 1991   9–2

Introduction.—Tumor necrosis factor (TNF) initiates its multiple effects on cell function by binding to specific high-affinity cell-surface receptors. There are 2 known molecular species of TNF receptors (TNF-Rs), the cell surface form and a soluble form. The soluble TNF-Rs have previously been detected in normal urine. The soluble forms of type I (p55) and type II (p75) TNF-R were measured in serum samples from patients with cancer and healthy controls.

Methods.—An enzyme-linked immunosorbent assay (ELISA) was used to measure soluble TNF-R levels in serum obtained from 59 patients with cancer and from 40 healthy controls. Colon cancer was present in 29 patients and various other solid tumors in 30. Serum levels of carcinoembryonic antigen, a commonly used cancer marker, were measured by radioimmunoassay. The in vitro cytocidal activity of TNF was determined using murine A9 cells as targets.

Results.—Increases in serum levels of TNF-R type I (TNF-RI) were abnormal in 40 (74%) patients with cancer, as were TNF-RII serum levels in 37 (68%) patients. The incidence and extent of the increase correlated with disease stage. Sera from patients with cancer markedly inhibited the in vitro cytocidal activity of TNF. This inhibition was proportional to the content of soluble TNF receptors. The inhibitory effect could be fully negated by the addition of specific antireceptor antibodies to the sera. Only 14 patients (25%) had increased serum carcinoembryonic antigen levels.

Conclusion.—Serum levels of soluble TNF-Rs in patients with cancer correlate with disease. Determination of serum levels of the soluble TNF-Rs may be useful in the early detection, follow-up, and prognosis of cancer.

▶ Whereas TNF is produced by tumor cells and by activated macrophages in response to tumor-induced inflammation, soluble TNF receptors in patients' sera block the antitumor and other effects of the TNF. The complex interactions of cytokines, tumors, and host defenses are still unclear.—O. Jonasson, M.D.

Evidence That Tumor Necrosis Factor Plays a Pathogenetic Role in the Paraneoplastic Syndromes of Cachexia, Hypercalcemia, and Leukocytosis in a Human Tumor in Nude Mice

Yoneda T, Alsina MA, Chavez JB, Bonewald L, Nishimura R, Mundy GR (Univ of Texas, San Antonio; Osaka Univ, Japan)

J Clin Invest 87:977–985, 1991

9–3

Background.—Paraneoplastic disorders such as cachexia and hypercalcemia are frequent accompaniments of neoplastic disease. Leukocytosis is also seen in this setting. A human squamous cell carcinoma of the maxilla, MH-85, was established. This carcinoma was associated with hypercalcemia, leukocytosis, and cachexia in the original patient and in nude mice. Marked splenomegaly was also observed in the mice.

Observations.—Splenomegaly in tumor-bearing mice paralleled tumor growth and was reversed by surgical removal of the tumor. Splenectomy, performed either 1 week before tumor inoculation or 6 weeks afterward, decreased tumor growth and limited the decrease in body weight and the increase in serum calcium. Injection of polyclonal neutralizing antibodies raised against murine tumor necrosis factor (TNF) led to a rapid decrease in blood calcium and suppression of osteoclast activity. Normal immune serum had no such effects. Specific antibody also increased body weight and decreased the white blood cell count. Tumor-bearing mice had plasma immunoreactive TNF levels that were nearly fourfold higher than those in control mice.

In Vitro Findings.—Spleen cells released an increased amount of TNF when cultured with MH-85 tumor-conditioned medium. The TNF activity, however, was not detected in MH-85 culture supernatants.

Conclusion.—Splenic cytokines may promote both the development of paraneoplastic syndromes and tumor growth.

▶ These are nice and logical experiments using the nude mouse, unable to reject a human tumor implant, to demonstrate the effects of soluble factors produced by certain human neoplasms. Nude mice with implants from a human tumor that had caused cachexia, leukocytosis, and hypercalcemia in the original patient also became cachexic and hypercalcemic. The source of these paraneoplastic manifestations was neatly pinpointed to normal spleen cells, apparently stimulated to secrete TNF by soluble factors from the tumor. Removing the spleen ameliorated the symptoms, and reinfusing normal spleen cells brought them back.—O. Jonasson, M.D.

The Local Effects of Cachectin/Tumor Necrosis Factor on Wound Healing

Salomon GD, Kasid A, Cromack DT, Director E, Talbot TL, Sank A, Norton JA
(Natl Cancer Inst, Bethesda, Md)

Ann Surg 214:175–180, 1991   9–4

Background.—Previous experimental studies have suggested both beneficial and detrimental effects of tumor necrosis factor (TNF) on wound healing. Recent work in a sponge matrix model indicated that TNF may occur in normal wound fluid but in minimal concentration.

Methods.—Doxorubicin-treated and control rats were given paired dorsal wounds and received local applications of either recombinant TNF, in a dose of .5, 5, or 50 µg, or vehicle for 1 or 2 weeks before the wounds were harvested and tested for bursting strength. Northern blot

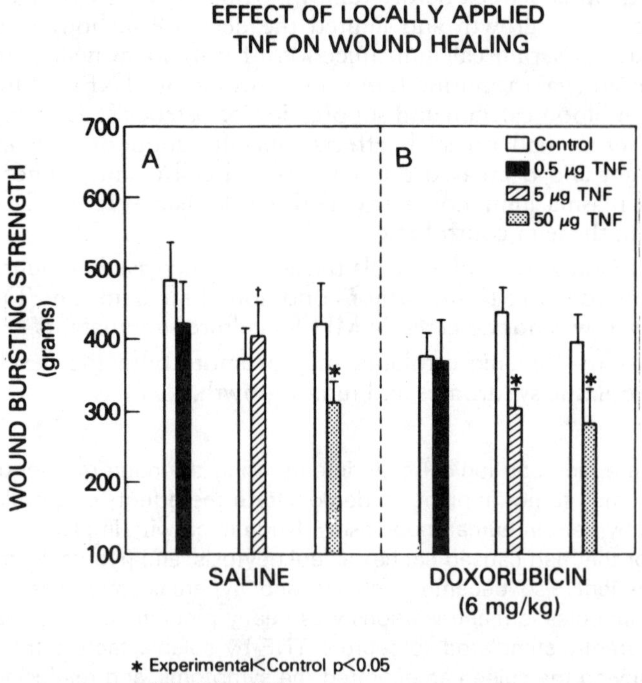

EFFECT OF LOCALLY APPLIED TNF ON WOUND HEALING

* Experimental<Control p<0.05
† Saline>D p<0.05

Fig 9–1.—Effect of locally applied tumor necrosis factor (TNF) on wound-bursting strength (WBS) of 7-day wounds. Rats were treated with either saline (**A**) or doxorubicin (**B**) and wounded. Either vehicle or recombinant TNF (.5, 5, OR 50 µg) was applied locally to paired wounds on the day of wounding. Wound bursting strength in grams was measured 7 days after wounding. *The local application of 50 µg of recombinant TNF in saline-treated rats significantly reduced WBS compared to vehicle-treated paired wounds (P < .05). *The local application of either 5 or 50 µg of TNF in doxorubicin-treated rats significantly reduced WBS compared to vehicle-treated paired wounds (P < .05). †Doxorubicin administration significantly decreased WBS in wounds treated locally with 5 µg of TNF (P < .05). (Courtesy of Salomon GD, Kasid A, Cromack DT, et al: *Ann Surg* 214: 175–180, 1991.)

methods were used to analyze the wounds for type 1 collagen and TNF gene activity.

Findings.—Application of recombinant TNF lowered wound bursting strength in the highest dose only (Fig 9–1). The 5-μg dose decreased wound strength in doxorubicin-treated animals at 1 week, but not 2 weeks after wound production. Doxorubicin treatment decreased the expression of collagen gene, and local TNF had the same effect in saline-treated rats. The gene for TNF was not detected in wounds of either normal or doxorubicin-treated animals at any interval. The gene was expressed in endotoxin-stimulated macrophages as a positive control.

Conclusions.—These findings do not support a significant role for TNF as an acute mediator of wound healing. The negative effects of exogenous TNF suggest that local application of the factor will not be helpful in correcting impaired wound healing.

▶ Tumor necrosis factor is not normally present in wounds, but in disease states such as cancer where, as demonstrated in the preceding paper, detectable levels of TNF may be found in patients with metastatic colon cancer, it may also be present in wounds. These experiments demonstrate that TNF impairs wound healing by suppressing expression of the gene for collagen synthesis. Some have suggested that TNF would accelerate wound healing because of its chemotactic and angiogenic effects, but this seems improbable.—O. Jonasson, M.D.

Effect of Intraperitoneal Recombinant Human Tumor Necrosis Factor Alpha on Malignant Ascites
Räth U, Kaufmann M, Schmid H, Hofmann J, Wiedenmann B, Kist A, Kempeni J, Schlick E, Bastert G, Kommerell B, Männel D (Ruprecht-Karls-Universität, Heidelberg; Universität Heidelberg; Institut für Immunologie und Genetik, Heidelberg; Knoll AG, Ludwigshafen, Germany)
Eur J Cancer 27:121–125, 1991   9–5

Introduction.—Recombinant human tumor necrosis factor-alpha (rhTNF-α) has produced tumor regression in various animal models. A group of 29 patients who had refractory malignant ascites caused by the peritoneal spread of adenocarcinoma received intraperitoneal infusions of 40–350 μg of rhTNF-α per m^2 per week) for 2 months. The ascites volume was measured ultrasonically. Ovarian, colorectal, gastric, and pancreatic adenocarcinomas were the most frequently occurring types.

Results.—Of the 28 evaluable patients, 22 had complete resolution of their ascites. All 10 patients with ovarian cancer responded. Two responders had recurrent ascites at the time of death. Patients with ovarian cancer had a median survival of 139 days from the start of treatment, compared with 56 days for those with gastrointestinal and other cancers. There was no significant change in TNF-α production by cultured mononuclear cells. In no patient did the side effects require withdrawal of treatment.

Implications.—Although no survival benefit was evident in this study, intraperitoneal TNF-α treatment had a substantial palliative effect in promoting the resolution of gross ascites. This approach should be studied in patients with smaller tumor burdens who have not been heavily pretreated.

▶ Although side effects of fever and chills, nausea and vomiting, malaise, and abdominal pain, typical of the cachectic effects known to be attributed to TNF, occurred in these patients, the rTNF was fairly well tolerated at high doses. Resolution of the ascites was usually achieved even though tumor cells could still be demonstrated, and survival was not prolonged. This innovative therapy might be most effective if the tumor implants were smaller. Trials are certainly in order.—O. Jonasson, M.D.

Specific Release of Granulocyte-Macrophage Colony-Stimulating Factor, Tumor Necrosis Factor-α, and IFN-γ by Human Tumor-Infiltrating Lymphocytes After Autologous Tumor Stimulation
Schwartzentruber DJ, Topalian SL, Mancini M, Rosenberg SA (Natl Cancer Inst, Bethesda, Md)
J Immunol 146:3674–3681, 1991   9–6

Introduction.—A variety of human tumors possess tumor-infiltrating lymphocytes (TIL). Some melanoma TIL have exhibited specific, major histocompatibility complex (MHC)-restricted recognition of autologous tumor cells in short-term lysis assays.

Objective.—Cytokine release by TIL was assessed as an indicator of specific tumor recognition. The TIL were cultured from metastatic tumors resected from 4 patients with melanoma and also from primary or metastatic lesions in 7 patients with breast carcinoma.

Observations.—The cultures of 2 of the 4 melanomas specifically released granulocyte-macrophage colony-stimulating factor, tumor necrosis factor-α, and interferon-γ after stimulation with autologous tumor cells. Of the 7 breast cancers, 1 was active. Studies of the lymphocytes from 2 melanoma patients indicated that virtually all of the specific cytokine secretion was promoted by the CD8+ cells. Specific cytokine release by CD8+ TIL was inhibited by monoclonal antibody against MHC class I antigen. Cytokine release from a CD4+ breast cancer TIL culture was inhibited by anti-MHC class II monoclonal antibody.

Implications.—High intratumoral levels of cytokines, which are above those that can be achieved by systemic administration, may be required to produce an antitumor effect in vivo. It may prove possible to use the selective tumor-homing properties of genetically modified TIL to deliver large amounts of cytokines directly to the tumor sites.

▶ Expression of histocompatibility antigens by tumor cells was found to be the condition under which the TIL were stimulated to release a number of cytokines. This phenomenon is known as MHC restriction. In the melanoma TIL cells, the CD8+ cells (the "cytotoxic-suppressor" population) responded to HLA class I antigens; in a case of breast cancer, CD4+ cells ("helper") responded similarly to HLA class II antigens. Because TIL cells "home" to the tumor when injected systemically, modification of the genes of the TIL to increase their cytokine production might allow large concentrations of cytokines to be produced directly within the tumor and cause tumor necrosis without intolerable systemic side effects. Expression of MHC antigens by tumor cells has important implications, as is discussed in the following papers.—O. Jonasson, M.D.

Elevated Circulating Interleukin-6 Is Associated With an Acute-Phase Response But Reduced Fixed Hepatic Protein Synthesis in Patients With Cancer

Fearon KCH, McMillan DC, Preston T, Winstanley FP, Cruickshank AM, Shenkin A (Royal Infirmary, Edinburgh; Royal Infirmary, Glasgow; Scottish Universities Research and Reactor Centre, East Kilbride)
Ann Surg 213:26–31, 1991   9–7

Introduction.—Most cancer patients with progressive disease become so emaciated that they appear to die primarily of cachexia. Cachectic cancer patients appear to have inappropriately elevated rates of whole-body protein turnover. It has been suggested that, as part of the inflammatory response to the presence of a tumor, a variety of cytokines are produced that induce hepatic synthesis of acute-phase proteins (APPs). Circulating interleukin-1 (IL-1), interleukin-6 (IL-6), and tumor necrosis factor (TNF) concentrations and fixed hepatic protein synthesis rates were compared in cancer patients and in healthy controls.

Patients.—The study was done in 6 patients with an established APP response secondary to hepatic metastasis from colorectal cancer and in 6 healthy controls. Fixed hepatic protein synthesis rates were measured after a primed, constant 20-hour infusion of labeled glycine. A liver biopsy was done at laparotomy. The APP response was assessed by serum C-reactive protein levels. Cytokines were assayed by immunoassay and bioassay.

Results.—Serum IL-6 levels in patients with advanced cancer and an ongoing APP response were significantly higher than those in controls. Three of the 6 cancer patients had detectable serum levels of tumor necrosis factor, which can elicit APP production. Interleukin-1 was not detected in the serum of patients or controls. Although the patients had 70% higher rates of whole-body protein synthesis than those in controls, rates of fixed hepatic protein synthesis were 30% lower than those in controls. Thus, although the synthesis of acute-phase export proteins can be increased in patients with hepatic metastasis, fixed protein synthesis is reduced in these patients. One cause of the increased rate of whole-body protein synthesis in cancer patients may be the production of inflammatory mediators in response to neoplasia.

Conclusion.—In patients with advanced cancer and weight loss, stimuli for cytokine production may reduce the overall protein synthesis in the hepatocyte. The role of IL-6 in changes in the distribution of hepatic protein synthesis requires further investigation.

▶ The inflammatory response to a cancer induces cytokines akin to the acute-phase response seen with sepsis. In these nice metabolic studies, IL-6 and tumor necrosis factor were found to be elevated in patients with metastatic colon cancer in association with reduced fixed hepatic protein synthesis and increased urinary nitrogen excretion. Cancer cachexia may be a result of these inflammatory cytokine-mediated events.—O. Jonasson, M.D.

Impairment of Natural Killer Functions by Interleukin 6 Increases Lymphoblastoid Cell Tumorigenicity in Athymic Mice

Tanner J, Tosato G (Ctr for Biologics Evaluation and Research, Bethesda, Md)
J Clin Invest 88:239–247, 1991   9–8

Introduction.—In vivo, B lymphocytes naturally infected with Epstein-Barr virus (EBV) are long-lived and subjected to immunoregulation to prevent their proliferation. In the presence of severe immunodeficiency, EBV-infected B cells can proliferate, giving rise to polyclonal or oligoclonal malignancies. The potential role for interleukin-6 (IL-6) in B cell lymphomagenesis was investigated.

Methods.—Interleukin-6 is a cytokine having a broad range of biological activities. It is an important factor in the establishment and maintenance of EBV-immortalized B cells. These virus-infected B cells secrete low levels of IL-6, express surface receptors for IL-6, and can use IL-6 as an autocrine growth factor. Experiments were conducted in vitro and in athymic mice. The tumors were lymphomas composed of the originally inoculated human lymphoblastoid cells.

Results.—The in vitro experiments showed that, at high concentrations, IL-6 markedly inhibited human lymphoblastoid cell killing by IL-2-activated murine splenocytes, suggesting that IL-6-related tumorigenicity might depend on IL-6 inhibiting cytotoxicity at the tumor site. In the in vivo experiments, parental and control virus-infected lymphoblastoid cells only rarely caused tumors in nude mice (7.5%). In contrast, tumors developed in 68% of the mice inoculated with IL-6 virus-infected lymphoblastoid cell lines. Neither tumor incidence nor the time of first tumor occurrence in mice correlated directly with the levels of IL-6 produced by IL-6 virus-infected cell lines.

Conclusion.—Lymphoblastoid cell lines that express IL-6 are highly tumorigenic in vivo. This effect is probably the result of IL-6-induced dysfunction of natural killer functions.

▶ The lymphomas of immunosuppressed transplant recipients and AIDS patients are derived from EBV-infected B lymphocytes whose proliferation escapes normal immune surveillance. The elegant experiments reported in this paper demonstrate that even in immune-compromised hosts, defenses against tumor cells exist, and these defenses are suppressed by IL-6 secreted by the tumor lymphocytes. Interleukin-6 has been used, especially in combination with TNF, in the treatment of advanced malignancies; this same suppression of natural killer cell function may occur, mitigating the desired effect.—O. Jonasson, M.D.

Enhanced Expression of Interleukin-6 in Primary Human Renal Cell Carcinomas

Takenawa J, Kaneko Y, Fukumoto M, Fukatsu A, Hirano T, Fukuyama H, Nakayama H, Fujita J, Yoshida O (Kyoto Univ; Nagoya Univ; Osaka Univ, Japan)
J Natl Cancer Inst 83:1668–1672, 1991   9–9

Introduction.—The pathogenesis of renal cell carcinoma is unknown. Reportedly, cultured renal cell carcinoma cells produce interleukin-6 (IL-6), which augments the growth of renal cell carcinoma cells in vitro. These findings suggest that IL-6 may function as an autocrine growth factor in renal cell carcinoma. The role of IL-6 in the pathogenesis of human renal cell carcinoma was investigated.

Methods.—Expression of the IL-6 receptor gene was studied by Northern blot analysis in primary renal cell carcinoma tissue specimens obtained surgically from 43 patients (aged 28–89 years) and in 8 normal kidney tissue specimens obtained from the normal portions of resected kidneys. The tissue specimens were also examined for expression of the IL-3 gene and presence of IL-6 receptor.

Results.—Northern blot analysis detected IL-6 gene expression in 22 of the 43 renal cell carcinoma tissue specimens and in 5 of the 7 renal cell carcinoma cell lines identified. In 10 (23%) renal cell carcinomas, there was as much as a 40-fold enhanced expression of IL-6. Patients with a high-level of IL-6 expression had a significantly higher incidence of lymph node metastasis and larger increases in serum C-reactive protein than those without it. To confirm that renal cell carcinoma cells, rather than vascular endothelial cells, were responsible for the expression of IL-6, immunohistochemical analysis was performed, which confirmed the expression of IL-6 by tumor cells. The IL-6 receptor was detected by Northern blot analysis in 11 of the 43 renal cell carcinomas, but in none of the 7 cell lines. However, use of the complementary DNA-polymerase chain reaction detected IL-6 receptor transcript in all

43 specimens and in all 7 cell lines. No expression of the IL-3 gene was identified in either the tumor specimens or cell lines.

Conclusion.—The IL-6 gene and its receptor may play a role in promoting transformation or proliferation of renal cell carcinoma and in the development of symptoms. The level of IL-6 expression could be used as a marker in predicting the patient's clinical course.

▶ In these observations in specimens of human renal cell carcinoma, IL-6 production by the tumor cells was demonstrated in half of the primary tumors and most renal cell carcinoma cell lines. As suggested in the preceding paper (Abstract 9–8), the effects of locally produced high concentrations of IL-6 may impede normal immune surveillance activities of lymphokine-activated natural killer cells rather than act as a growth factor for the tumor. Also, as noted in Fearon's paper (Abstract 9–7), increased acute-phase proteins were found in the patients whose tumors produced IL-6; tumor cachexia may be correlated.—O. Jonasson, M.D.

Frequent Down-Regulation of Major Histocompatibility Class I Antigen Expression on Individual Micrometastatic Carcinoma Cells
Pantel K, Schlimok G, Kutter D, Schaller G, Genz T, Wiebecke B, Backmann R, Funke I, Riethmüller G (Universität München; Ludwig-Maximilians Universität, Munich; Medizinische Klinik II, and Pathologisches Institut in Zentralklinikum, Augsburg, Germany)
Cancer Res 51:4712–4715, 1991   9–10

Introduction.—In many patients with small primary cancers, occult metastases are a major cause of late relapse. Marrow aspirates from patients with colon carcinoma have indicated an extremely high rate of micrometastatic cells, despite the rarity of skeletal metastasis. This observation raises questions about the malignant potential of such cells.

Objective and Methods.—The expression of major histocompatibility complex (MHC) class I antigens on marrow micrometastases was examined in 54 patients with primary adenocarcinoma of the breast, stomach, or colon. The disseminated tumor cells were identified using the immunoalkaline phosphatase technique with monoclonal antibody to the epithelial differentiation antigen cytokeratin 18 (CK-18). The specimens with CK-18-positive cells were colabeled with a monoclonal antibody (W6/32) directed to a framework antigenic determinant of MHC class I heavy chains associated with β_2-microglobulin.

Findings.—Class I expression was found in 35% of the CK-18-positive cells from patients with breast cancer, compared with 71% to 73% of the cells from patients with colon or stomach cancer—a significant difference (table). Class I expression was nearly twice as frequent in the patients with moderately differentiated primary tumors as in those with

MHC Class I Expression on CK-18-Positive Cells in Bone
Marrow and the Origin of the Primary Tumor

Origin of primary tumor	No. of patients/ group	No. of patients with MHC class I*CK-18+ cells in marrow		
		Positive	Positive/negative **	Negative
Breast	26	9 (34.6) †	4 (15.4)	13 (50.0)‡
Colon	17	12 (70.6)	1 (5.9)	4 (23.5)
Stomach	11	8 (72.7)	2 (18.2)	1 (9.1)
Total	54	29 (53.7)	7 (13.0)	18 (33.3)

*As defined with monoclonal antibodies CK2 and W6/32 in the double-labeling procedure.
**Both types of CK-18+ cells (class I positive and negative) occurred in the marrow sample of the same patient.
† The *numbers in parentheses* indicate the percentage of the total number of patients in the particular group.
‡ The differences between breast cancer patients and patients with carcinomas of the colon ($P < .05$) and stomach ($P < .02$) were statistically significant (χ^2 test) comparing the ratios of the positive and negative expressors.
(Courtesy of Pantel K, Schlimok G, Kutter D, et al: *Cancer Res* 51:4712–4715, 1991.)

poorly differentiated tumors. No significant correlation was found between class I expression and tumor stage.

Implication.—This approach may prove useful for identifying cancer patients with minimal residual disease who are nevertheless at a relatively high risk of having metastatic disease. Such patients may benefit from treatment with MHC class I-inducing agents such as interferon-γ or tumor necrosis factor-α.

▶ Micrometastases in the bone marrow are a frequent finding in patients with breast cancer; that bone marrow micrometastases are also present in patients with colon cancer is a surprise, because overt bone metastasis is rare in this disease. These investigators found that the micrometastases from colon cancer most often express MHC antigens, whereas those from breast cancer usually do not. They hypothesize that lack of MHC expression protects breast cancer micrometastases from cytotoxicity by the abundant cytotoxic cell population in the marrow. These are interesting observations, but the speculation that MHC expression or lack thereof is responsible for overt metastatic growth is less appealing, especially because tumor cells are readily identified in so many colon cancer patients. If these are so vulnerable, why are they present at all? Nonetheless, the suggestion that administration of cytokines known to upregulate MHC expression may be useful in order to facilitate cytotoxicity is interesting, although the MHC loss of expression may be permanent.—O. Jonasson, M.D.

Relation Between Skin Cancer and HLA Antigens in Renal-Transplant Recipients

Bouwes Bavinck JN, Vermeer BJ, van der Woude FJ, Vandenbroucke JP, Schreuder GMTh, Thorogood J, Persijn GG, Claas FHJ (University Hosp Leiden; Eurotransplant Found, Leiden; Leiden Univ, The Netherlands)
N Engl J Med 325:843–848, 1991   9–11

Background.—Renal allograft recipients have an increased risk of skin cancer. Those who are homozygous for HLA antigens are also at an increased risk for certain cancers, as are those recipients who are mismatched with their donors for these antigens. The relationship between skin cancer in renal transplant recipients and HLA homozygosity and mismatching was studied.

Methods.—A group of 764 renal transplant recipients were enrolled in a case-control study. The transplantations were done between 1966 and 1988. A total of 66 patients had squamous cell or basal cell carcinoma of the skin after transplantation. Assessment of HLA homozygosity was done in all 66 patients, and HLA mismatching was assessed in 39. The results were then compared with those of the 124 transplant recipients without skin cancer. Also studied was the relationship between skin cancer and the use of immunosuppressive drugs, as well as the effect of exposure to the sun and keratotic skin lesions.

Results.—Recipients who were mismatched for HLA-B antigens had an increased risk of squamous cell carcinoma; the relative risks of 1 and 2 antigen mismatching were 2.6 and 5, respectively, compared with no mismatching. Mismatching for HLA-A or HLA-DR antigen had no effect on the risk of squamous cell carcinoma. There were no associations between the mismatches at any of the HLA loci and the occurrence of basal cell carcinoma. Total azathioprine and prednisone doses were unrelated to the occurrence of skin cancer or HLA matching. Both sunlight exposure and keratotic skin lesions were strongly related to skin cancer but not to HLA mismatching. Homozygosity for HLA-DR occurred more frequently among patients with squamous cell carcinoma and among those with 100 or more keratotic skin lesions.

Conclusions.—Both HLA-B mismatching and HLA-DR homozygosity are significantly associated with the risk of squamous cell carcinoma in renal transplant recipients. These findings cannot be explained by indirect effects, nor does exposure to sunlight or the number of keratotic lesions account for this observation.

▶ Looked at from another aspect, HLA homozygosity has been found to be associated with an increased frequency of cancers. It is proposed that homozygosity, which halves the different major histocompatibility complex class I and II determinants, limits the possibilities of interaction with antigens such as tumor antigens and lessens immune surveillance. Organ transplant recipients are at a notoriously high risk for the development of skin cancer, the most frequent malignancy in this population. Immunosuppression, exposure to sunlight, and constant exposure to antigens from the transplanted organ seem to be additive effects. The finding that squamous cell cancers were more frequent in recipients who were homozygous for HLA alleles and were mismatched for their organs is a logical outcome of these observations.—O. Jonasson, M.D.

Active Specific Immunotherapy in Patients With Melanoma: A Clinical Trial With Mouse Antiidiotypic Monoclonal Antibodies Elicited With Syngeneic Anti-High-Molecular-Weight-Melanoma-Associated Antigen Monoclonal Antibodies
Mittelman A, Chen ZJ, Kageshita T, Yang H, Yamada M, Baskind P, Goldberg N, Puccio C, Ahmed T, Arlin Z, Ferrone S (New York Med College, Valhalla)
J Clin Invest 86:2136–2144, 1990   9–12

Introduction.—Anti-idiotypic antibodies are antibodies to determinants expressed on the variable region of antitumor-associated antigens (anti-TAA). Anti-idiotypic antibodies bear the mirror image of TAA and elicit or enhance anti-TAA responses. The results of 2 clinical trials of a mouse anti-idiotypic monoclonal antibody (MAb) in patients with stage IV malignant melanoma were reviewed.

Trial I.—Seven women and 9 men aged 38–72 years with a median performance status of 70% were enrolled. After an initial dose-finding phase, the anti-idiotypic MAb MF11-30 was injected subcutaneously on days 0, 7, and 28. Additional injections were given if anti-anti-idiotypic antibodies did not develop or if the titer decreased. A dose of 2 mg per injection effectively induced anti-anti-idiotypic antibodies. Although anti-mouse Ig antibodies could be detected even before treatment was initiated, none of the patients had any toxic, allergic, or anaphylactic reactions. In 3 patients there were minor responses lasting for 34–83 weeks.

Trial II.—Studies were made in 11 men and 10 women aged 27–74 years with a mean performance status of 70%. The MAb MF11-30 was given at a dose of 2 mg per injection. The average duration of treatment was 34 weeks. Two patients could not be evaluated. None of the patients had toxic or allergic reactions. In 1 patient, a complete remission was achieved, with disappearance of multiple abdominal lymph nodes; this lasted for 95 weeks; 3 other patients had minor responses lasting for 14–77 weeks. The 7 patients in whom anti-anti-idiotypic antibodies developed with a titer of at least 1:8 without changes in the level of serum high-molecular-weight-melanoma-associated antigen (HMW-MAA) had an average survival of 55 weeks. In contrast, 12 patients with a titer of 1:4 or less who had an increase in the serum level of HMW-MAA had an average survival of 19 weeks. The difference was statistically significant.

Conclusion.—Mouse anti-idiotypic MAb that bear the internal image of HMW-MAA may be useful in the immunotherapy of patients with malignant melanoma.

▶ A tumor vaccine prepared in mice against a mouse monoclonal antibody to a melanoma tumor antigen has been used in patients with advanced melanoma. In these early studies, toxicity was not observed and partial responses of increased immunity occurred, including a single dramatic remission. Human antibodies may be more effective.—O. Jonasson, M.D.

Immunization With Haptenized, Autologous Tumor Cells Induces Inflammation of Human Melanoma Metastases
Berd D, Murphy G, Maguire HC Jr, Mastrangelo MJ (Thomas Jefferson Univ; Univ of Pennsylvania)
Cancer Res 51:2731–2734, 1991   9–13

Introduction.—Evidence is accumulating that human cancer cells have tumor-associated antigens. Immunization of patients with cancer against these antigens, however, has proven difficult. Experimental studies suggest that immunization with tumor cells conjugated to helper determinants augments cell-mediated immunity to the tumor-associated antigens. The results of a clinical trial of a hapten-conjugated autologous tumor cell vaccine were reviewed in 24 patients with metastatic, surgically incurable melanoma.

Methods.—The patients were sensitized to dinitrophenyl (DNP) with 1% dinitrofluorobenzene in acetone-corn oil applied topically on 2 consecutive days. Because cyclophosphamide heightens the immune response, a low dose of cyclophosphamide was given 3 days before sensitization; 2 weeks later the patients were given an injection of DNP-conjugated melanoma vaccine after additional pretreatment with cyclophosphamide. Low-dose cyclosphosphamide pretreatment and vaccine injections were repeated every 28 days.

Results.—In 14 patients vaccine treatment induced a striking inflammatory response in superficial metastases. In 10 of these patients, biopsy specimens were obtained from the inflamed tumors and analyzed by immunohistochemistry. Melanoma cells were infiltrated with T lymphocytes, and most of these were CD8+ and HLA-DR+ T lymphocytes. In contrast, biopsy specimens of melanoma metastases obtained before vaccine treatment showed only rare scattered T cells. The remaining 10 patients did not have clinically evident inflammation at tumor sites. Histochemical analysis of specimens from all 7 patients who underwent biopsy showed lymphocytic infiltration of the tumor masses similar to that seen in the first 14 patients.

Conclusion.—Because the inflammatory response occurred in metastatic tumors but not in normal tissue, the T-cell-mediated immune response against melanoma-associated antigens appears to have been facilitated by the helper effect of the antihapten response. Immunization with a haptenized autologous tumor cell vaccine induces T cell infiltration in human melanoma metastases.

▶ Enhancement of melanoma antigenicity was achieved directly in these experiments by mixing the irradiated tumor cells with BCG and conjugation to DNP. When inoculated with this autologous vaccine, cutaneous metastases were clearly the site of a delayed hypersensitivity reaction with CD8+ cells, but they rarely regressed. In work reported by others using "internal image" antibodies as a skin test, the DTH infiltrate was largely composed of CD4+ cells; the significance of these differences is not clear.—O. Jonasson, M.D.

Detection of Melanoma Cells in Peripheral Blood by Means of Reverse Transcriptase and Polymerase Chain Reaction

Smith B, Selby P, Southgate J, Pittman K, Bradley C, Blair GE (St James's Univ Hosp; Univ of Leeds, England)
Lancet 338:1227–1229, 1991 9–14

Objective.—The small numbers of cells from solid tumors that are required for hematogenous metastasis have proved difficult to detect. Reverse transcriptase was used to make complementary (c)DNA from peripheral blood messenger RNA, and the polymerase chain reaction (PCR) technique was used to amplify DNA specific for a gene that is actively transcribed only in tumor tissue.

Methods.—Complementary DNA was prepared from the peripheral blood of 7 patients who had malignant melanoma, 4 who had other metastatic cancers, and 4 healthy subjects. Several melanoma-derived cell lines also were analyzed. The PCR method served to amplify the gene for tyrosinase, which is a tissue-specific gene in melanocytes. Normal melanocytes do not circulate in the peripheral blood. The level of detection was much improved by amplification with nested primers; RNA equivalent to less than 1 cell was detectable.

Observations.—The method proved to be highly sensitive, detecting a single melanoma cell in 2 mL of normal blood. Blood from 4 of 7 patients with melanoma gave positive results (Fig 9–2), whereas all control specimens were negative. Restriction enzyme digestion confirmed that the PCR product was homologous with tyrosinase cDNA.

A B C D E F G H I J K L M N O P Q R S

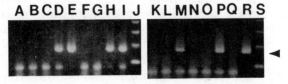

Fig 9–2.—Detection of tyrosinase messenger RNA in blood of patients with cancer. Lanes *D, E, M,* and *P* = positive malignant melanoma patients; lanes *C, F,* and *G* and *N* (same patient) = negative malignant melanoma patients; lanes *A, B, K, L, O,* and *Q* = negative controls (2 healthy subjects and 4 other cancers); lanes *H, I,* and *R* = positive controls (tyrosinase RNA and complementary DNA). (Courtesy of Smith B, Selby P, Southgate J, et al: *Lancet* 338:1227–1229, 1991.)

Implications.—It may be possible using this approach to diagnose primary cancers by demonstrating inappropriate cells in the peripheral blood, precluding the need for more invasive methods. The method might help in assessing the prognosis, as well as in detecting residual disease after treatment.

▶ The technique of PCR is exquisitely sensitive. In these studies, 1 melanoma cell added to 2 mL of normal blood could be detected. Given the data that circulating cancer cells can be found in the bone marrow even in early colon cancer, the technique of PCR may be a useful diagnostic modality and, especially, could pinpoint patients who would likely benefit from additional systemic treatment.—O. Jonasson, M.D.

Expression of HLA-A2 Antigen in Human Melanoma Cell Lines and Its Role in T-Cell Recognition

Pandolfi F, Boyle LA, Trentin L, Kurnick JT, Isselbacher KJ, Gattoni-Celli S (Massachusetts Gen Hosp, Boston; Harvard Med School, Charlestown, Mass)
Cancer Res 51:3164–3170, 1991   9–15

Background.—Previous studies have shown that expression of HLA-A2 antigen by human melanoma plays an important role in tumor cell recognition by autologous T lymphocytes. Many human tumors, especially those of epithelial origin, express greatly reduced levels of HLA-I antigens.

Objective and Methods.—The role of HLA-A2 expression was assessed in the response of cytotoxic T lymphocytes against autologous melanomas. Pairs of tumor-infiltrating lymphocytes and autologous melanoma cell lines were derived from 4 HLA-A2-positive patients with malignant melanoma that had metastasized.

Findings.—All 4 lymphocyte cultures expressed HLA-A2 antigen, but only 2 of the melanoma cell lines did so. The cells from the other 2 patients exhibited neither surface expression of the antigen nor corresponding messenger RNA. The loss of HLA-A2 expression correlated to some degree with the level of c-*myc* transcription. Although tumor-infiltrating lymphocytes obtained from patients whose tumor cell lines expressed HLA-A2 were normally able to lyse autologous melanoma cells, those lymphocytes obtained from other patients had virtually no cytotoxic activity. The ability to lyse tumor cells was not restored by preincubating the melanoma cells with interferon.

Conclusions.—Downregulation of expression of the HLA-A2 antigen by melanoma cells may be one way in which tumor cells escape immunologic recognition by lymphocytes. Transfection studies have indicated that merely restoring HLA-A2 antigen expression may not trigger an effective cytotoxic response.

▶ The most common HLA-A phenotype in Caucasians in North America is HLA-A2. These studies demonstrate that HLA-A2 (or perhaps other HLA-A alleles) function to present the melanoma-associated antigens to cytotoxic T cells. The investigators propose that loss of HLA expression by tumor cells may render these cells invisible to immune surveillance, or, more fundamentally, cause failure of the tumor to generate or attract cytotoxic CD8+ tumor-infiltrating lymphocytes. In a highly sophisticated set of experiments, the ability to express HLA-A2 was reintroduced into melanoma clones that had lost this capability. Only a partial response was obtained and cytotoxicity was not enhanced. Although A2 was clearly most important in initiating the activation and recruitment of appropriate cytotoxic cells, other factors such as major histocompatibility complex determinants, may also play an important role.—O. Jonasson, M.D.

Identification of p53 as a Sequence-Specific DNA-Binding Protein
Kern SE, Kinzler KW, Bruskin A, Jarosz D, Friedman P, Prives C, Vogelstein B (Johns Hopkins Univ)
Science 252:1708–1711, 1991   9–16

Introduction.—The tumor-suppressor gene p53 is the most commonly mutated gene identified in human cancers. Missense mutations occur in numerous human malignancies, including tumors of the colon, lung, breast, ovary, and bladder. However, the biochemical properties of p53 and how mutation affects these properties are unknown. A study was conducted to determine whether p53 binds to specific DNA sequences within the human genome, and whether that ability could be a functional target of p53 mutations.

Methods.—To identify a sequence-specific DNA binding site within the human genome, cloned DNA sequences were screened with an immunoprecipitation technique. Two classes of clones were tested. The first group consisted of 400 clones containing inserts of 300–1,000 basic proteins obtained randomly from the human genome. The second class consisted of cosmid and plasmid clones selected because they contain sequences that might be important in normal growth control. Each clone was digested with a restriction endonuclease, end-labeled with ^{32}P, and incubated with lysates of vaccinia-virus-infected cells that synthesize wild-type p53. Labeled DNA fragments that bound to p53 were then recovered by immunoprecipitation with anti-p53 monoclonal antibodies.

Results.—A DNA sequence in the human genome that binds specifically to wild-type human p53 protein in vitro was identified. As few as 33 base pairs were sufficient to confer specific binding. Proteins encoded by either of 2 missense p53 mutants commonly found in human tumor cells were unable to bind significantly to this sequence.

Conclusion.—The fragments identified will most likely not be the only ones in the human genome with the ability to bind p53. The putative target sequences that mediate the biological actions of p53 in tumor suppression will be identified in future studies. Human p53 protein binds to specific DNA sequences in the human genome, and this binding activity is altered by mutations that occur in human tumors.

▶ How the gene product of p53 acts to suppress tumor formation is unknown. Using sophisticated molecular techniques, these investigators identified a DNA sequence to which p53 protein binds, and fails to bind if mutation has occurred. Further investigations into the nature of the specific DNA sequences will provide insight into the nature of tumorigenesis.—O. Jonasson, M.D.

Direct Sequencing From Touch Preparations of Human Carcinomas: Analysis of p53 Mutations in Breast Carcinomas
Kovach JS, McGovern RM, Cassady JD, Swanson SK, Wold LE, Vogelstein B, Sommer SS (Mayo Clinic and Found, Rochester, Minn; Johns Hopkins Univ)
J Natl Cancer Inst 83:1004–1009, 1991   9–17

Introduction.—Mutations in the p53 gene are commonly found in many cancers. Loss of p53 gene function by mutation or deletion is associated with cell transformation in vitro and with fully developed human cancers. A new method was developed for characterizing mutations in genomic DNA in very small samples of cellularly heterogeneous human cancer tissue. Mutations in the p53 gene in breast carcinomas were used as a model system.

Methods.—Grossly malignant tissue was dissected from 11 breast carcinomas. Touch preparations were prepared by pressing the cut surface of the tissue specimen against the clean surface of standard microscopic slides. The slides were stained in a standard mixture of toluidine blue and methylene blue. Freshly stained, tightly adherent cell clusters of 10-50 malignant cells were transferred with a micropipette into microfuge tubes. The cells then were processed for polymerase chain reaction amplification to increase the amount of target gene sequence sufficiently to permit direct sequencing of the p53 gene.

Results.—The cell clusters in the touch preparations contained only malignant cells, as confirmed by direct microscopic observation and by the absence of normal DNA sequences. The touch preparation technique also worked well for adenocarcinomas from other organs.

Conclusion.—The touch preparation technique is simple, rapid, and selective for carcinoma cells. Standard histochemical stains can be used. The p53 gene amplified is being sequenced from multiple carcinoma cell clusters. Because the touch preparations were made of various portions of primary and metastatic human breast cancers, it is expected that the technique will disclose molecular heterogeneity of p53 mutations within primary and metastatic lesions.

▶ The importance of p53 gene mutations in the genesis of human cancers is being realized through these elegant and extraordinarily sensitive techniques. As an accompanying editorial (1) points out, detection of p53 mutations may be a useful diagnostic tool.—O. Jonasson, M.D.

Reference

1. Cossman J, Schlegel R: *J Natl Cancer Inst* 83:980, 1991.

Her-2/neu and INT2 Proto-Oncogene Amplification in Malignant Breast Tumors in Relation to Reproductive Factors and Exposure to Exogenous Hormones
Olsson H, Borg Å, Fernö M, Ranstam J, Sigurdsson H (Univ Hosp, Lund; Malmö Gen Hosp, Sweden)
J Natl Cancer Inst 83:1483–1487, 1991   9–18

Introduction.—Extended use of oral contraceptives (OCs) at an early age has been associated with an increased risk of premenopausal breast cancer, and tumors developing in these patients have shown a more aggressive behavior. Gene amplification is a major mechanism of proto-oncogene activation in human breast cancer. The Her-2/neu and the INT2 genes are of prognostic importance in breast cancer. Amplification of the Her-2/neu and INT2 genes was correlated with a number of reproductive risk factors for breast cancer.

Methods.—Within 2 months of the primary diagnosis, 72 premenopausal women with primary breast cancer for whom tumor specimens were available were interviewed. Reproductive risk factors analyzed included starting age and duration of OC use, early and late abortion, parity, progestin use, age at diagnosis, and age at first full-term pregnancy. Gene amplification was analyzed by Southern blot and slot blot techniques. The effects of different hormonal and reproductive risk factors on gene amplification were assessed.

Results.—The Her-2/neu gene was amplified in 22 patients (31%) and the INT2 gene was amplified in 8 patients (11%). Amplification of the Her-2/neu gene was more common among early OC users, defined as use starting at or before age 20 years, than among nonusers or late users of OCs. Amplification of INT2 in early and late OC users did not differ significantly. However, the likelihood of INT2 amplification was greater among progestin users and women with a history of early abortion (i.e., before the first full-term pregnancy). There was no significant relationship between gene amplification and parity, age at first full-term pregnancy, or late abortion.

Conclusion.—Among premenopausal women with breast cancer, early OC use is significantly associated with Her-2/neu amplification, whereas early abortion and progestin use is associated with INT2 amplification. Both results are biologically plausible.

▶ In these observations, the connection is drawn between exogenous hor-

mone contraceptive use at an early age, the activation of 2 important oncogenes, and the development of aggressive breast cancers.—O. Jonasson,
M.D.

**Tumor Angiogenesis and Metastasis—Correlation in Invasive Breast
Carcinoma**
Weidner N, Semple JP, Welch WR, Folkman J (Brigham and Women's Hosp;
Children's Hosp, Boston)
N Engl J Med 324:1–8, 1991   9–19

Objective and Methods.—There is considerable experimental evidence
that tumor growth is critically dependent on angiogenesis. Whether the
extent of angiogenesis is correlated with metastases was investigated in
human breast cancers. A group of 49 primary invasive breast cancers was
sampled, and the endothelial cells were stained immunocytochemically
for factor VIII. The microvessels were counted and their density graded.
A total of 30 patients had distant disease.

Findings.—Both the microvessel counts and density grades correlated
with the presence of metastatic disease. Microvessels were more than
tiwce as frequent in patients with metastatic disease. By itself, the density
of microvessels provided the best estimate of the relative risk of metastasis.

Implications.—Counting microvessels in invasive breast cancers may
provide an independent predictor of metastatic disease, either in axillary
nodes or at distant sites. Quantifying tumor angiogenesis may therefore
help in selecting those patients with early breast cancer who should receive aggressive treatment.

▶ Angiogenesis marks the onset of rapid tumor growth and metastatic
spread. In these elegant observations, new vessel growth in breast cancer
specimens was strongly correlated with the overt onset of metastatic disease. The authors suggest that identification of active angiogenesis in breast
cancer specimens may select patients at risk for metastases and, therefore,
those whose adjuvant therapy should be aggressive.—O. Jonasson, M.D.

**Synthetic Analogues of Fumagillin That Inhibit Angiogenesis and
Suppress Tumor Growth**
Ingber D, Fujita T, Kishimoto S, Sudo K, Kanamaru T, Brem H, Folkman J
(Children's Hosp, Brigham and Women's Hosp, Boston; Takeda Chemical In-
dustries Ltd, Osaka, Japan)
Nature 348:555–557, 1990   9–20

Background.—Neovascularization is a critical process in tumor growth and a predominant feature of various angiogenic disorders such as diabetic retinopathy and hemangioma. Studies of capillary endothelial cells in culture have revealed a fungal contaminant that produces local cell rounding, which is possibly an antiproliferative effect. Established angiogenesis inhibitors produce this effect as part of their action in vivo.

Objective.—An attempt was made to isolate the contaminating fungus and characterize its action. The endothelial effects were studied in the growing chick chorioallantoic membrane.

Observations.—The fungus was identified as *Aspergillus fumigatus* fresenius, and its active fraction was identified as fumagillin, an antibiotic used to treat amebiasis. The purified fumagillin totally prevented endothelial cell proliferation in the presence of basic fibroblast growth factor. Fumagillin suppressed angiogenesis in the chorioallantoic membrane model and neovascularization in the mouse dorsal air sac; however, marked weight loss also occurred. The fumagillin analogues were synthesized, producing strong angiogenesis inhibitors with relatively few side effects. One of these analogues, AGM-1470, inhibited the growth of various solid tumors when given systemically to mice; it did not produce weight loss.

Conclusion.—Synthetic angiogenesis inhibitors may prove useful in treating tumors and other angiogenic diseases that require long-term therapy.

▶ In these studies, tumor growth was conclusively slowed when angiogenesis was inhibited. Folkman's group has carried these studies further and demonstrated inhibition of the establishment of hematogenous metastases as well, as reported in the *Surgical Forum* (1). The effect of "angioinhibins" on wound healing must also be investigated, but the prospect of prevention of establishment of new malignant growth is quite intriguing.—O. Jonasson, M.D.

Reference

1.   Brem H, et al: *Surg Forum* 42:439, 1991.

Expression of Blood-Group Antigen A—A Favorable Prognostic Factor in Non-Small-Cell Lung Cancer
Lee JS, Ro JY, Sahin AA, Hong WK, Brown BW, Mountain CF, Hittelman WN (Univ of Texas–MD Anderson Cancer Ctr, Houston)
N Engl J Med 324:1084–1090, 1991   9–21

Background.—Tumor stage is the most important prognostic factor in patients with non–small-cell lung cancer. The prognostic value of altered expression of ABH blood group antigens was studied in tumor cells to find a possible alternative indicator for treatment. The tumor samples were taken from 164 patients who underwent curative surgery for non–small-cell lung cancer between 1980 and 1982.

Methods.—Paraffin-embedded tumor samples that were representative of the primary tumor were used for immunohistochemical assessment. Monoclonal antibodies were used to detect the A and B antigens. The blood group H antigens were detected with *Ulex europaeus* agglutinin I.

Results.—The 28 patients with blood type A or AB who had primary tumors negative for blood group antigen A had a median survival of 15 months; the 3-year and 5-year survival rates were 22% and 15%, respectively. The 43 patients with antigen A-positive tumors had a 71-month median survival rate, with 3-year and 5-year rates of 74% and 59%, respectively. The median survival of the 93 patients with type B or type O blood was 39 months, with 3-year and 5-year survival rates of 51% and 38%, respectively. Disease progressed significantly earlier in those patients with tumors negative for antigen A. The loss of blood group antigen B or H did not correlate with a disadvantage for survival in patients with type B, AB, or O blood. The expression of blood group antigen A in tumor cells added significantly to the prediction of overall survival provided by other known prognostic factors in patients with blood type A or AB.

Discussion.—The expression of blood group antigen A in tumor cells appears to suggest an improved prognosis for patients with non–small-cell lung cancer. The fact that the expression of blood group antigen B or H in tumor cells did not correlate with survival in patients with type B or O blood suggests that simple retention or loss of blood group antigen is not the important variable. The expression of blood group antigen A should be considered in the design of future trials of therapy.

▶ In these studies, a striking correlation was found in expression of A blood group antigen and survival in lung cancer. Although loss of expression of A antigen may be a manifestation of poorly differentiated malignancies, no correlation was found with B or H (blood group O) antigen expression. Loss of blood group A antigens appears to correlate with aggressive tumor behavior, an unexplained phenomenon.—O. Jonasson, M.D.

Tumor Cell Adhesion to Endothelial Cells: Endothelial Leukocyte Adhesion Molecule-1 as an Inducible Adhesive Receptor Specific for Colon Carcinoma Cells
Lauri D, Needham L, Martin-Padura I, Dejana E (Istituto di Ricerche Farmacologiche Mario Negri, Milan; British Biotechnology Ltd, Oxford)
J Natl Cancer Inst 83:1321-1324, 1991   9–22

Background.—Tumor cell adhesion to the vascular endothelium is a key event in the metastatic process. The 2 inflammatory mediators interleukin-1 (IL-1) and tumor necrosis factor (TNF) activate endothelial cells, which strongly increases tumor cell adhesion. Cytokine treatment of endothelial cells in vitro induces cell-surface expression of molecules that augment adhesion. One of these interactions was characterized using a monoclonal antibody specific for endothelial leukocyte adhesion molecule-1 (ELAM-1).

Methods and Findings.—In several tumor cell lines that were tested, ELAM-1 was the major, if not only, mediator of colon carcinoma cell adhesion to activated endothelial cells. Seven colon carcinoma cell lines were sensitive to ELAM-1 antibodies. The time course of ELAM-1 expression paralleled that of the HT29 tumor cell adhesion to activated endothelial cells. The anti-ELAM-1 monoclonal antibody blocked this effect any time after endothelial cell activation by IL-1. The ELAM-1 antibody did not affect adhesion of melanoma, osteosarcoma, or lung, cervix, or kidney carcinoma cell lines to IL-1-treated endothelial cells.

Conclusions.—Apparently, ELAM-1 is selectively recognized by colon carcinoma cells. These findings also suggest that different and specific mechanisms may mediate adhesion of tumor cells to activated endothelial cells.

▶ An initiating event in metastasis is adherence of circulating tumor cells to vascular endothelium, followed by invasion of the vessel wall and angiogenesis. Selection of metastatic sites by specific tumors may be influenced by the presence of adhesion molecules on the endothelium of that organ. In these nice experiments, colon cancer cells were found to adhere to the ELAM-1 molecule of endothelial cells, but other cancer cells did not. The authors speculate that endothelial cells in the liver may express increased levels of ELAM-1 in response to cytokines liberated during inflammation or by the tumor cells themselves, thus promoting tumor cell adhesion and invasion.—O. Jonasson, M.D.

Retardation of Metastatic Tumor Growth After Immunization With Metastasis-Specific Monoclonal Antibodies

Reber S, Matzku S, Günthert U, Ponta H, Herrlich P, Zöller M (German Cancer Research Ctr, Heidelberg; Univ of Karlsruhe; Kernforschungszentrum, Karlsruhe, Germany)
Int J Cancer 46:919–927, 1990   9–23

Introduction.—High doses of monoclonal antibodies (MAbs) may benefit patients with solid tumors. Four mechanisms by which therapeutic efficacy is achieved have been proposed. Antitumor MAbs may function via an antibody-dependent cellular cytotoxicity; they may induce an internal image-type anti-idiotypic response against which the organism again responds by following the idiotypic (ID) cascade; they may function as a site-directed attractor for effector cells and molecules; and they may block receptors at the cell surface that are important for the settlement of metastasizing cells in secondary tissues. A study was undertaken to distinguish among these 4 possibilities.

Methods.—The influence on metastatic spread of 4 murine MAbs directed against surface determinants of a metastasizing rat adenocarcinoma was evaluated and compared to their in vivo binding and to induction of a humoral anti-MAb response. Special attention was given to the development of anti-ID antibodies of the internal image type.

Results.—In a protocol of explicit immunization, all 4 murine MAbs transiently inhibited metastatic growth. Survival was prolonged with only 1 of the 4 MAbs. With another MAb, metastatic growth was actually accelerated after transient retardation. Retardation of metastatic growth correlated with the humoral anti-MAb response.

Interpretation.—The MAb-induced inhibition of metastatic spread may be based on 2 independent mechanisms: blockade of metastasis-associated epitopes and induction of an antimouse immunoglobin (Ig) response. In the latter case, whether the response is isotype-specific or idiotype-specific would be irrelevant.

▶ These complicated experiments were designed to determine the mechanisms by which MAbs retard tumor growth and metastasis. In contrast to the following papers, which attempt to utilize the anti-idiotypic "mirror image" antibodies to enhance host immunity through a more effective means of presenting the tumor antigen, these experiments show that the mirror image antibodies actually enhance metastasis. The mechanism for this effect is proposed to be a blocking of the antigen sites of the tumor that serve as sites for adhesion to endothelium and invasion into tissues. The vagaries of the immune response to tumors and general lack of effect in established tumors remain a challenge.—O. Jonasson, M.D.

Induction of Delayed Hypersensitivity to Human Tumor Cells With a Human Monoclonal Anti-Idiotypic Antibody
Austin EB, Robins RA, Baldwin RW, Durrant LG (Nottingham Univ, England)
J Natl Cancer Inst 83:1245–1248, 1991   9–24

Introduction.—Heterologous anti-idiotypic antibody-induced antitumor antibodies can induce immunity to human cancer. However, after repeated immunization with a foreign antibody, the immune response may become dominated by antibodies to the constant regions of heterologous antibody with no further therapeutic effect. A human monoclonal anti-idiotypic antibody, 105AD7, directed against the anti-tumor antibody 791T/36 was developed. The ability of antibody 105AD7 to induce cellular immune responses to human tumor cells was assessed in experimental animals.

Methods.—The 3 human tumor cell lines used were the osteogenic sarcoma cell line 791T, which expresses high levels of gp72; the bladder carcinoma cell line T24, which expresses low levels of gp72; and the colorectal carcinoma cell line Colo 205, which is negative for gp72. Cell-mediated immunity to tumors induced by the human anti-idiotypic antibody 105AD7 was investigated by induction of a delayed-type hypersensitivity response. Mice or rats were primed by subcutaneous injection of antibody and challenged 5 days later with the different tumor cells.

Results.—Mice primed with the human monoclonal anti-idiotypic antibody 105AD7 mounted a delayed-type hypersensitivity reaction when challenged with gp72 antigen bearing human osteosarcoma cells, but not when challenged with low-level gp72 human bladder cancer cells or gp72-negative colon cancer cells. The difference between the cellular immune responses was highly significant.

Conclusion.—It is probable that the human monoclonal anti-idiotypic antibody 105AD7 can induce cellular immune responses to tumors in patients with cancer. A phase I clinical trial of immunization with 105AD7 in patients with advanced cancer is being designed.

▶ Using a rodent tumor model, delayed hypersensitivity was demonstrated using tumor cells as a challenge after treating the animals bearing the tumor with a specific antitumor monoclonal antibody. In addition, this effect was successfully transferred with peritoneal exudate cells, demonstrating conclusively that internal image (ab2) antibodies generated anti-anti-idiotypic cells (and antibodies) that were reactive to the tumor cells themselves. The use of ab2 as a tumor vaccine to induce active cellular immunity with effector cells against the tumor gains more credence.—O. Jonasson, M.D.

Patients Treated With a Monoclonal Antibody (ab$_1$) to the Colorectal Carcinoma Antigen 17-1A Develop a Cellular Response (DTH) to the "Internal Image of the Antigen" (ab$_2$)

Mellstedt H, Frödin J-E, Biberfeld P, Fagerberg J, Giscombe R, Hernandez A, Masucci G, Li S-L, Steinitz M (Karolinska Hosp, Stockholm)
Int J Cancer 48:344–349, 1991   9–25

Introduction.—The antitumor effector functions of unconjugated mouse monoclonal antibodies (MAbs) used as cancer therapy are not well understood. It has been hypothesized that the infused antibody (ab$_1$) may elicit an antibody response (ab$_2$) against idiotopes on the V region of the heavy and light chains of the ab$_1$. Some ab$_3$s have the same binding specificity as ab$_1$, and these ab$_3$s may have a direct antitumor cell effect. There may also be a T cell response against the idiotopes of ab$_1$ and ab$_2$ in patients treated with MAb. Inducible anti-ab$_2$-reacting T cells may also bind to tumor cells and exert a cytotoxic/cytostatic effect.

Patients.—Human monoclonal ab$_2$s that mimic the tumor-associated antigen (TAA) CO17-1A of colorectal carcinoma (CRC) cells, or the "internal image" of the antigen, were produced and injected intradermally in 12 patients with metastatic CRC who had been treated with MAb 17-1A (ab_1).

Results.—Five of the 12 patients had a specific delayed-type hypersensitivity (DTH) skin reaction, indicating induction of an anti-ab_2 idiotype cellular response after treatment with MAb (ab_1) directed against a TAA. The reaction was most likely a specific response against idiotopes located in the variable region of the ab_2. Untreated patients had no DTH skin reaction. Part of the DTH was presumably mediated by T cells specifically recognizing idiotypic structures on the ab_2 molecules. Activation of specific antigen-sensitized T cells is one of the most characteristic features of this type of DTH. Serum ab_3 was demonstrated in 4 patients who had a DTH reaction and in 4 patients who did not have a skin reaction.

Conclusion.—The treatment of CRC patients with the unconjugated MAb 17-1A induces an idiotypic cascade at both the humoral and the cellular level. Generation of such an idiotypic response may be interpreted as an active antitumor "vaccination" and should be considered in future therapeutic strategies.

▶ The observations in humans with CRC in this paper are in contrast to those reported in Abstract 9–24, in which a rat pancreatic cancer known to metastasize seemed to be protected by certain internal image antibodies. Humans with metastatic colorectal cancer, when treated with an MAb directed against a TAA (ab_1), also developed an immune response to the antigen-binding sites of ab_1 (anti-idiotypic antibodies, ab_2, the "internal image") but then developed antibodies to these antibodies (anti-anti-idiotypic antibodies, ab_3) together with effector cells. These ab_3 cells and antibodies have similar specificity to the original antitumor monoclonal antibody. Demonstration of the presence of effector lymphocytes by a skin test with ab_2 is validation of the hypothesis of a tumor vaccine—immunizing with ab_2 carrying the internal image of the tumor antigen in order to produce antigen-reactive effector cells.—O. Jonasson, M.D.

10 Skin and Subcutaneous Tissue

A Bilayer "Artificial Skin" Capable of Sustained Release of an Antibiotic

Matsuda K, Suzuki S, Isshiki N, Yoshioka K, Okada T, Hyon S-H, Ikada Y
(Kyoto Univ, Japan)
Br J Plast Surg 44:142–146, 1991

10–1

Introduction.—The most frequent complication of a bilayer "artificial skin" is infection beneath it. A mechanism for sustained release of antibiotics was successfully incorporated in a new type of artificial skin.

Material.—The artificial skin has a lower sponge sheet of collagen that is converted spontaneously into new connective tissue. Microspheres of poly-L-lactic acid are used as carriers of tobramycin (M-TOB), an aminoglycoside. Tobramycin was selected because its antibacterial spectrum includes the bacteria commonly found in infections under artificial skin. The collagen sheet containing M-TOB is attached to a silicone layer, creating a combined sheet. The upper silicone sheet has a water vapor permeability comparable to normal skin (Fig 10–1). Sustained release of tobramycin continued for at least 2 weeks in laboratory studies (Fig 10–2).

Results.—The artificial skin with continuously released tobramycin was used to treat 6 patients with burns or nevi. Three weeks after the artificial skin was applied, the silicone layer was peeled off and a thin split-thickness skin graft grafted onto the newly synthesized dermis-like tissue. No local infection occurred in any of the 6 patients. By comparison, artificial skin without antibiotic resulted in infection in 5 of 13 regions in 12 patients.

▶ Synthetic skin substitutes continue to be improved. One problem has been a high rate of infection, especially in excised full-thickness burns. This slow-release antibiotic modification is a major step forward. One can imagine slow-release anti-inflammatory agents or slow-release peptide growth factors being combined with skin substitutes in the future. If this Japanese product can pass FDA standards, possibly trials could begin in the United States to finally allow an "artificial skin" to be clinically available in this century.—M.C. Robson, M.D.

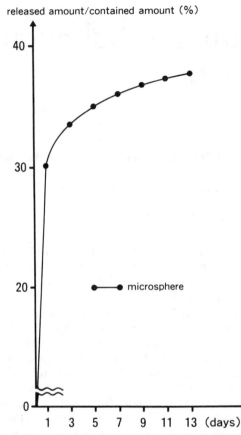

Fig 10–1.—Sustained release of tobramycin into saline from M-TOB continuing until 13th day. (Courtesy of Matsuda K, Suzuki S, Isshiki N, et al: *Br J Plast Surg* 44:142–146, 1991.)

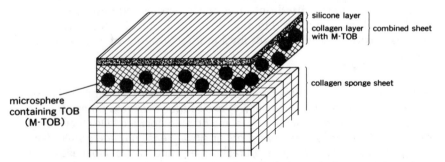

Fig 10–2.—Structure of "artificial skin" capable of sustained release of tobramycin; silicone layer attached to collagen layer as reservoir of M-TOB. (Courtesy of Matsuda K, Suzuki S, Isshiki N, et al: *Br J Plast Surg* 44:142–146, 1991.)

Prognosis After Initial Recurrence of Cutaneous Melanoma
Markowitz JS, Cosimi LA, Carey RW, Kang S, Padyk C, Sober AJ, Cosimi AB
(Massachusetts Gen Hosp, Boston; Harvard Med School)
Arch Surg 126:703–708, 1991   10–2

Introduction.—Malignant melanoma is increasingly common. Approximately 30% to 35% of patients with malignant melanoma will have recurrence, but the clinical course and prognosis of these patients are not well documented. The records of 231 patients with melanoma recurrence after surgical therapy for clinical stage I cutaneous melanoma were reviewed retrospectively.

Management.—Treatment for recurrent disease included aggressive surgical extirpation for all resectable lesions, including visceral recurrences. Patients with unresectable disease received adjuvant systemic chemotherapy/immunotherapy or regional hyperthermic perfusion. Patients with nonresectable brain or other isolated symptomatic metastases received radiation therapy. The mean interval to recurrence was 32 months (range, 1–218 months). The mean follow-up after recurrence was 43 months (range, 1–250 months).

Outcome.—The overall 5-year survival rate was 36%, and the median survival, 2.1 years. Multivariate analysis showed 3 independent risk factors: the anatomical site of initial recurrence, stage of primary disease, and gender. Only 11% of patients whose initial recurrence was in a visceral organ achieved prolonged remission, whereas patients with soft tissue or nodal recurrence had 5-year survival rates of 49% and 38%, respectively. Furthermore, survival rates were better after successful complete eradication of gross disease by surgical excision or intensive chemotherapy, with 25% of patients with visceral recurrence surviving for at least 5 years after aggressive treatment. Men were 1.4 times more likely to die than women, but the difference was of marginal significance. The thickness, anatomical location, and pathologic type of the primary lesion and interval to recurrence were not predictive of outcome.

Discussion.—Given the prolonged remission of cutaneous melanoma in patients with visceral recurrence after aggressive therapy, the philosophy of aggressive surgical excision combined with systemic therapy appears justified in patients with recurrent disease, excluding those with multiple metastases to brain or liver.

Surgical Prophylaxis of Malignant Melanoma
Cohen MH, Cohen BJ, Shotkin JD, Morrison PT (Washington Hosp Ctr Cancer Inst, Washington DC; Mid-Atlantic Pigmented Lesion Clinic, Washington, DC; George Washington Univ)
Ann Surg 213:308–314, 1991   10–3

Introduction.—Prophylactic removal of pigmented skin lesions is of debatable merit in the prevention of malignant melanoma.

Patients.—Among 250 melanoma patients seen in a 4-year period, 75 with a history of localized melanoma and 3 with controlled regional melanoma had multiple skin lesions removed prophylactically. In addition, about 1,000 patients with pigmented lesions and no history of melanoma were seen; 112 of them had lesions removed prophylactically. Nearly one third of these patients had a first-degree relative with melanoma. Typically, up to 3 lesions were removed in an office setting.

Findings.—Abnormalities ranging from hyperplasia to melanoma were found in 28% of the lesions removed from patients with a history of melanoma. Nine patients had unsuspected in situ melanoma, and 3 were found to have invasive melanoma. An estimated 4–6 melanomas were prevented by removing precursor lesions. Hyperplasia, atypia, or dysplasia was found in 22% of the lesions removed from patients with no personal history of melanoma. Three in situ melanomas were found, and an estimated 3–5 further melanomas were prevented. No patient seen during this study had recurrent disease or died of a primary cutaneous melanoma that was not apparent at the time of the initial visit.

Conclusion.—A balance must be struck between routine excision of all pigmented lesions and purely observational management. The benefits of excising selected lesions at an early stage may well outweigh the disadvantages.

▶ These 2 papers (Abstracts 10–2 and 10–3) on malignant melanoma should be read by all surgeons who deal with the disease, but for very different reasons. The first, by Markowitz et al. (Abstract 10–2), is one of the best papers available describing a series of patients treated for recurrence of malignant melanoma. The authors show that aggressive treatment of the recurrence is justified and can result in prolongation of life and palliation. The second paper (Abstract 10–3) purports to justify prophylactic removal of nevi. The paper is flawed in that it does not adequately describe the selection criteria for excision, and the numbers are biased toward support of prophylactic excision because hundreds of patients are excluded from the final analyses. One should read the entire paper carefully before concurring with the conclusions.—M.C. Robson, M.D.

Progress in Flap Surgery: Greater Anatomical Understanding and Increased Sophistication in Application
Lamberty BGH, Cormack GC (Addenbrooke's Hosp, Cambridge, England; Bangour Gen Hosp, Edinburgh)
World J Surg 14:776–785, 1990   10–4

Background.—Local pedicled skin flaps and tube pedicles have been used since the early 20th century, but the greatest advance in the past decade was the discovery of the fasciocutaneous or septocutaneous system of vessels and the flaps based on them. Behan and Wilson described an angiotome as "any area of skin that can be cut as a flap which is supplied by an axial vessel but may be extended via its communication with branches of an adjacent vessel." Pontén first described the use of flaps based on the fasciocutaneous system of vessels in 1981.

Findings.—Below the knee, the fascial plexus is fed by perforators that reach the deep fascia by passing along the intermuscular fascial septa and between the flexor digitorum longus and soleus. Because the greater functional length of vessels in the deep fascia is along the long axis of

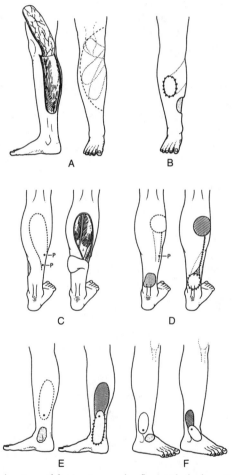

Fig 10–3.—A, general pattern of fasciocutaneous leg flaps with the base containing several vessel branches at the level of the deep fascia. The arc of rotation on the anterior leg is demonstrated. **B,** skin island with subcutaneous pedicle of fat and deep fascia based proximally. **C,** retrograde flap based laterally on a peroneal artery (P) perforator. **D,** retrograde flap pedicled subcutaneously. The perforator is from the peroneal artery (P). **E,** medial island flap based distally and rotated through 180 degrees around its perforator from the posterior tibial artery and accompanying venae comitantes. **F,** lateral island flap based on the terminal branch of the peroneal artery that pierces the interosseous membrane. (Courtesy of Lamberty BGH, Cormack GC: *World J Surg* 14:776-785, 1990.)

the limb, fasciocutaneous flaps with long length-to-breadth ratios can be raised (Fig 10–3). In the lateral thigh, the fasciocutaneous perforators emerge along the lateral intermuscular septum and divide into branches running obliquely anterosuperiorly and anteroinferiorly. Superior, middle, and lower posterolateral thigh flaps can be oriented over the vessels. True fasciocutaneous perforators exist on the trunk where the branches of the circumflex scapular artery emerge from between teres major and teres minor at the lateral border of the scapula.

Conclusions.—Refinement of the flap graft has led to greater reliability and less donor site morbidity. Free flaps have been used successfully in early coverage of upper and lower extremity injuries and in breast and mandibular reconstruction.

▶ Although review articles are seldom chosen for inclusion in the YEAR BOOK by this reviewer, this article is an exception. These authors have done such exemplary work identifying the vascular bases for fasciocutaneous and septocutaneous flaps that a single review of their work complete with references seems useful reading for the anatomist, vascular physiologist, and reconstructive surgeon. The flaps demonstrated in Figure 10–3 are all for defects previously believed to require staged procedures or free tissue transfer with microvascular anastomoses.—M.C. Robson, M.D.

Effects of Sodium Pentobarbital Anesthesia on Blood Flow in Skin, Myocutaneous, and Fasciocutaneous Flaps in Swine

Thomson JG, Kerrigan CL, Abrahamowicz M (Royal Victoria Hosp, Montreal; McGill Univ)
Plast Reconstr Surg 88:269–274, 1991   10–5

Background.—Nitrous oxide and halothane significantly depress cardiac function in several species, including pigs. Sodium pentobarbital has similar effects, but its influence on cutaneous and muscle and blood flow is uncertain.

Methods.—The effects of pentobarbital anesthesia on blood flow were studied in white Landrace pigs using the microsphere technique. Flow was measured in normal skin and at 2-cm intervals along 7 forelimb skin flaps, 7 forelimb fasciocutaneous flaps, 14 arterial buttock flaps, and 14 latissimus dorsi flaps as surgical anesthesia was maintained with sodium pentobarbital.

Findings.—Flow in all flaps was significantly greater during pentobarbital anesthesia than when the animals were awake. At the same time, pentobarbital exerted a cardiac depressant effect. No changes in flow were evident in control skin or control muscle.

Implication.—Further work is needed to find the optimal anesthetic agent for use in studies of acute changes in flap blood flow.

▶ Many drugs affect blood flow in the skin. Among these are various anesthetics. The authors show a previously unreported increase in blood flow of flaps caused by sodium pentobarbital. If these experimental observations made in pigs occur in humans, they could have clinical consequences. A flap raised on a precarious borderline blood supply may appear adequate at the time of surgery, only to appear ischemic when the patient awakes and the effect of the anesthetic wears off.—M.C. Robson, M.D.

The Five-Year Cure Rate Achieved by Cryosurgery for Skin Cancer
Kuflik EG, Gage AA (New Jersey Med School, Newark; State Univ of New York, Buffalo)
J Am Acad Dermatol 24:1002–1004, 1991   10–6

Introduction.—Cryosurgery has been used for more than 20 years to treat nonmelanotic skin cancer. The cure rates in a 20-year span and a more recent 5-year period were examined.

Data Analysis.—From 1971 to 1989, cryosurgical techniques were used to treat 3,540 new skin cancers, with a cure rate of 98.4%. Because some of these patients have been treated too recently for sufficient follow-up, and cryosurgical techniques were just beginning to evolve in the 1970s, a closer look was taken at the 684 nonmelanotic skin cancers treated with cryosurgery between 1980 and 1984.

Results.—Of the 684 new skin cancers, there were 628 basal cell carcinomas, 52 squamous cell carcinomas, and 4 basosquamous cell carcinomas. Basal cell carcinomas had a 5-year cure rate of 99% squamous cell carcinomas, 96.1%, and basosquamous cell carcinomas did not recur at all during the follow-up period. The overall cure rate for the 5-year study was 98.8%.

Conclusions.—The failure rate in this study compares to that reported for other treatment modalities. Others have reported that cryosurgery is the quickest to perform, is cost effective, and yields the best cosmetic results. Further investigation should study case selection and technique and attempt to lower the recurrence rate.

▶ Cryosurgery has often been considered adjunctive or palliative. This large series shows that it is curative for nonmelanotic skin cancers. The cure rate for basal cell carcinomas is the same as for other modalities, e.g., excision or radiation. The follow-up of the series is good. It would be nice to have an evaluation of esthetic results, because cryotherapy has not always been associated with esthetically acceptable scarring.—M.C. Robson, M.D.

Use of the Carbon Dioxide in Treating Multiple Cutaneous Neurofibromas
Becker DW Jr (Twin Falls Clinic and Hosp, Idaho)
Ann Plast Surg 26:582–586, 1991   10–7

Introduction.—There are reports that the carbon dioxide laser is helpful in removing cutaneous neurofibromas in the office using local anesthesia. This modality may be able to destroy neurofibromas rapidly with minimal blood loss and postoperative discomfort. General anesthesia may be preferred because of the unpleasant smoke smell consequent to the treatment of a large number of lesions.

Technique.—If a pedunculated lesion is present, 10–15 W are applied to the stalk at the base, cauterizing the base at the same time the growth is excised. Sessile tumors are vaporized above the skin using a slightly defocused beam at 35–60 W. Subcutaneous lesions are treated with a focused beam to open the skin before vaporizing the bulk of the tumor under direct vision. Sutures are avoided except when a large skin defect remains. Antibiotic ointment is applied after treatment.

Conclusion.—Pending a cure for neurofibromatosis, the carbon dioxide laser is useful for minimizing the cutaneous deformity associated with this disorder.

▶ This technique using the CO_2 laser to remove hundreds of neurofibromas at a single sitting would appear simple, efficient, and time saving.—M.C. Robson, M.D.

The Value of Micrographic Surgery for the Management of Eyelid Tumours
Downes RN, Collin JRO, Walker NPJ (Princess Mary's RAF Hosp, Aylesburg, Bucks, England; Moorfields Eye Hosp, London; St Thomas' Hosp, London)
Orbit 9:223–229, 1990   10–8

Introduction.—At no site more than the periocular tissues are basal cell epitheliomas more dangerous. The goal of surgery is to eradicate disease while preserving as much healthy tissue as is possible. The fresh tissue technique of micrographic surgery, an adaptation of the fixed tissue technique described by Mohs, was developed for these situations.

Patients.—Forty-one patients treated since late 1987 were followed prospectively after undergoing micrographic surgery for periocular basal cell epithelioma of the eyelid. One patient had 2 separate tumors that were treated by micrographic surgery. The average age of the 25 women and 16 men was 63 years. Twenty-three tumors were primary and 19 were recurrent basal cell epitheliomas. Nine patients previously had conventional surgery without frozen-section control.

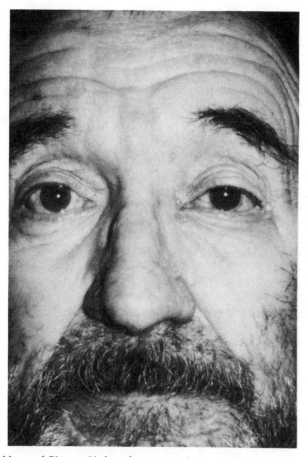

Fig 10–4.—Man aged 70 years 90 days after micrographic surgery for eyelid tumor. (Courtesy of Downes RN, Collin JRO, Walker NPJ: *Orbit* 9:223–229, 1990.)

Outcome.—About half of the tumors extended beyond a 4-mm margin. A significant part of the lacrimal apparatus was preserved in 14 of 20 patients, and a significant portion of the posterior lamella of the eyelid was preserved in 6 of 10 patients. In 1 man the lacrimal apparatus was preserved without epiphora (Fig 10–4). No recurrences were noted during an average follow-up of 17 months; all patients were followed for at least 6 months. Two procedures ended prematurely because of patient intolerance, and 2 were terminated for logistic reasons.

Discussion.—Micrographic surgery represents a considerable advance over conventional surgical management or radiation therapy. It is, however, expensive and time consuming, and it may be arduous for the patient. The results to date have been encouraging. Micrographic surgery may be the best approach to medial canthal and extensive or poorly defined upper lid tumors, as well as recurrent periocular basal cell epitheliomas.

▶ An indication for micrographic surgery with which most surgeons can agree is the basal cell carcinoma of periocular tissue origin. This series of 41 patients demonstrates its utility in such patients. One might argue with the authors that some of the primary smaller lesions might have been controlled just as well with excision, but the recurrent lesions and those involving deeper structures seem to be well treated by the described technique.—M.C. Robson, M.D.

The Effects of Ultraviolet Radiation on Wound Healing
Davidson SF, Brantley SK, Das SK (Univ of Mississippi)
Br J Plast Surg 44:210–214, 1991   10–9

Introduction.—Despite increasing concern over ultraviolet (UV)-induced skin cancer, many persons still expose themselves to high doses of solar radiation and to artificial UV radiation (Fig 10–5). A hairless guinea pig model was used to determine the changes in skin structure and wound tensile strength consequent to exposure to UVA and UVB radiation.

Methods.—Guinea pigs were irradiated with UVA (80 J/cm²) or UVB (.46 J/cm²) on alternate days for 16 weeks. After treatment a dorsal wound was made in each animal and allowed to heal; it was mechanically tested to failure at 3 weeks. Serial punch biopsy specimens were acquired at 2- to 4-week intervals.

Findings.—Wound tensile strength was significantly lower in irradiated than in control animals. Both UVA and UVB radiation compromised wound strength. Irradiation produced "sunburn" cells, swollen vascular endothelial cells, and perivascular hemorrhage in the papillary dermis.

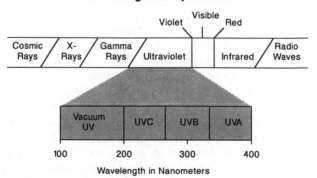

Fig 10–5.—Divisions of the electromagnetic spectrum. (Courtesy of Davidson SF, Brantley SK, Das SK: *Br J Plast Surg* 44:210–214, 1991.)

Ultraviolet B radiation led to focal eosinophilic infiltration. Dermal collagen and the elastic fibers were unaltered.

Implications.—Ultraviolet radiation impairs the reparative capacity of the skin through mechanisms that remain to be clarified. The changes caused by environmental levels of UVA radiation suggest that tanning beds be avoided and sunscreens that protect against UVA radiation be used.

▶ The message from this article is twofold. It describes the pathologic changes of skin secondary to UVA and UVB light, and also shows a decrease in the tensile strength of healing incisions in UV light-injured skin. Ultraviolet radiation obviously causes much greater skin injury than the more commonly recognized UV-induced skin cancer.—M.C. Robson, M.D.

11 The Breast

Prognostic Factors in Cystosarcoma Phyllodes: A Clinicopathologic Study of 77 Patients

Cohn-Cedermark G, Rutqvist LE, Rosendahl I, Silfverswärd C (Karolinska Hosp, Stockholm)

Cancer 68:2017–2022, 1991   11–1

Objective.—Cystosarcoma phyllodes (CSP) is an infrequent fibroepithelial breast tumor making up fewer than 1% of all breast tumors. Seventy-seven cases of CSP recorded since 1958 in the Swedish Cancer Registery were studied. The patients (median age, 50 years) were followed for a median of 8 years.

Findings.—By the last follow-up, 21% of the patients had died of CSP, 23% had died without evidence of disease, and 56% were alive without evident disease. Fifteen patients (20%) had locally recurrent disease and 21% had distant metastases, all within 5 years of primary surgery. Local recurrence was less frequent after simple or radical mastectomy than after local tumor excision. All local recurrences were excised radically. Atypical mitoses and degree of stromal cellularity were not significant prognostic factors. On multivariate analysis, prominent stromal overgrowth was associated with the outcome but not significantly.

▶ The prognostic factors related to cystosarcoma phyllodes have been difficult to define. In this series the incidence of distance metastases was quite high. Palmer et al. (1) reviewed 31 patients with this rare tumor. Metastatic lesions developed in 4. Local recurrence occurred in 6 women; no patients younger than 30 years had a recurrence. The authors indicated that neither the histologic appearance nor the size of the tumor could predict clinical behavior. In general, wide surgical excision rather than mastectomy should suffice; nodal dissection appears necessary only when the axillary nodes are clinically suspicious.—S.I. Schwartz, M.D.

Reference

1. Palmer ML, et al: *Surg Gynecol Obstet* 170:193, 1990.

Biopsy of the Breast for Mammographically Detected Lesions

Franceschi D, Crowe J, Zollinger R, Duchesneau R, Shenk R, Stefanek G, Shuck JM (Case Western Reserve Univ)

Surg Gynecol Obstet 171:449–455, 1990   11–2

Introduction.—Mammography is used increasingly to screen asymptomatic women and, as a result, many patients with impalpable breast lesions undergo biopsy. A prospective study was made of 718 women (mean age, 57 years) who had biopsy. In all, 825 mammographically suspicious breast lesions were biopsied. Patients with a benign outcome were younger than those with malignancy. More than half of the biopsies were done solely because of the presence of a mass lesion and more than a third because of calcifications alone.

Findings.—Malignancy was unrelated to the Wolfe mammographic pattern. Mammography became more accurate as the degree of suspicion of malignancy increased. One fourth of all lesions were malignant. When a mass was associated with calcifications, about a third of lesions were in fact malignant. Malignancy correlated with a linear or branching pattern of calcifications, small calcifications, and more than 15 calcifications. A stellate configuration was highly suggestive of malignancy. Invasion was much more frequent in patients with mass lesions than when suspicious calcifications were present.

Conclusions.—Because screening mammography is not sufficiently specific, an aggressive approach is warranted when a suspicious mass and/or calcification is observed. Few clinical characteristics reliably identify those patients who are most likely to have early breast cancer.

▶ This article focuses on an issue of increasing concern to surgeons. The corollary of the office findings, namely, that 25% of the specimens taken at biopsy contained carcinoma, is that 75% of the biopsies were carried out for known malignant lesions. Eddy et al. (1) pointed out that the present practice of encouraging all women to have mammograms and treating suspicious lesions by needle localization and open biopsy is not cost effective. There is evidence that breast cancer screening, using both mammography and physical examination, reduces the mortality from breast cancer in women older than 50 years of age. This effect has not been demonstrated for younger women. Meyer et al. (2) reported that in a 1-year period, 53 patients scheduled for biopsy at their hospital had the procedure cancelled on the scheduled day because the radiologists designated to do the localization found that the breast abnormalities did not warrant biopsy. At this point, the problem of too many biopsies being performed remains rampant.—S.I. Schwartz, M.D.

References

1.   Eddy DM, et al: *Ann Intern Med* 111:389, 1989.
1.   Meyer JE, et al: *Radiology* 169:629, 1989.

Complications Associated With Needle Localization Biopsy of the Breast
Rappaport W, Thompson S, Wong R, Leong S, Villar H (Univ of Arizona)
Surg Gynecol Obstet 172:303–306, 1991   11–3

Introduction.—Needle-directed breast biopsy is increasingly being used for histologic assessment of the breast, but little attention has been given to complications of this method. Data were reviewed on 144 consecutive needle localization biopsies of the breast performed from December 1985 through June 1989.

Complications.—Twenty-seven patients had a total of 34 complications, including 11 wound infections. The use of drains may have been a factor in wound infection. Seven patients had an electrocautery burn that required local wound care, and 4 of them later had wound infection. In 4 instances the breast lesion was not removed at the initial attempt. When methylene blue was used, only 1 of 53 patients required more than 1 biopsy. Four patients had cardiovascular complications that required overnight admission to the hospital.

Recommendations.—Wound infection after needle localization biopsy of the breast can be limited by the cautious use of electrocautery and by avoiding the use of drains. Postexcision mammograms appear to be necessary because of occasional failure to remove the lesion.

▶ The article is selected to bring into focus the fact that the procedure is associated with complications and, therefore, efforts should be made to refine radiographic techniques and interpretations so that the incidence of negative biopsies is reduced. It is difficult to accept the statement that the infection rate could be lessened by cautious use of electrocautery, although it would be hard to refute the fact that gentle handling of wounds and avoiding drains are appropriate.—S.I. Schwartz, M.D.

Breast Cancer in Women Under 35 Years of Age
Schmidt RT, Tsangaris TN, Cheek JH (Baylor Univ Med Ctr, Dallas)
Am J Surg 162:197–201, 1991   11–4

Background.—Only a small percentage of breast cancers occur in women younger than 35 years of age. No clear conclusions have been reached as to the natural history of disease in these patients. A 25-year review was made of women younger than 35 years with breast cancer, including the clinical and pathologic characteristics and how they affect survival.

Patients.—Of 1,995 breast cancer patients seen in a private practice from 1960 to 1987, 206 were younger than 35 years, a rate of 11.3%. The average age was 31.3 years, and the youngest patient was 19 years old. Sixty-four percent of patients had upper outer quadrant lesions, and

93% had infiltrating duct carcinomas. Lymph nodes were negative in 60%. Of those with positive nodes, about half had 4 or more. Treatment was radical mastectomy in 45%, modified radical mastectomy in 40%, and a breast-conserving procedure in 10%. Fifty percent of the patients were followed for at least 5 years.

Outcome.—On restaging, 32% of the patients had stage I and 55% had stage II disease. The overall 5-year survival was 72% and the 10-year survival, 54%. There were 26 pregnant or postpartum patients, 27% of whom had stage I and 42% of whom had stage II disease. Their 5-year and 10-year survival rates were 67% and 57%, being worse for those with stage II disease. Twenty-three stage II node-positive patients received chemotherapy and 41 did not; the 5-year survival rate was 69% for those who had chemotherapy and 68% for those who did not. Ten-year survivals were 33% and 23%. Overall, 68 patients died of the disease.

Conclusions.—These young women have many of the same tumor types, locations, sizes, and nodal involvement found in older patients. Those with stage I or II disease and negative axillary lymph nodes had survival rates comparable to those of older patients, but young women with stage II disease and positive nodes appear to have decreased survival compared to older patients.

▶ The data fail to support the role of aggressive chemotherapy in premenopausal patients with carcinoma of the breast. Improved survival after adjuvant chemotherapy has not been noted for patients with stage II, node-positive disease. The authors' findings are substantiated by Rosen et al. (1), who could not demonstrate a survival advantage for young patients who received adjuvant chemotherapy. The reported survival of node-negative young patients is comparable to that previously reported by Memorial Hospital for node-negative older patients (2).—S.I. Schwartz, M.D.

References

1. Rosen PP, et al: *Ann Surg* 199:133, 1984.
2. Schottenfeld D, et al: *Cancer* 38:1001, 1976.

Paget's Disease of the Nipple
Dixon AR, Galea MH, Ellis IO, Elston CW, Blamey RW (City Hosp, Nottingham, England)
Br J Surg 78:722–723, 1991   11–5

Introduction.—In 1874, James Paget first recognized the relationship between chronic eczema of the nipple and underlying impalpable breast carcinoma. The mechanism of the large, clear intraepidermal Paget cell is thought to be derived from an underlying breast carcinoma with migration upward to the epidermis along the mammary ducts. To determine the optimal surgical approach to this malignancy, data were reviewed on 48 patients with Paget's disease without palpable lumps.

Methods.—The 48 women (median age, 62 years) had nipple eczema containing Paget cells but without a palpable lump. The history was usually unilateral nipple discharge, crusting, bleeding, or erythema. All patients underwent nipple biopsy followed by simple mastectomy; node biopsy was done in 37 patients. Conservative surgery (excision of the nipple-areola complex and a cone of underlying breast tissue) was performed in 10 patients; 1 patient was treated with tamoxifen alone.

Results.—Ductal carcinoma in situ (DCIS) was found in 96% of the operative specimens, with associated invasion in 8 patients. The DCIS was predominantly large cell solid/comedo in type and was multifocal in 7 patients. Of the 10 patients treated with cone excision, local recurrence developed in 4 within a median follow-up of 56 months; 2 of these patients also had metastases. Of the 37 patients who underwent mastectomy, 2 who had invasive foci at their first operation experienced locoregional recurrences but remained disease free at 8 years.

Conclusion.—Mammography was not reliable in the diagnosis of Paget's disease. Of 34 patients with histologic evidence of an underlying carcinoma, 11 had a normal mammogram. Conservative surgery led to a 40% recurrence rate. The high rate of invasive components found and the extensive DCIS of mastectomy specimens support the use of simple mastectomy for Paget's disease of the nipple.

▶ The authors' caveat that improvement or temporary healing of nipple eczema does not preclude a nipple biopsy is in order for all patients. It is now generally accepted that Paget's disease constitutes 1% of all breast carcinomas and is a primary carcinoma of the mammary ducts of the nipple. Robbins and Berg's study (1) of 89 cases indicated that a third of the patients had noninfiltrating carcinoma and, in this group, the survival rate was 100% after 5 years. It is hard to argue against simple mastectomy in the face of the 40% recurrence rate following conservative therapy.—Seymour I. Schwartz, M.D.

Reference

1. Robbins GF, Berg J: *World J Surg* 1:284, 1977.

Long-Term Results of a Combined Modality Approach in Treating Inflammatory Carcinoma of the Breast
Elias EG, Vachon DA, Didolkar MS, Aisner J (Univ of Maryland)
Am J Surg 162:231–235, 1991   11–6

Background.—Inflammatory carcinoma of the breast accounts for up to 4% of all primary cancers. If untreated, it will ulcerate and fungate through the skin, often within a few weeks. Treatment with mastectomy alone yields a 5-year survival rate of 2.4%; radiation improves local control, but the 5-year survival rate remains less than 5%. Twenty-eight patients with inflammatory breast carcinoma were managed initially by induction chemotherapy.

Patients and Treatments.—Median age was 50 years, and all 28 patients had erythema and edema of the entire breast. All had palpable breast masses with enlarged axillary lymph nodes; 17 had no distant metastases and 11 had overt metastases. Median estrogen and progesterone receptor values were 0 fmol/mg protein. All of the women had the same initial treatment in the single-arm, nonrandomized study: 3 courses of combination cyclophosphamide, doxorubicin hydrochloride, and 5-fluorouracil. Responders were given the same regimen postoperatively. Nonresponders were given radical radiation therapy followed by combination chemotherapy with cyclophosphamide, methotrexate, 5-fluorouracil, vincristine sulfate, and prednisone. If chemotheraphy failed during follow-up, radiation and/or combined mitomycin-C and vinblastine were given as necessary.

Results.—Twenty-two patients had a local-regional response to initial chemotherapy, including 16 of those without distant metastases and 6 with overt metastases. For the most part, breast masses and axillary lymph nodes decreased by less than 50%. There was significant hematologic toxicity, with white blood cell counts up to 3,900/mm³. Doxorubicin caused nausea and vomiting, and all patients had alopecia. Twenty-one of the responders underwent mastectomy. There was no residual tumor in 2 of the surgical specimens, and all had residual metastases in the axillary lymph nodes. Of the patients without distant metastases, the median disease-free survival was 30 months and the median survival overall was 32 months. The 5-year survival rate was 18%. In patients with distant metastases, the maximum overall survival was 14 months.

Conclusions.—In some patients with stage III inflammatory carcinoma of the breast, initial systemic chemotherapy, followed by local-regional cytoreductive and systemic therapy, might have some survival benefit. More effective chemotherapy is needed to control distant metastases and, potentially, to aid in local and regional control. Chemotherapy must be continued in patients with residual, recurrent, or metastatic disease.

Results of Radical Radiotherapy for Inflammatory Breast Cancer

Lamb CC, Eberlein TJ, Parker LM, Silver B, Harris JR (Harvard Med School; Brigham and Women's Hosp; Dana-Farber Cancer Inst, Boston)
Am J Surg 162:236–252, 1991   11–7

Background.—Published reports disagree as to the efficacy of radiotherapy in the clinical syndrome of inflammatory breast cancer. Mastectomy appears to be important in the local treatment of these patients.

Sixty-five patients with nonmetastatic clinical inflammatory breast carcinoma were treated with radical radiotherapy as the sole local treatment, focusing on factors that might predict local failure.

Methods.—The patients were treated during an 18½-year period. The median age was 49 years, and 31 patients were postmenopausal. Eighteen patients, most of them treated in the first 6 years of the series, received radiotherapy alone. Forty-seven had chemotherapy in addition to radiotherapy. Total dose (median, 6,984 cGy) was influenced by the size of the tumor. In survivors, the median follow-up was 41 months.

Results.—There was a 17%, 5-year actuarial probability of relapse-free survival and an overall survival of 28%. There were 30 treatment failures in breast, skin, or draining lymph nodes; this yielded a crude, uncensored local recurrence rate of 46%. The only factor that predicted local recurrence was the response to initial chemotherapy—none of the 3 patients who achieved a complete response had local recurrence, compared to 12 of 17 patients with less than a partial response.

Conclusions.—Even at high doses, conventional radial radiotherapy is insufficient for local tumor treatment in unselected patients with inflammatory breast cancer. The best treatment at this time appears to be combined chemotherapy, surgery, and radiotherapy. The prognosis remains poor, and further investigation is needed.

▶ These 2 articles (Abstract 11–6 and 11–7) emphasize the continued poor survival rate associated with inflammatory carcinoma of the breast. Inflammatory breast cancer remains a distinct clinical entity with an ominous course. Donegan et al. (1) also reported a 5-year survival rate of 20%. If mastectomy was included in the treatment, the 5-year survival was 28% compared with 23%. There is little question that chemotherapy should be initiated before local therapy, as evidenced by a 5-year survival rate of 40% of the former group compared to 0% for the few patients who received local therapy first. The role of mastectomy in achieving local control merits further investigation.—S.I. Schwartz, M.D.

Reference

1. Donegan WL, et al: *Arch Surg* 125:578, 1990.

Mastectomy Following Preoperative Chemotherapy: Strict Operative Criteria Control Operative Morbidity
Broadwater JR, Edwards MJ, Kuglen C, Hortobagyi GN, Ames FC, Balch CM (Univ of Texas MD Anderson Cancer Ctr, Houston)
Ann Surg 213:126–129, 1991   11–8

Introduction.—Overall response rates to preoperative chemotherapy in patients with locally advanced primary breast cancer have exceeded

90%, with most patients undergoing mastectomy subsequently. An experience with preoperative chemotherapy was reviewed to learn whether this treatment adversely affects postoperative recovery and to determine whether a delay in beginning postoperative chemotherapy affects survival.

Patients.—The records of 106 patients with T3, T4, and/or N2, N3 breast cancer were reviewed. These patients received preoperative chemotherapy followed by total mastectomy with axillary dissection, postoperative chemotherapy, and external beam radiation. They were compared with 91 patients who had mastectomy alone for the end points of wound infection, wound necrosis, seroma, and delay in resuming postoperative chemotherapy. The surgery was timed according to strict operative criteria.

Findings.—Wound infection rates were 7% in the group having chemotherapy and 4% in the mastectomy-only group, and the incidence of wound necrosis was 11% and 6%, respectively. These differences were not significant. However, the chemotherapy group had a 15% rate of seroma formation, compared with 28% in the mastectomy-only group. Thirty percent of patients given chemotherapy had delayed postoperative chemotherapy, compared with 20% in the mastectomy-only group. This difference was not significant, but patients whose postoperative chemotherapy was delayed more than 30 days had a significant decrease in overall survival (Fig 11–1).

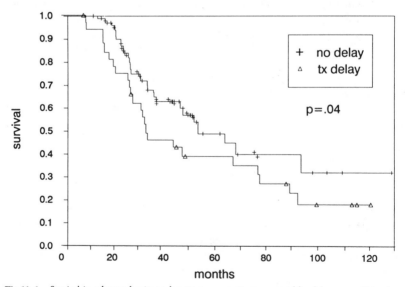

Fig 11–1.—Survival in advanced primary breast cancer patients grouped by delay vs. no delay in resuming systemic therapy after mastectomy. (Courtesy of Broadwater JR, Edwards MJ, Kuglen C, et al: *Ann Surg* 213:126–129, 1991.)

Conclusions.—Intensive preoperative chemotherapy and mastectomy can be given to patients with advanced breast cancer without causing increased morbidity. Postoperative chemotherapy should be given within 30 days to maximize survival. Mastectomy can be done without increasing surgical complication rates by the use of strict operative criteria.

▶ The use of preoperative chemotherapy in patients with advanced primary breast cancer and inflammatory cancer of the breast represents an advance. The fact that intensive preoperative chemotherapy, followed by mastectomy, can be performed without an increase in morbidity is an important one. A small series suggests that the combination of chemotherapy, radiation therapy, and mastectomy may augment the cure rate of inflammatory breast cancer (1).—S.I. Schwartz, M.D.

Reference

1. Knight CD, et al: *Surgery* 99:385, 1986.

Breast Reconstruction: Progress in the Past Decade
Elliott LF, Hartrampf CR Jr (Atlanta Plastic Surgery PA, Atlanta, Ga)
World J Surg 14:763–775, 1990   11–9

Background.—There have been significant improvements in the results of breast reconstruction in women who have undergone mastectomy. Breast reconstruction does not interfere with extirpative surgery, nor does it delay any necessary postoperative adjuvant therapy. Increasing numbers of women therefore are electing immediate as opposed to delayed breast reconstruction.

Methods.—The most radical change in reconstructive procedures in the past decade has been the use of autogenous tissue. The first such technique introduced was the transverse rectus abdominis myocutaneous (TRAM) flap, which quickly became the leading technique of autogenous tissue breast reconstruction (Fig 11–2). Although they require the use of microsurgical techniques, the lateral transverse thigh flap (LTTF) and the buttock flap are important alternatives for patients who elect autogenous tissue breast reconstruction. Introduction of tissue expanders has been a major technological advance. Tissue expanders reduce the risk of overlying skin necrosis and implant extrusion, and allow some degree of ptosis if necessary. There have also been significant improvements in the area of nipple-areola reconstruction. Use of the tissues of the breast mound itself avoids the transfer of grafts from distant sites, which do not usually maintain their size and projection.

Conclusions.—Of the recent advances in breast reconstruction, the use of autogenous tissue grafting, tissue expanders, and improvements in nipple-areola reconstruction are the most important.

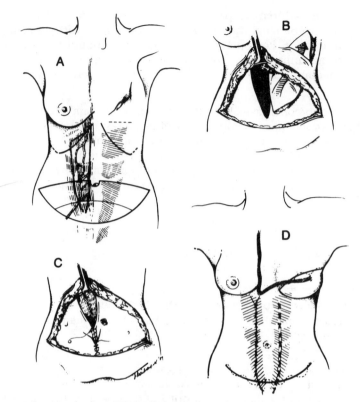

Fig 11–2.—Drawing of unilateral TRAM flap operation. **A,** depiction of preoperative planning of the flap on the lower abdomen. Superior epigastric vasculature depicted within the right rectus muscle for left breast reconstruction. **B,** flap being passed behind upper abdominal skin to left chest. **C,** direct closure of abdominal wall defect. **D,** postoperative result showing direct closure of right abdominal wall with plication of left anterior rectus sheath for abdominal wall balance. (Courtesy of Elliott LF, Hartrampf CR Jr: *World J Surg* 14:763–775, 1990.)

▶ The article is a summary of the favored procedures of breast reconstruction. It provides the general surgeon with a complete overview of the applicability, techniques, and consequences of the various flap procedures and the improvements related to implants. The issue of breast reconstruction, either immediate or delayed, will likely increase in importance in the ensuing years.—S.I. Schwartz, M.D.

12 The Head and Neck

Development of a New In Vivo Model for Head and Neck Cancer
Dinesman A, Haughey B, Gates GA, Aufdemorte T, Von Hoff DD (Albuquerque, NM; Washington Univ; Univ of Texas, San Antonio)
Otolaryngol Head Neck Surg 103:766–774, 1990   12–1

Background.—None of the xenograft models for studying human carcinomas in vivo are adequate for long-term studies because of size contraints and eventual transplant rejection. A model for head and neck carcinoma that exhibits significant local invasion and metastatic activity should be valuable in the study of human tumor kinetics and immunobiology; it may allow more meaningful studies of the effectiveness of antineoplastic treatment methods. Such a model was developed using nude mice.

Methods.—Tumor cells from the Hep-2 or HLaC-79 laryngeal squamous cell carcinoma cell lines were injected into the floor of the mouth in 42 nude mice. The critical volume was .07 cc, which contained 5.25 × 10⁶ cells; given more than this volume, animals died by a mechanism similar to that of Ludwig's angina. The animals were killed and examined microscopically when the tumor burden became large enough to cause severe cachexia.

Results.—In the group given Hep-2 cells, the average tumor size was 10.34 mm² and the mean growth period was 48 days. All animals had soft tissue invasion, 94% had bony invasion, 82% had angioinvasion, and 65% had neural invasion. The average HLaC-79 tumor size was 11.17 mm², and the average time until killing was 58 days. Soft tissue invasion occurred in 96%, bone invasion in 80%, neural invasion in 76%, angioinvasion in 92%, and pulmonary metastases in 44%.

Conclusions.—A new, metastasizing model of head and neck carcinoma shows not only the locally invasive properties of malignant neoplasms but also parallels the results of studies of the percent of end-stage and autopsy patients with pulmonary metastases. The rarity of regional neck node metastasis (in 2 of 42 mice) is a major deviation from the behavior of the tumors in human beings.

▶ Athymic and athymic/asplenic mice or rats have proved to be outstanding models in the study of explanted human tissue (both normal and diseased). This model of human laryngeal carcinoma should be no different. It should provide an excellent opportunity to examine tumor biology and therapeutic interventions.—M.C. Robson, M.D.

Incisional or Excisional Neck-Node Biopsy Before Definitive Radiotherapy, Alone or Followed by Neck Dissection

Ellis ER, Mendenhall WM, Rao RV, McCarty PJ, Parsons JT, Stringer SP, Cassisi NJ, Million RR (Univ of Florida)
Head Neck 13:177–183, 1991   12–2

Introduction. —Open diagnostic cervical node biopsy before definitive resection of squamous cell carcinoma of the head and neck is controversial because surgical violation of diseased nodes may enhance tumor dissemination. However, no adverse effect of open neck-node biopsy has been reported for patients who undergo radiation therapy, either alone or combined with resection. Whether surgical violation of the neck compromises the results of subsequent definitive radiation therapy, either alone or followed by resection, was investigated.

Patients. —During a 21-year period, 508 patients were treated for head and neck squamous cell carcinoma and clinically positive neck nodes in 660 heminecks; 457 were treated with radiation therapy alone and 203 received radiation therapy followed by neck dissection. Sixty-six patients had incisional or excisional biopsy of a positive neck node before the start of radiation therapy. All patients were observed for at least 2 years or until death. The prognostic factors analyzed included biopsy status of the neck, node stage, treatment, node mobility and location, tumor stage, primary site, and control of disease above the clavicles.

Findings. —Overall comparison of the Kaplan-Meier hemineck control curves for the biopsy and non-biopsy groups did not show a statistically significant difference between the groups for any of the 4 neck stages. In 3 of the 4 node stages the results actually favored those who underwent neck biopsy before treatment.

Conclusion. —The data do not support a potential adverse effect from violating the neck before definitive treatment in patients with head and neck squamous cell carcinoma and positive neck nodes who undergo radiation therapy as the next step of treatment.

▶ These data are useful for proving that node biopsy is not harmful to the patient who will be treated definitively with radiation therapy. However, the data beg the question somewhat. The biopsy may be performed to determine the need for radiation therapy or before an informed consent for radiation therapy has been obtained. In such a case, the positive biopsy may lead to wound implantation, if resection turns out to be the only modality.—M.C. Robson, M.D.

Characterization, Quantification, and Potential Clinical Value of the Epidermal Growth Factor in Head and Neck Squamous Cell Carcinomas

Santini J, Formento J-L, Francoual M, Milano G, Schneider M, Dassonville O,

Demard F (Centre Antoine-Lacassagne, Nice, France)
Head Neck 13:132–139, 1991

12–3

Objective.—Epidermal growth factor (EGF) promotes the growth of several epithelial tissues and possesses potent mitogenic activity that is mediated by its cell surface receptor (EGFR). An attempt was made to characterize EGFR and quantify it in biopsy specimens from 70 patients with head and neck tumors.

Methods.—A miniaturized competition technique employing radiolabeled ligand was used to evaluate functional EGFR. Four tumor samples and 1 control sample served to characterize the EGF findings.

Findings.—A single family of high-affinity binding sites was identified. Similar EGF-binding characteristics were found when comparing tumor tissue with nontumoral tissues. Levels of EGFR were higher in tumor tissue than in controls in 59 of 60 instances, and the EGFR level correlated significantly with tumor size and stage. Tumors containing more than 100 fmol of EGFR per milligram of protein were more likely to respond completely to chemotherapy than were EGFR-negative tumors.

Implications.—Epidermal growth factor receptor may prove to be a useful biological marker for head and neck cancer. It is possible that high EGFR levels secondary to stimulation by EGF and transforming growth factors - α confer proliferative activity on tumor cells, making them more sensitive to cytotoxic drug treatment.

▶ This paper evaluates the possible effect of growth factor receptor levels on tumor cell biology. If the data demonstrated for this small number of tumors hold when applied to a great many tumors, it may prove to be useful marker in head and neck cancers, most of which are of epidermal origin.—M.C. Robson, M.D.

Functional Results After Total or Near Total Glossectomy With Laryngeal Preservation
Weber RS, Ohlms L, Bowman J, Jacob R, Goepfert H (Univ of Texas MD Anderson Cancer Ctr, Houston)
Arch Otolaryngol Head Neck Surg 117:512–515, 1991

12–4

Background.—Because treatment of advanced carcinoma of the tongue often involves total glossectomy together with laryngectomy, the functional outcome may be poor. Laryngeal preservation in patients requiring total or near-total glossectomy was reviewed, along with the effectiveness of this approach in controlling the cancer and allowing speech and deglutition rehabilitation.

Patients.—Between 1982 and 1989, 27 of 39 patients undergoing total or near-total glossectomy were able to have the larynx preserved. Twelve of these patients had laryngeal suspension to elevate the larynx and improve deglutition. A palatal augmentation prosthesis, designed to improve deglutition and speech quality, was prepared for 18 patients.

Results.—At a median follow-up of 18 months, speech rehabilitation was judged to be good in 7 patients, fair in 14, poor in 4, and unintelligible in 1. The quality of speech was not assessed in the remaining patient. Deglutition was accomplished after surgery in 18 patients. The remaining 9 patients were either fed by a nasogastric tube or required a gastrostomy. Nearly half of the patients (48%) experienced locoregional failures. The 2-year survival in 24 patients eligible for 2-year follow-up was 51%. Although no patient undergoing total or near-total glossectomy for salvage was a long-term survivor, 65% of the previously untreated patients were alive in 18 months.

Conclusion.—In selected patients with advanced tongue cancer, total glossectomy with laryngeal preservation may be a successful procedure. Postoperative videofluoroscopic studies aid in rehabilitation by providing information regarding aspiration and deglutition.

▶ The dogma that laryngectomy is required when total or near-total glossectomy is performed has always escaped this reviewer. For the past 20 years, I have preserved the larynx whenever possible. The bulk of the reconstructive tissue is key. With the advent of musculocutaneous flaps and composite free flaps, necessary bulk is easily attainable. Therefore, it was refreshing to review this paper, which demonstrates laryngeal preservation in 27 of 39 patients undergoing total or near-total glossectomy.—M.C. Robson, M.D.

A Modified Neoglottis Procedure: Update and Analysis
Brandenburg JH, Cragle SP, Rammage LA (Univ of Wisconsin)
Otolaryngol Head Neck Surg 104:175–181, 1991   12–5

Rationale.—More than 12,000 persons will have a diagnosis of laryngeal cancer this year in the United States, and half of them will undergo laryngectomy. Optimal rehabilitation of the voice can promote reentry into a productive and satisfying life, whereas failure to achieve adequate speech may condemn a patient to an isolated dependent state.

Objective.—A rigid neoglottis, used in a preliminary series to construct an epithelium-lined tract from the upper tracheal rings, was constructed in 22 additional patients requiring surgery for T_3 or T_4 squamous cell cancer of the larynx.

Results.—All but 2 patients were initially able to produce a voice, and 76% of the group were still using the neoglottis an average of 52 months after surgery or when they died. Fourteen of 19 neoglottic voices were rated excellent or good and 5, fair. In 2 patients stenosis of the neoglottis developed after postoperative irradiation. Three fourths of the patients required revision of the neoglottis for symptomatic aspiration; the average number of revisions was 1.7. Four patients had regionally persistent or recurrent tumor and 3 had local recurrences. Complications of surgery included 2 hypopharyngeal/cutaneous fistulas and 3 wound infections.

Conclusions.—The rigid neoglottis is created relatively easily and combines adequate tumor control with good speech intelligibility. The procedure should be considered in all patients who require total laryngectomy for glottic cancer.

▶ Many attempts at neoglottis construction have been reported. Most have not stood the test of time and are associated with long-term problems. The neoglottis described by Brandenberg in 1980(1) has now been used in 22 additional patients. All 34 patients were reviewed and the series spans 12 years. It appears that this neoglottis is excellent, allowing 32 of 34 patients to speak initially and 76% to continue to use it for an average of 52 months.

Reference

1. Brandenberg JA: *Arch Otolaryngol* 106:688, 1980.

Analysis of the Morbidity Associated With Immediate Microvascular Reconstruction in Head and Neck Cancer Patients

Schusterman MA, Horndeski G (Univ of Texas MD Anderson Cancer Ctr, Houston)
Head Neck 13:51–55, 1991   12–6

Objective.—Free tissue transfers are frequently used for reconstructive procedures in patients with head and neck cancer, but some surgeons continue to be concerned about the added time needed to perform free flap reconstruction. In an attempt to determine whether morbidity actually is increased by the added time, 20 consecutively treated patients undergoing immediate microvascular free flap reconstruction after tumor excision were compared with 20 others treated by primary closure, skin grafting, or a pedicle flap procedure.

Observations.—Postoperative medical events were comparably frequent in the 2 surgical groups. Surgical complications also were similar. Hospitalization averaged 13½ days for controls and 16 days for those having free flap reconstruction, not a significant difference; surgery lasted significantly longer, however, in the latter patients (11 vs. 7 hours).

Conclusion.—A longer operating time should not in itself determine whether immediate microvascular flap reconstruction is undertaken after excision of head and neck cancer.

▶ This kind of analysis of results is important to prove the efficacy of free flap reconstruction. Advantages such as pliability, lack of tethering pedicles, and earlier mobilization have previously been shown. In this reviewer's hand, time has not been increased with free flap reconstruction when a 2-team approach is used routinely.—M.C. Robson, M.D.

Oromandibular Reconstruction Using Microvascular Composite Free Flaps: Report of 71 Cases and a New Classification Scheme for Bony, Soft-Tissue, and Neurologic Defects

Urken ML, Weinberg H, Vickery C, Buchbinder D, Lawson W, Biller HF (Mount Sinai Med Ctr, New York)
Arch Otolaryngol Head Neck Surg 117:733–744, 1991   12–7

Background.—Restoring normal oral function after ablative surgery or trauma relies on various factors, including the reconstruction of complex osseous, dental, and soft tissue anatomy. A variety of classification schemes have been proposed for segmental mandibular defects. A series of patients underwent reconstruction using microvascular composite free flaps. A new classification scheme was proposed for bony, soft tissue, and neurologic defects.

Methods.—Seventy-one patients underwent oromandibular reconstruction. The new classification system was applied in the description of each case.

Results.—The overall flap success rate was 94%. Most (97%) of the patients had mandibular reconstruction with free vascularized bone flaps. Implant-borne dental prostheses were used to rehabilitate 15 patients. Sixteen patients had primary repair of discontinuity defects of the inferior-alveolar nerve using a variety of nerve grafts.

Conclusions.—Vascularized composite free flaps can clearly be transferred to the oral cavity with a high degree of consistency and an acceptable complication rate. Primary oromandibular reconstruction is now so refined that it can be offered to virtually any patient who must undergo ablative surgery for oral carcinoma, but for optimum success, an interdisciplinary team should guide the patient's rehabilitation.

▶ Classifications are usually helpful in categorizing procedures, results, or complications. The one presented by the authors serves little purpose. Knowing the exact amount of tissue needed for reconstruction does not aid significantly in choice of donor site or gaining informed consent. Possibly, it will aid in communication among professionals when discussing patients. Despite this reviewer's failure to see the purpose of the classification, the paper does present a significant series of composite free flaps for ormandibular reconstruction. The authors are beginning to use nerve grafts to restore sensation to the lower lip to decrease postoperative drooling. To date, this has not resulted in hyperesthesia to the lip and painful neuroma formation, but the reinnervation procedures are few, with shorter follow-up than the rest of the procedures.—M.C. Robson, M.D.

Anterior Ischemic Optic Neuropathy Causing Blindness in the Head and Neck Surgery Patient

Wilson JF, Freeman SB, Breene DP (Naval Hosp, Portsmouth, Va)
Arch Otolaryngol Head Neck Surg 117:1304–1306, 1991   12–8

Introduction.—Anterior ischemic optic neuropathy (AION) is characterized by painless, sudden loss of vision that rarely is reversible. A patient had classic AION as a complication of head and neck surgery.

Case Report.—Man, 48, had hypertension and a T_2, N_1, M_0 epiglottic squamous cell carcinoma. He refused surgery and received external-beam irradiation totaling 64 Gy to the primary site and both sides of the neck. Residual disease progressed rapidly, making total laryngectomy and left radical dissection necessary. A year later the patient underwent total glossectomy and dissection of the right side of the neck for recurrent tumor, but complete resection was not possible. Nearly 4 liters of blood were lost during the 13-hour operation. Significant facial and eyelid edema was noted, and the patient was unable to see on awakening 6 hours postoperatively. The optic nerves were pale and edematous, and the retinal vessels were patent. Complete blindness persisted despite aggressive treatment that included bilateral canthotomies and inferior cantholyses. Follow-up funduscopy affirmed bilateral optic disk atrophy. The patient died of recurrent cancer 9 months after surgery.

Discussion.—The patient's markedly edematous lids and conjunctivas filled the bubbles of the eye protectors that adhered to the orbital rim, possibly transmitting pressure to the globe and raising the intraocular pressure. Treatment should be directed toward lowering the intraocular pressure, if necessary by canthotomy and cantholysis.

▶ This case is of importance to head and neck surgeons. Staging neck dissections has been thought to decrease the risk of the devastating complication of blindness. Possibly, the radiation given previously to both sides of the neck decreased collateral vessel formation. Aggressive therapy appeared to be of little help in this case.—M.C. Robson, M.D.

Fibrosarcoma of the Head and Neck: The UCLA Experience

Mark RJ, Sercarz JA, Tran L, Selch M, Calcaterra TC (Univ of California, Los Angeles)
Arch Otolaryngol Head Neck Surg 117:396–401, 1991   12–9

Background.—Because there have been few reports of the prognostic factors and optimal management for the rare lesion of fibrosarcoma, a series of 29 patients with fibrosarcoma of the head and neck was reviewed.

Methods.—Between 1955 and 1987, 15 men and 14 women (median age, 35 years) were evaluated; 9 of the patients were children. The series

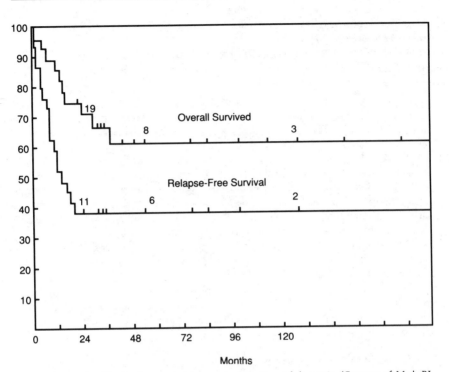

Fig 12–1.—Life-table showing survival in months from time of diagnosis. (Courtesy of Mark RJ, Sercarz JA, Tran L, et al: *Arch Otolaryngol Head Neck Surg* 117:396–401, 1991.)

excluded patients with fibrous tumors distinguishable from fibrosarcoma. The treatment was individualized according to tumor size, location, extent of disease, and histologic grade. There were 17 low-grade and 11 high-grade lesions. Grade was not assigned in 1 patient. The median follow-up was 66 months.

Results.—The absolute 5-year survival was 62%. Of the 17 patients who initially had surgery alone, local control and long-term survival were achieved in 5 low-grade lesions. Postoperative radiation was given in 5 cases because of positive surgical margins. Three of these patients, all of whom had low-grade lesions, achieved a disease-free state. Four of the 6 patients who had primary radiation therapy received additional chemotherapy; 2 of the 6 were disease free after more than 5 years. Surgery with and without adjuvant therapy salvaged 5 of the 12 patients with local recurrence. Only 8% of patients with high-grade lesions were ultimately rendered disease free, compared with 80% of those with low-grade lesions. Of the patients with local recurrence, 72% were known to have positive surgical margins, and 68% had high-grade lesions and/or a tumor larger than 5 cm. The median survival time was 152 months (Fig 12–1).

Conclusions.—The most important prognostic feature in patients with fibrosarcomas of the head and neck is tumor grade, followed by tumor size and status of the surgical margins. Surgery alone appears to be beneficial for patients with low-grade lesions and adequate surgical margins. Adjuvant treatment is needed for those with high-grade lesions or positive surgical margins.

▶ In describing one of the largest series of head and neck fibrosarcomas, this paper demonstrates several useful points. The first is that grading is useful prognostically, and that low-grade lesions do well, even when this initial resection is inadequate. It also demonstrates a better response to radiation therapy than is generally accepted for this lesion.—M.C. Robson, M.D.

Patient-Controlled Analgesia (PCA) in Head and Neck Surgery
Cannon CR (Jackson, Miss)
Otolaryngol Head Neck Surg 103:748–751, 1990   12–10

Background.—The management of pain, whether from trauma, surgery, or medical illness, is a complicated issue. In the hospital setting, conservative nursing practices may prevent a patient's ready access to analgesics ordered by the physician. The value of a patient-controlled analgesia (PCA) infusion device was assessed in patients who had undergone head and neck surgery.

Technique.—The Abbott Patient-Controlled Infuser allows the patient to deliver a predetermined narcotic analgesic by pressing a button attached to the infuser. The infuser is then "locked out" for an interval of time before another dose can be delivered. Patients selected for PCA should be of a suitable age, mentally alert, and without a history of allergic reaction to narcotics or drug addition. Pregnant or nursing women are also ineligible.

Results.—The records of 75 consecutive patients who had undergone head and neck procedures were reviewed. Only 2 complications were associated with PCA; 1 patient had a rash caused by morphine, and another—a terminal cancer patient treated at home—became obtunded. There were no reports of excessive nausea or vomiting, narcotic withdrawal symptoms, or equipment malfunction.

Conclusion.—Significant pain is associated with head and neck surgery. A small intravenous bolus of opioid analgesic provides more pain relief at lower dosages than intramuscular administration of the drug. The good results of the PCA system and its acceptance by patients and nursing staff recommended its use for pain relief.

▶ Patient-controlled analgesia has been used successfully whenever it has been tried. Despite this, it has not caught on very widely in the United States, compared to other countries, e.g., Australia. This series of patients whose pain was adequately controlled without increased complications would suggest that PCA be more likely used for head and neck surgery patients.—M.C. Robson, M.D.

13 The Thorax

"Directed" Emergency Room Thoracotomy: A Prognostic Prerequisite
for Survival
Ivatury RR, Kazigo J, Rohman M, Gaudino J, Simon R, Stahl WM (New York
Med College, Lincoln Med & Mental Health Ctr, Bronx)
J Trauma 31:1076–1082, 1991   13–1

Background.—The literature shows that emergency department resuscitative thoracotomy (ERT), although providing a modest survival in a small group of moribund patients, is futile in most. Patient selection for this procedure is therefore important to maximize cost effectiveness. Experience with ERT was evaluated in an attempt to define appropriate patient selection.

Methods.—The results of ERT in 163 patients were analyzed. Forty-nine patients had stab wounds; 85, gun shot wounds; and 29, blunt trauma. One patient had been shot with a shotgun. Revised Trauma Scores (RTSs) ranged from 0 to 3 in 138 patients, 4 to 8 in 21 patients, and more than 8 in 4.

Outcomes.—None of the 29 patients who sustained blunt trauma survived. Twelve patients with stab wounds and 4 with gun shot wounds were discharged eventually, for an overall survival of 9.8%. Eight survivors had not vital signs on arrival at the emergency department; 1 had signs of life only at the scene of injury. The best survival was achieved when the site of penetration was thoracic and ERT was directed at potential cardiac injury. Sixty-six percent of these patients had cardiac wounds with tamponade, and 21.4% survived. Of the remaining 28 patients, only 2 were salvaged. Both had pulmonary injury. The survival rate was significantly lower in patients with head and neck, abdominal, or multiple site injuries when ERT was not directed. Two of the 5 patients with vascular injuries of an extremity survived after ERT successfully restored cardiac rhythm.

Conclusions.—In patients with no vital signs, ERT directed at potential cardiac injury based on thoracic penetration is an important prerequisite for patient survival. The procedure was not beneficial in victims of blunt trauma in this series. The role of ERT in patients with penetrating abdominal injuries remains uncertain.

▶ Experiences with ERT in 163 patients are described in this report. None of the 29 patients with blunt trauma survived. Survival rates were 25% after a stab wound and 5% after a gunshot wound. The best survival occurred with cardiac injuries (56 patients), especially when resuscitation was directed primarily toward the potential cardiac injury. The authors concluded that ERT is not indicated in blunt trauma.—F.C. Spencer, M.D.

Reappraisal of Emergency Room Thoracotomy in a Changing Environment
Esposito TJ, Jurkovich GJ, Rice CL, Maier RV, Copass MK, Ashbaugh DG (Harborview Med Ctr, Seattle)
J Trauma 31:881–887, 1991   13–2

Background.—The benefit of resuscitative emergency room thoracotomy (ERT) has been questioned, especially in victims of blunt trauma. The wide use of this technique may not be cost effective, and for medical personnel the risk of exposure and lethal infection during ERT is great. The policy of performing ERT on all moribund patients with penetrating torso injuries and all those with blunt injuries with any evidence of cardiac electrical activity was assessed by analyzing patient charts over a 4-year period. Of 112 patients undergoing ERT, 24 had penetrating injuries and 88 had blunt injuries.

Outcomes.—The overall survival was 1.8%. Patients with penetrating injuries had a 4.2% survival rate, and those with blunt injuries had a 1.1% survival rate. There were no survivors among patients who had cardiopulmonary resuscitation (CPR) started at the scene and required it throughout transport. Patients with blood pressure and spontaneous respirations in the field had had a survival rate of 11.8%. Those with sinus rhythm or ventricular fibrillation on emergency department arrival had a 6.4% survival. There were no survivors among the patients arriving at the hospital with an idioventricular rhythm or asystole. Total hospital charges for patients having ERT were $59,565 more than reimbursement. Hepatitis and HIV screening could be documented in only 2 patients, both of whom had negative tests.

Conclusions.—This liberal policy for performing ERT had dismal results, incurring monetary losses and increasing the risk of exposure to lethal infection in hospital personnel. Resuscitative ERT is warranted only when vital signs or resuscitatible cardiac rhythm exists in the field or emergency department and deteriorates shortly before the procedure. Such a policy would maximize survival while reducing inappropriate expenditures and risks.

▶ This important paper describes experiences with 112 emergency room thoracotomies performed in a period of 4 years. Eighty-eight patients (79%) had a blunt injury, with a survival of only 1.1%. No patient who required CPR during transport survived. If a patient had a detectable blood pressure and spontaneous respiration before arrival, survival was about 12%, whereas among those who had either fibrillation or sinus rhythm on arrival, it was only 6%. Idioventricular rhythm or asystole was uniformly fatal. These data strongly indicate that ERT should not be performed unless vital signs are clearly present near the time of arrival in the emergency room.—F.C. Spencer, M.D.

Early Tracheostomy for Primary Airway Management in the Surgical Critical Care Setting

Rodriguez JL, Steinberg SM, Luchetti FA, Gibbons KJ, Taheri PA, Flint LM (State Univ of New York, Buffalo; Univ of Michigan; Tulane Univ)
Br J Surg 77:1406–1410, 1990   13–3

Background.—Tracheostomy is one of the most common operations in the critical care unit, yet there are few data on the effect of its timing on the duration of mechanical ventilation or duration of stay. A 1-year prospective study was done to compare results in multiple-injury patients who had early and late tracheostomy.

Methods.—Of the 264 patients with multiple injuries who required mechanical ventilation, 46% were disengaged from the ventilator and 14% died. This left 106 patients for analysis. On an alternate-day basis, 51 patients were randomized to receive tracheostomy within 7 days of admission, and 55 received tracheostomy for 8 or more days after admission. Admission factors, operative procedures, ventilatory needs, and outcomes, were analyzed to define the effect of early tracheostomy. Morbidity and mortality also were analyzed.

Results.—The group having early tracheostomy had a significantly shorter duration of mechanical ventilation. They also had a lower incidence of pneumonia and required fewer days of ventilation after the diagnosis of pneumonia. Early tracheostomy was also associated with shorter stays in the intensive care unit and hospital. Tracheostomy caused no deaths, and the overall rate of morbidity was 4%.

Conclusions.—The overall risk with early tracheostomy is equivalent to that with endotracheal intubation. Early tracheostomy appears to shorten the duration of ventilation use as well as intensive care unit and hospital stays. Early tracheostomy should probably be considered for all intensive care patients likely to need more than 7 days of ventilation.

▶ This important study randomized 106 intubated patients receiving ventilatory support after multiple injuries. Fifty-one had tracheostomy between 1 and 7 days, and 55 had a tracheostomy at a late date. Early tracheostomy had an overall morbidity of only 4% identical to prolonged intubation. However, the frequency of pneumonia, duration of mechanical ventilation, and duration of stay in the intensive care unit were shorter. Pneumonia was especially decreased if tracheostomy was performed within 48 hours.

The authors emphasize that the 1989 Consensus Conference regarding early tracheostomy reached their recommendations on outmoded data that are not relevant to current practice. Clearly, a well-performed tracheostomy permits better evacuation of pulmonary secretions. An additional advantage of fiberoptic bronchoscopy is its increasing use to facilitate removal of tenacious secretions if suction is ineffective. Let's hope that this paper will generate more frequent performance of tracheostomy rather than reliance on long periods of intubation for fallacious reasons.—F.C. Spencer, M.D.

Infant Tracheotomy: Endoscopy and Decannulation
Benjamin B, Curley JWA (Royal Alexandra Hosp for Children, Sydney, Australia)
Int J Pediatr Otorhinolaryngol 20:113–121, 1990   13–4

Introduction.—The indications for tracheotomy in young children have changed in recent years, partially because of the survival of premature infants of low birth weight. It has been suggested, however, that some infants may become physiologically and psychologically dependent on the tracheotomy.

Methods.—The records of 73 children aged 24 months or younger who had undergone a tracheotomy during a 10-year period were reviewed retrospectively. Nineteen infants were premature. Laryngoscopy and bronchoscopy were performed before tracheotomy in all children. Indications for tracheotomy were diverse. The first tube change and a follow-up endoscopic examination were conducted under general anesthesia 7–10 days after the initial procedure. The decannulation procedure was performed when the patient had a clear airway after treatment of granulations or suprastomal collapse at the tracheotomy site. It usually occurred within 24–48 hours after endoscopy and under general anesthesia.

Results.—Of the 73 children, 49 underwent decannulation—38 within 12 months and 11 after 12 months; 15 patients continued with their tracheotomy. Six infants died soon after the tracheotomy procedure of unrelated causes, and 3 others were lost to follow-up. Suprastoma collapse from a flap of anterior tracheal wall cartilage located above the stoma was observed in 10 patients at endoscopy. Five of these patients were treated with a nasotracheal tube for internal support of the flap or by placement of a suture during endoscopy. The initial attempt at decannulation was not successful in 15 children but was so on the second procedure in 14. Nine children experienced complications.

Conclusions.—Unexplained dependence on the tracheotomy did not occur in this patient population. Tracheotomy remains a safe procedure for both the short and long term in children in this age group. Decannulation should be based on clinical readiness and endoscopic assessment.

▶ This report from Sydney contains a large amount of valuable data that substantiate the safety of tracheotomy in infants. Seventy-three infants undergoing tracheotomy in a 10-year period were reviewed. Endoscopic evaluation of the airway before decannulation showed granulations or suprastomal collapse of the anterior trachael wall to be the most common problems hampering decannulation. Once the primary airway problem was corrected, the tracheostomy was removed satisfactorily in all of the children, clearly refuting the myth that a tracheostomy in an infant may be "permanent" for the first year of life.—F.C. Spencer, M.D.

The Effect of Muscle-Sparing Versus Standard Posterolateral Thoracotomy on Pulmonary Function, Muscle Strength, and Postoperative Pain
Hazelrigg SR, Landreneau RJ, Boley TM, Priesmeyer M, Schmaltz RA, Nawarawong W, Johnson JA, Walls JT, Curtis JJ (Univ of Missouri)
J Thorac Cardiovasc Surg 101:394–401, 1991   13–5

Introduction.—The standard posterolateral thoracotomy produces significant pain and, as a result, can compromise pulmonary function.

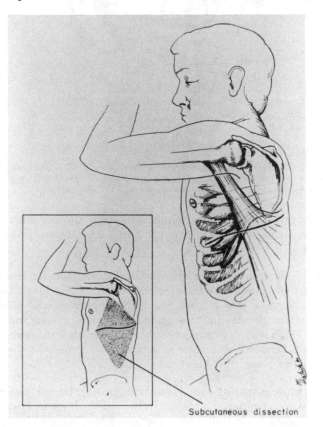

Subcutaneous dissection

Fig 13–1.—The *stippled area of the inset* represents the generous subcutaneous dissection that allowed adequate mobilization of the latissimus dorsi and serratus anterior musculature. (Courtesy of Hazelrigg SR, Landreneau RJ, Boley TM, et al: *J Thorac Cardiovasc Surg* 101:394–401, 1991.)

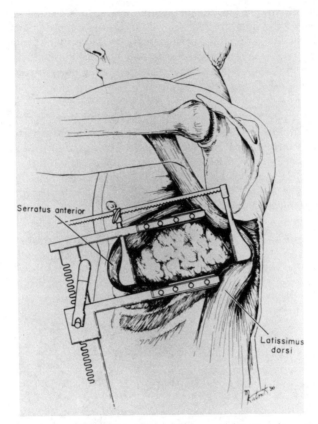

Fig 13–2.—After the chest had been entered, one rib retractor was positioned to retract the ribs and a second retractor separated the serratus anterior and latissimus dorsi muscles. (Courtesy of Hazelrigg GR, Landreneau RJ, Boley TM, et al: *J Thorac Cardiovasc Surg* 101:394–401, 1991.)

Several surgeons now advocate muscle-sparing thoracotomy to limit postoperative pain, preserve lung function, and lessen postoperative complications.

Technique.—The entire anterior border of the latissimus dorsi is freed from its superior aspect in the axilla toward its inferior insertion (Fig 13–1). The border of the serratus anterior than is freed, and the intercostal muscles incised using retractors to retract the ribs and to separate the serratus anterior and latissimus dorsi muscles (Fig 13–2). A 1-cm segment of the lower rib at the intercostal incision is resected. Pericostal absorbable sutures are used around the ribs. Two soft closed suction drains are left in the subcutaneous space.

Results.—Muscle-sparing and standard posterolateral thoracotomy techniques were compared prospectively in 50 patients. Postoperative pulmonary function and shoulder motion were comparable in the 2 groups, as was the extent of lung resection. Patients had significantly less pain after the muscle-sparing procedure and required less narcotics. Shoulder girdle strength was better preserved with the muscle-sparing technique, but muscle strength did not differ after 1 month. Seromas developed only in those patients having muscle-sparing surgery.

Conclusion.—The muscle-sparing thoracotomy technique provides adequate exposure and limits postoperative pain. Seroma formation is its chief disadvantage.

▶ This prospective, randomized study of 50 patients undergoing thoracotomy compared standard posterolateral thoracotomy with the muscle-sparing technique. There was no difference in postoperative pulmonary function, shoulder range of motion, mortality, or hospital stay. There was less pain after the muscle-sparing procedure, although there was a 23% frequency of seromas. Shoulder girdle strength was decreased at 1 week in the standard incision group but was at preoperative levels at 1 month. Hence the month-sparing incision is a reasonable alternative, even though it does not result in any dramatic significant long-term difference.—F.C. Spencer, MD

Thoracoplasty: Current Application to the Infected Pleural Space
Horrigan TP, Snow NJ (Case Western Reserve Univ; Cleveland Metropolitan Gen Hosp)
Ann Thorac Surg 50:695–699, 1990   13–6

Introduction.—Thoracoplasty was performed in 13 patients in 1976–1989. These patients represented about one fifth of all patients treated for pleural space infection complicated by unexpandable or absent lung tissue during this period. There were postresection spaces in 8 patients, usually after lobectomy or removal of giant apical bullae; 5 others had apical empyema without previous lung resection.

Technique.—The 1-stage procedure begins with subperiosteal rib resection to expose the thickened pleural membrane. The empyema cavity is entered and the intercostal muscles, neurovascular bundles, and the empyema cavity wall resected. Electrocautery is used liberally. The first rib is consistently resected. Bronchopleural fistulas are occluded with small slips of viable muscle, sutured into the openings with fine silk. Adjacent muscle is sutured to the apical lung tissue over the fistula repair.

Results.—In 2 patients, revision was required because of inadequate space obliteration. A patient with extensive atypical tubercular infection of the residual lung required tracheostomy and prolonged ventilatory support. The infectious process was eventually controlled in all patients, and there were no late recurrences.

Conclusions.—Thoracoplasty remains a useful means of treating the infected pleural space in selected patients. All of the present patients have some degree of scoliosis, but this has not been severe or caused symptoms. The cosmetic results have been acceptable. Severe deformity is avoided by limiting rib removal below the third rib to the more posterior aspect of the chest.

▶ This paper describes excellent results in 13 patients undergoing thoracoplasty in a period of 13 years. Eight had previous pulmonary resections. Eleven of the 13 had bronchopleural fistulas. A type of Schede thoracoplasty was done, excising the wall of the empyema cavity with resection of both ribs and intercostal muscles. The first rib was resected routinely, as were the transverse processes. Muscle was then brought into the wound and used to meticulously close any fistulous openings. All patients survived with cures of both their infection and bronchopleural fistulas. No repeat operations were required.

All patients had some scoliosis afterward, but in none was it severe. Hence the cosmetic defect was accepted for the curative procedure.

With increasing demonstration of the efficacy of muscle flaps, thoracoplasy is seldom necessary. Both the Mayo Clinic and the Emory Clinic, in recent publications, state that they seldom, if ever, use thoracoplasy. However, the problem of bronchopleural fistula is clearly not solved. The fact that the thoracoplasty in these 13 patients was 100% percent effective is a significant one to consider in deciding on the appropriate course of therapy.—F.C. Spencer, M.D.

The Role of Extrapleural Pneumonectomy in Malignant Pleural Mesothelioma: A Lung Cancer Study Group Trial
Rusch VW, Piantadosi S, Holmes EC (Mem Sloan-Kettering Cancer Ctr, New York; Johns Hopkins Oncology Ctr, Univ of California, Los Angeles)
J Thorac Cardiovasc Surg 102:1–9, 1991   13–7

Background.—Malignant pleural mesothelioma is usually fatal. The mainstay of treatment has been surgery because chemotherapy and radiation are relatively ineffective. The choice of surgery is still debated. Some have advocated extrapleural pneumonectomy, because it allows complete gross tumor removal and has been associated with long-term survival. This procedure was evaluated in a prospective multi-institutional trial.

Methods.—Between 1985 and 1988 a total of 83 eligible patients were enrolled. All had biopsy-proved, previously untreated malignant pleural mesothelioma. Criteria for extrapleural pneumonectomy were unilateral disease that was potentially completely resectable according to the CT scan, a predicted postresection forced expiratory volume in 1 second of more than 1 L, and the absence of other major medical problems. Those who were not candidates for the procedure underwent more limited surgery with or without adjuvant treatment, or they were treated nonsurgically.

Outcomes.—Only 20 patients (24%) underwent extrapleural pneumonectomy; 3 died after surgery. Recurrence-free survival was significantly longer for those undergoing extrapleural pneumonectomy than for those in the other 2 groups. However, overall survival in the 3 groups did not differ significantly. According to univariate analyses, epithelial as opposed to sarcomatoid and mixed histologic findings, and platelet counts of less than 400,000, predicted a better overall survival. Performance status of less than 80 on the Karnofsky scale predicted recurrence. Extrapleural pneumonectomy was associated with a higher chance of relapse in distant sites than were the other 2 treatment strategies.

Conclusions.—Only a small percentage of patients with malignant pleural mesothelioma are candidates for extrapleural pneumonectomy. This procedure is associated with significant surgical mortality and apparently does not improve overall survival. It does alter patterns of relpase. In a multivariate analysis, neither histologic findings, sex, age, extrapleural pneumonectomy, weight loss, nor performance status had a significant impact on survival.

▶ This extensive multi-institutional study clearly demonstrates the limited value of extrapleural pneumonectomy for malignant pleural mesothelioma. The 2-year survival was 33%, with a median survival for the entire group of 10 months. Quite significant is the fact that the 2-year results were about the same with less extensive operations such as pleurectomy followed by radiation. The operative mortality with extrapleural pneumonectomy was 15%, but was only 2% at Memorial Sloan-Kettering with more limited operations. Hence the data seem clear that extrapleural pneumonectomy should be undertaken only in good-risk patients in whom low operative mortality is expected.—F.C. Spencer, M.D.

National Survey of the Pattern of Care for Carcinoma of the Lung
Humphrey EW, Smart CR, Winchester DP, Steele GD Jr, Yarbro JW, Chu KC, Triolo HH (American College of Surgeons, Chicago; Natl Cancer Inst, Bethesda, Md; Information Management Services, Silver Spring, Md)
J Thorac Cardiovasc Surg 100:837–843, 1990   13–8

Background.—Most diagnostic and therapeutic decisions for patients with lung cancer are made in community hospitals. The Commission on Cancer of the American College of Surgeons conducted a national survey to determine patterns of care for cancer patients in United States hospitals.

Methods.—The survey included 34,293 patients in 941 hospitals. The long-term portion of the survey included 15,219 patients with cancer diagnosed during 1981; the short-term portion, 19,074 patients with cancer diagnosed in 1986. The ratios of men to women were 2.2 in 1981 and 1.9 in 1986.

Table 1.—Preoperative Biopsy Results

Tumor size (cm)	Total No. of cancers of this size	Percutaneous needle biopsy		Transbronchial biopsy	
		No. biopsied	Percent positive	No. biopsied	Percent positive
0.0-2.0	3484	721	82	607	64
2.1-3.0	3961	1031	85	837	65
3.1-4.0	3280	875	87	757	67
4.1-5.0	2578	696	85	613	68
5.1-6.0	3581	937	89	889	69
>6.1	1533	401	88	323	74

(Courtesy of Humphrey EW, Smart CR, Winchester DP, et al: *J Thorac Cardiovasc Surg* 100:837–843, 1990.)

Results.—Most cancers occurred in the upper lobes, particularly of the right lung. Adenocarcinoma was the most prevalent histologic type in smokers and nonsmokers younger than age 55; squamous carcinoma was more prevalent in smokers older than age 55. The accuracy of biopsy results increased as tumor size increased, but not greatly so (Table 1). Mediastinoscopy was done in 17.6% of patients. Of those who had mediastinoscopy with no report of enlarged lymph nodes, lymph node biopsy was positive in 27%. Of the patients with cancer diagnosed in 1981, 30.5% had resection, compared to 28.1% in 1986. The only change in resectional procedures performed was for tumors measuring 1 cm or less, for which the proporation of wedge or segmental resection increased from 21% to 34%. Lobectomy was still the most common operation. There was no change in the prevalence of postoperative complications. The 5-year survival for all 1981 patients was 14.4%. Survival was best in patients with stage I bronchoalveolar cancers (Table 2). There was little change in the use of adjuvant irradiation; it was done in about half of patients with stage III disease. Adjuvant chemotherapy was little used (4% of patients in 1981 and 3% in 1986).

Conclusions.—Survival with lung cancer seems to be improving; it is unknown whether this is a true improvement or a reflection of an unrecognized change in the pattern of care. There is a continuing trend toward more conservative resections.

▶ This epidemiologic report is a valuable reference source for data on long-term trends with carcinoma of the lung. It provides data from more than 15,000 patients whose disease was first diagnosed in 1981. No dramatic changes in the biological nature of the malignancy were evident. Percutaneous biopsy was uniformly highly accurate—more than 80%. Mediastinoscopy was primarily beneficial after CT showed enlarged mediastinal nodes. In such patients, 73% of the nodes were positive, whereas without a positive CT scan, only 27% were positive. Overall resectability remained near 30%

Table 2.—Actuarial Survival Estimates by Stage in All Patients Undergoing Resection in 1981

Pathologic AJC stage	Squamous cell		Adenocarcinoma		Bronchoalveolar		Small cell		Large cell	
	No. of patients	5-year survival (%)	No. of patients	5-year survival (%)	No. of patients	5-year survival (%)	No. of patients	5-year survival (%)	No. of patients	5-year survival (%)
Stage I	848	51.9	757	53.7	287	61.7	68	30.9	155	44.3
Stage II	290	32.2	176	21.9	43	21.9	23	8.7	46	16.4
Stage III	548	13.6	394	14.1	70	15.8	99	6.1	128	4.6

(Courtesy of Humphrey EW, Smart CR, Winchester DP, et al: J Thorac Cardiovasc Surg 100:837–843, 1990.)

with 5-year survival of 50% for patients with stage I lesions, decreasing to 30% for those with stage II and 13% for those with stage III, respectively. The role of radiation and chemotherapy, except for small cell carcinoma, remains uncertain.—F.C. Spencer, M.D.

Bronchogenic Carcinoma With Chest Wall Invasion

Allen MS, Mathisen DJ, Grillo HC, Wain JC, Moncure AC, Hilgenberg AD
(Massachusetts Gen Hosp, Boston)
Ann Thorac Surg 51:948–951, 1991   13–9

Series.—Fifty-two patients (37 men) seen consecutively from 1973 to 1988 underwent resection of bronchogenic carcinoma with chest wall involvement. The average age was 63 years. In about one fourth of the patients the finding of a lesion on chest roentgenography was incidental. Half of the patients had lobectomy and 6 underwent pneumonectomy. Nine patients received radiotherapy preoperatively.

Outcome.—Hospital mortality was 4%. Ten percent of patients had prolonged air leakage that did not require surgical treatment. Four patients contracted pneumonia, and 2 had nonfatal pulmonary embolism. Survival at 2 years was 41% and at 5 years, 26%. The absolute 5-year survival rate was 29% for patients with negative nodes and 11% for those with positive N1 nodes. Survival at 5 years was 25.5% for patients with squamous cell carcinoma and 30.5% for those having adenocarcinoma.

Recommendations.—Full-thickness resection of the chest wall is appropriate in these patients. Extrapleural dissection alone is not adequate. The indications for radiotherapy in patients with chest wall involvement remain uncertain, but radiotherapy is administered preoperatively when tumor occurs at a site where it would be difficult to achieve an adequate margin. Radiotherapy is given postoperatively if positive nodes are found or the margins are close.

▶ Experiences with 52 bronchogenic carcinomas invading the chest wall, treated in a period of more than 15 years, are described. Chest wall invasion is a well-recognized grim prognostic factor but, as the authors' data indicate, it is not automatically "incurable." One to 6 ribs were removed, but only 2 required chest wall reconstruction. Patients with negative nodes had a 5-year survival near 30%, whereas those with N_1 nodes had a survival rate of only 11%.—F.C. Spencer, M.D.

Carinal Resection for Bronchogenic Carcinoma

Mathisen DJ, Grillo HC (Massachusetts Gen Hosp, Boston)
J Thorac Cardiovasc Surg 102:16–23, 1991   13–10

Background.—Carinal resection and reconstruction is technically challenging. Successful surgical outcomes rely on careful patient selection, thorough preoperative assessment, careful anesthetic management, strict attention to surgical technique, and compulsive care postoperatively. Carinal resection and reconstruction for bronchogenic cancer were evaluated.

Methods.—Thirty-seven carinal resections for bronchogenic carcinoma have been done since 1973 at 1 center. There were 21 right carinal penumonectomies, 7 carinal resections, 7 carina plus lobe resections, and 2 carina plus pneumonectomy stump resections. Five patients had diseased N_2 nodes, and 13 had disease N_1 nodes.

Outcomes.—Pulmonary complications occurred in 8 cases, vocal cord paresis in 3, atrial fibrillation in 9, anastomotic stenosis in 4, and anastomotic separation in 3. Three patients (8%) died early in the postoperative period. All deaths were related to adult respiratory distress syndrome. These patients did not respond to aggressive treatment. Four late postoperative deaths occurred between 2 and 4 months, for an incidence of 10.9%. All of the late deaths were related to anastomotic complications. There were 5 absolute 5-year survivors. The acturial 5-year survival rate was 19%.

Conclusions.—Carinal resection of bronchogenic carcinoma involving the carina should be done only at institutions having sufficient experience to minimize operative mortality. A dedicated team of thoracic surgeons, anesthesiologists, and persons skilled in postoperative care is mandatory. If operative mortality can routinely be kept under 10% and 5-year survival rates routinely reach 25%, inclusion of carinal involvement by bronchogenic cancer in the state III-A classification should be considered.

▶ This report of cumulative experiences by Grillo's group at the Massachusetts General Hospital describes experiences with 37 carinal resections performed in a period of 18 years. The early operative mortality rate was about 8%; 11% of deaths occurred in the next 2–4 months as a result of anastomotic complications. The actuarial 5-year survival rate was 19%. In the discussion of this report, Dr. Faber commented that his group in Chicago had performed about 36 carinal pneumonectomies with an overall mortality of 28% and a survival rate of about 20%. Hence this radical procedure is clearly indicated in selective cases, but it requires detailed planning and technical expertise because of the serious problems resulting from anastomotic complications.—F.C. Spencer, MD

Surgical Treatment for Limited Small-Cell Lung Cancer: The University of Toronto Lung Oncology Group Experience
Shepherd FA, Ginsberg RJ, Feld R, Evans WK, Johansen E (Toronto Gen Hosp; Princess Margaret Hosp, Toronto; Mount Sinai Hosp, Toronto)
J Thorac Cardiovasc Surg 101:385–393, 1991   13–11

Background.—Interest in surgical treatment for some patients with small cell lung cancer (SCLC) has revived with the finding that $1_1 N_0$ tumors have a projected 5-year survival of 60%. Although 80% of patients may respond to chemotherapy, less than 15% will be alive after 2 years.

A series of 119 patients underwent combined chemotherapy and surgery for SCLC in a 10-year period.

Patients.—Surgery was done first in 79 patients, 58 men and 21 women (median age, 63 years). Adjuvant chemotherapy was used in 67 of these patients. Chemotherapy was done first in 40 patients, 27 men and 13 women (median age, 59 years). Of these, 94% had at least a partial response before surgery. Preoperatively, there were 69 stage I, 27 stage II, and 23 stage III tumors. Lobectomy was done in 88 patients, pneumonectomy in 26, and no resection in 5. On postoperative pathologic examination, SCLC alone was found in 95 patients, non–SCLC in 3, mixed findings in 17, and no residual tumor in 4. Postoperatively, there were 35 stage I, 36 stage II, and 48 stage IIIa tumors.

Outcome.—The overall median survival was 111 weeks, and the projected 5-year survival was 39%, with no difference between those who had chemotherapy before and after surgery. The median survivals were 82 weeks for patients with stage II disease and 83 weeks for those with stage III disease. Projected 5-year survivals were 51%, 28%, and 19% for patients with stage I, stage II, and stage III disease, respectively. Of 12 patients who received no chemotherapy, 7 were alive after as many as 4 years. Sixty-seven patients died, 11 with no evidence of disease. Only 10 patients had relapse at the primary site alone, 7 at primary and distant sites, and 39 at distant sites only.

Conclusions.—In patients with SCLC, resection appears to improve control at the primary site. Combination therapy can achieve long-term survival and cure in many patients with stage I disease. In patients with stage II and IIIa SCLC, survival is similar to that in patients with surgically treated stage IIIa non–SCLC.

▶ This report reviews experiences over 13 years with 119 patients who had SCLC undergoing both surgery and chemotherapy. Projected survival for pathologic stage I disease was 51%, whereas stages II and III had projected survivals of only 28% and 19%, respectively.

Although the data do not show significant differences between patients who received chemotherapy before operation and those who received it later, for reasons explained in the manuscript the authors recommend that patients initially have chemotherapy, with surgical resection reserved for those who respond initially to chemotherapy. This combination has been more effective than surgery alone, which results in a survival rate of only about 5%. Routine radiotherapy has not improved survival. Hence these studies identify a small percentage of patients with SCLC who may significantly benefit from the combination of surgical resection and chemotherapy.—F.C. Spencer, MD

Primary Cysts and Tumors of the Mediastinum
Cohen AJ, Thompson L, Edwards FH, Bellamy RF (Walter Reed Army Med

Ctr, Washington, DC; Uniformed Services Univ of the Health Sciences)
Ann Thorac Surg 51:378–386, 1991   13–12

Introduction.—Changes over time in the occurrence of primary cysts and tumors of the mediastinum were examined in 230 patients, 84 of them first seen from 1944 to 1969 and 146 seen from 1970 to 1989. The 138 men and 92 women had a mean age of 29 years, and 54 of them were younger than 18 years.

Trends.—The prevalence of malignancy rose significantly from 17% in the earlier period to 47% in the later one. Numbers of lymphomas and malignant neurogenic tumors increased significantly. Both anterior and paravertebral tumors were more prevalent in the later period. Also, more ancillary diagnostic studies were done in the later period. More than three fourths of the patients with malignant disease and fewer than half of those with benign disease were symptomatic.

Outcome.—Tumor was totally excised in 141 patients, all but 10 of the benign tumors being totally removed. Six perioperative deaths occurred, 5 in patients with malignant disease. None of 95 patients with benign disease who were followed had recurrence or malignant change. Of 62 patients with malignant disease, 17 died of their disease during follow-up.

Conclusions.—Malignant mediastinal masses have increased in frequency in the past 2 decades, as have anterior compartment tumors and, particularly, lymphomas. Surgical resection of benign lesions and aggressive multimodality treatment of malignant lesions are recommended.

▶ A retrospective analysis was performed on 230 patients evaluated at the Walter Reed Army Medical Center in a period of 45 years. A comparison was made between those seen in the past 20 years and those seen earlier. The frequency of malignancy rose to 47% from 17%, primarily because of an increase in the number of lymphomas and neurogenic tumors.

Among the 230 patients, the 5 most common tumors, in descending order of frequency, were as follows: thymic (56), cyst (45), neurogenic (39), lymphomas (36), and germ cell (22).—F.C. Spencer, M.D.

14 Congenital Heart Disease

Long-Term Outcome After Surgical Repair of Isolated Atrial Septal Defect: Follow-Up at 27 to 32 Years
Murphy JG, Gersh BJ, McGoon MD, Mair DD, Porter CJ, Ilstrup DM, McGoon DC, Puga FJ, Kirklin JW, Danielson GK (Mayo Clinic and Found, Rochester, Minn; Univ of Alabama)
N Engl J Med 323:1645–1650, 1990   14–1

Introduction.—Long-term survival is poorly documented in patients treated some time ago for atrial septal defect. A 3-decade follow-up was made of 123 patients undergoing repair of an isolated septal defect in 1956–1960. The mean age at surgery was 26 years. Three fourths of the patients were symptomatic at the time of operation.

Outcome.—The 30-year actuarial survival rate was 74% compared with 85% for age- and sex-matched controls. The perioperative mortality rate was 3.3% in this series. Long-term survival was compromised only for patients aged 25 years and older at the time of surgery. Apart from age, pulmonary artery systolic pressure was a significant independent predictor of long-term survival. Late heart failure, stroke, and atrial fibrillation all occurred more often in older patients. Atrial fibrillation/flutter persisted in 13 of 19 patients after operation. Of 104 patients in sinus rhythm preoperatively, 77% remained so during long-term follow-up.

Conclusions.—Patients operated on for atrial septal defect before age 25 years have an excellent outlook. Invalon sponge no longer is considered suitable for patch closure of atrial septal defects. All patients should be monitored for late atrial arrhythmia.

▶ This important paper analyzed the late results in 123 patients older than 25 years after operation at the Mayo Clinic. In patients operated on before 25 years of age, there was no significant difference in late results compared with control patients. Those operated on between 25 and 40 years of age had a significant increase in late mortality, 16% vs. 9% in controls; those operated on after 41 years of age had an even larger difference—60% late mortality vs. 41% in controls. In addition, late cardiac events, especially atrial fibrillation and stroke, were far more common in the older group.

The difference in mortality was clearly not simply the result of pulmonary artery pressure. Age exerted an independent significant influence for unknown reasons. Late death was attributable to a cardiac cause in 48% of patients and to a stroke in 19%. The serious influence of atrial fibrillation is clearly shown by the fact that all of the late deaths from stroke occurred in patients with atrial fibrillation or flutter. The vast majority of these patients were in atrial fibrillation before operative repair.

Hence, as the operative risk of closure of an atrial septal defect is near zero, there would seem to be little or no justification for postponing operation in patients with a significant atrial defect, even though completely asymptomatic. Apart from the decreased life expectancy, the simple hazard of permanent atrial fibrillation, per se, is sufficient justification to indicate prompt operation. The authors are to be congratulated for this important study.—F.C. Spencer, M.D.

Methods for Repair of Simple Isolated Ventricular Septal Defect

McGrath LB (Deborah Heart and Lung Ctr, Browns Mills, NJ; Univ of Medicine and Dentistry of New Jersey, New Brunswick)
J Cardiac Surg 6:13–23, 1991   14–2

Introduction.—A total of 115 consecutive patients had various types of simple isolated interventricular communication repaired in 1985-1989 without the need for ventriculotomy. Twelve patients had previous surgery. About three fourths of the group had a perimembraneous septal defect.

Technique.—Surgery is done under cardiopulmonary bypass at a nasal temperature of 28° C. In closing a simple perimembraneous defect, the patch is at-

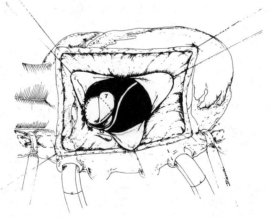

Fig 14–1.—Transatrial repair of perimembranous ventricular septal defect (VSD) using a standard oblique right atriotomy incision. Stay sutures are placed on the right atrial wall and on the tricuspid valve to arrange the exposure. Direct caval vein cannulation is used. Care is taken to avoid injury to the penetrating and branching portions of the His bundle that is located on the posteroinferior rim of the VSD. (Courtesy of McGrath LB: *J Cardiac Surg* 6:13-23, 1991.)

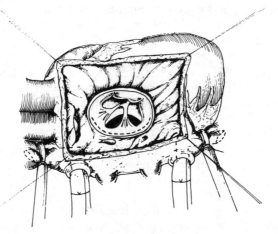

Fig 14–2.—If exposure of the ventricular septal defect (VSD) via the tricuspid valve is obscured by aneurysm formation of the membranous septum or chordal attachments close to the edge of the VSD, the base of the septal leaflet of the tricuspid valve may be detached to facilitate the exposure. (Courtesy of McGrath LB: *J Cardiac Surg* 6:13–23, 1991.)

tached inferiorly to the infundibular and trabecular septum; in the area of the His bundle, the suture line is directed 7–10 mm away from the edge of the defect (Fig 14–1). If the defect edges are not seen clearly, the septal leaflet may be detached and reflected upward (Fig 14–2). A continuous monofilament suture technique is used.

Results.—A Sauvage Dacron patch was used in 94% of the patients. Operative mortality was .9%. One fifth of the patients had associated procedures. In no case was late reoperation necessary.

Conclusion.—Virtually any isolated interventricular communication may be repaired by this approach with a low risk of adverse events. The risks of hospital death and surgically induced complete atrioventricular dissociation both are close to zero.

▶ This short technique paper describes the outcome in 115 consecutive patients undergoing repair of an isolated ventricular septal defect. The results are impressive. A ventriculotomy was not required in any patient, and there were no instances of heart block or reoperation. One operative death occurred. Repair was accomplished by the transatrial approach in 104 patients, by the transaortic approach in 3, and via the pulmonary artery in 8. If exposure was inadequate through the tricuspid valve, the septal leaflet of the tricuspid valve was temporarily detached to facilitate exposure. The illustrations are excellent.—F.C. Spencer, M.D.

Complete Repair of Atrioventricular Septal Defect

Merrill WH, Hammon JW Jr, Graham TP Jr, Bender HW Jr (Vanderbilt Univ)
Ann Thorac Surg 52:29–32, 1991   14–3

Background.—Without surgery, children with complete atrioventricular (AV) septal defect have a poor prognosis. Repair of complete AV septal defect was carried out between 1971 and 1990 in 103 children who had no other major cardiovascular malformation. Ninety-one of the children were younger than 18 months.

Procedure.—Treatment involved deep hypothermia and circulatory arrest. The 12 older patients (mean age, 40 months) underwent repair using moderate hypothermia and cardiopulmonary bypass. The single-patch technique was used.

Outcomes.—Two children died during surgery. Four of the younger patients needed repeat repair to control residual or recurrent mitral regurgitation. Two older patients required late reoperation to replace 1 or both AV valves. Of 3 younger patients who had pulmonary banding initially, 1 died after complete repair. Two of 3 children undergoing initial pulmonary artery banding died. The survivor needed pulmonary artery reconstruction, which was subsequently repeated. After 1977 the policy was to do primary definitive repair when possible. Since then, 2 children have died of unrelated causes. Most children had no or only minimal symptoms at the most recent follow-up.

Conclusions.—Primary complete repair of AV septal defects should be done in symptomatic children with congestive heart failure and failure to thrive. Early primary repair is preferred to continued medical treatment or preliminary pulmonary artery banding. The key features of such repair are surgery before pulmonary vascular obstructive disease develops, careful assessment of the anatomical details, and precise reconstruction of AV valvular functional integrity and closure of the septal defects.

▶ Experiences with 103 consecutive children undergoing repair of a complete AV septal defect in a period of 19 years are described in this report. Most of the patients (91) were less than 18 months of age. The younger patients were operated on with deep hypothermia and circulatory arrest. There were 15 perioperative deaths.

The policy of primary definitive repair, rather than palliative pulmonary artery banding, has been followed since 1977, because results with pulmonary artery banding were both unpredictable and inconsistent. Late results in most patients were quite good. Significant residual mitral regurgitation required repeat operation in 6 patients, 4 of whom were treated by reconstruction; the other 2 required valve replacement.—F.C. Spencer, M.D.

Neonatal Repair of Tetralogy of Fallot With and Without Pulmonary Atresia

Di Donato RM, Jonas RA, Lang P, Rome JJ, Mayer JE Jr, Castenada AR (Children's Hosp, Boston; Harvard Med School)
J Thorac Cardiovasc Surg 101:126–137, 1991   14–4

Background.—The arterial switch operation can yield excellent results when done on an elective basis in neonates with tetralogy of Fallot (TOF). Previously, this operation was performed in neonates only when severe persistent cyanosis or cyanotic spells were present. Data were reviewed on nonelective repairs in 27 neonates treated during a 15-year period.

Patients.—The 19 boys and 8 girls had a mean age of 8 days and a mean weight of 3 kg at the time of operation. Fourteen had TOF and 13 had TOF with valvar pulmonary atresia. Four patients had had unsuccessful Blalock-Taussig shunts placed at other centers. Indications were persistent hypoxemia, less than 70% arterial oxygen saturation, in 22 patients and hypoxic spells in 5. The right ventricular outflow tract was reconstructed with a transannular patch in 25 patients and a conduit in 2.

Outcome.—Five patients died in the hospital, 3 because of avoidable technical problems; all 5 of these patients had a pulmonary artery index of less than 150 mm^2/m^2. Absent pulmonary valve-type syndrome was present after operation in a child who weighed 2.3 kg; death resulted from respiratory complications caused by aneurysmal branch pulmonary arteries.

The 5-year actuarial survival was 74%, with the danger of death approaching zero at 1.5 years after operation. The 5-year actuarial freedom from repeat surgery was 76%. Fifteen long-term survivors had postoperative catheterization; in all cases but 2, the right ventricular pressure was less than 70% systemic. All survivors were well and in sinus rhythm a mean of 5 years after operation.

Conclusions.—Early mortality for neonates with symptomatic TOF is high, although freedom from reoperation is relatively low. The best age for operative repair remains controversial. If mortality of repair is lower in infants without symptoms, elective repair of TOF during the first months of life should be a realistic goal.

▶ This report analyzes the experiences at the Boston Children's Hospital over a period of 15 years when neonatal repair of tetralogy of Fallot was necessary because of severe anoxia. Elective operations were not performed. The mean age of operation was near 8 days, and 27 neonates were operated on. The right ventricular outflow tract was reconstructed with a transannular patch in the majority. Five deaths occurred, 3 of which were said to be caused by avoidable technical problems. Long-term results were excellent, with an actuarial survival at 5 years near 74%. From these data, the authors' conclusion that elective repair of tetralogy can be undertaken at an early age seems reasonable.—F.C. Spencer, M.D.

Comparison of the Aortic Homograft and the Pulmonary Autograft for Aortic Valve or Root Replacement in Children

Gerosa G, McKay R, Davies J, Ross DN (Natl Heart Hosp, London; Royal Liverpool Children's Hosp, UK)
J Thorac Cardiovasc Surg 102:51–61, 1991   14–5

Introduction.—A total of 146 pediatric patients underwent aortic valve or aortic root replacement from 1964 to 1990. An aortic homograft was given to 103 patients, whose mean age was 12 years. Forty-three others (mean age, 14 years) had their own pulmonary valve transferred to the aortic position. The homografts included 54 valve and 49 aortic root replacements. Autografts replaced 36 valves and 7 aortic roots. Homografts were followed for a total of 867 patient-years and autografts for 297 patient-years.

Observations.—Hospital mortality was 15.5% in patients receiving homograft valves and 11.6% in those receiving autografts. The respective late mortality rates were 16.7% and 13.2%. Twenty-four surviving patients with homografts and 6 with pulmonary autografts required reoperation. Primary tissue failure complicated 19 aortic homografts and possibly 1 pulmonary autograft. Freedom from death and all valve-related complications was comparable in the homograft and autograft groups. None of the patients was anticoagulated and none had thromboembolism. Surviving patients had excellent exercise tolerance.

Conclusions.—Pulmonary autografting is the procedure of choice in children who require replacement of the aortic valve or root. If root autografts grow as well as valves, it may be possible to solve the problem of aortic valve disease in early life, thereby conserving left ventricular function. Aortic homografts may be preferable for children who have associated cardiac defects or a history of cardiac infection. An autograft then can be used to replace a homograft that degenerates.

▶ During a period of 25 years, aortic homograft or pulmonary autograft valves were implanted into the left ventricular outflow tract of children. Early operative mortality was high, but no fatalities have occurred after valve replacement since 1975. In long-term survivors, the pulmonary autograft showed a surprising susceptibility to endocarditis, more so than the homograft. However, it was quite striking that, to date, more than 15 years since the early operations, there has been no valve degeneration in any pulmonary autograft. Hence the pulmonary autograft may be the ideal operation for aortic valve replacement in children.

No patient received anticoagulation in either group, and there were no episode of thromboembolism.—F.C. Spencer, M.D.

The Myth of the Aortic Annulus: The Anatomy of the Subaortic Outflow Tract

Anderson RH, Devine WA, Ho SY, Smith A, McKay R (Natl Heart and Lung

Moving?

I'd like to receive my *Year Book of Surgery* without interruption.

Please note the following change of address, effective: _____

Name: _____

New Address: _____

_____

City: _____ State: _____ Zip: _____

Old Address: _____

_____

City: _____ State: _____ Zip: _____

Reservation Card

Yes, I would like my own copy of the *Year Book of Surgery*. Please begin my subscription with the current edition according to the terms described below.* I understand that I will have 30 days to examine each annual edition. If satisfied, I will pay just $59.95 plus sales tax, postage and handling (price subject to change without notice).

Name: _____

Address: _____

City: _____ State: _____ Zip: _____

Method of Payment

❏ Visa   ❏ Mastercard   ❏ AmEx   ❏ Bill me   ❏ Check (in US dollars, payable to Mosby-Year Book, Inc.)

Card number _____ Exp date _____

Signature _____

LS-0907

*Your *Year Book* Service Guarantee:

When you subscribe to the *Year Book*, we'll send you an advance notice of future volumes about two months before they publish. This automatic notice system is designed to take up as little of your time as possible. If you do not want the *Year Book*, the advance notice makes it quick and easy for you to let us know your decision; and you will always have at least 20 days to decide. If we don't hear from you, we'll send you the new volume as soon as it's available. And, of course, the *Year Book* is yours to examine free of charge for 30 days (postage, handling and applicable sales tax are added to each shipment).

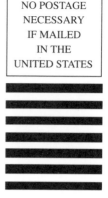
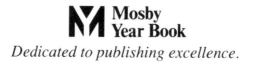

Mosby Year Book

Dedicated to publishing excellence.

Inst, London; Children's Hosp of Pittsburgh; Univ of Liverpool, England)
Ann Thorac Surg 52:640–646, 1991   14–6

Background.—Much attention has been given to describing the "annulus" of the arterial valves and ascertaining the best way of enlarging the structure when treating a stenotic or obstructive subarterial outflow tract. In reality, the leaflets do not attach in a ringlike manner around the circumference of the ventricular outlet, and it may well not be appropriate to describe the semilunar attachments in terms of an annulus.

Observations.—Experience with normal hearts suggests that aortic valve leaflets attach to the left ventricular outflow tract in the manner of 3 half-moons. The interleaflet triangles extending beneath the commissural apices are incorporated as extensions of the ventricular outflow tract. In critical aortic stenosis of infancy, the entire pattern of leaflet formation is distorted. There is a relatively circular arrangement of attachment of what is in effect a single leaflet. In these hearts, the attachment of the leaflets is much more annular than normal; formation of the fibrous triangles is deficient.

Conclusion.—The concept of an annulus impedes the understanding of normal and abnormal valve function. Instead, emphasis should be placed on appreciating the semilunar attachment of the valve leaflets.

▶ This short paper by Anderson, an internationally recognized authority on cardiac anatomy in congenital heart disease, was selected for its elegant description of the anatomy of the subaortic outflow tract in both normal and abnormal hearts. It should be studied in detail by those working with the difficult problem of the small aortic root in infants and children.—F.C. Spencer, M.D.

Aortic Regurgitation After Left Ventricular Myotomy and Myectomy
Brown PS Jr, Roberts CS, McIntosh CL, Clark RE (Natl Heart, Lung, and Blood Inst, Bethesda, Md)
Ann Thorac Surg 51:585–592, 1991   14–7

Background.—The most common surgical procedure for left ventricular outflow tract obstruction is transaortic left ventricular myotomy and myectomy (LVMM). This procedure, however, is associated with a risk of aortic regurgitation. To evaluate the incidence and cause of aortic regurgitation as a complication of LVMM, 30 years of experience were reviewed.

Technique.—After exposure, institution of cardiopulmonary bypass, and vertical aortotomy, the septum is exposed by retracting the right coronary leaflet anteriorly with a cloth-covered retractor placed into the aortic root (Fig 14–3). The initial ventricular myotomy incision begins 2–3 mm to the right of the midpoint of the leaflet, the second 10–15 mm to the left and parallel, and the third trans-

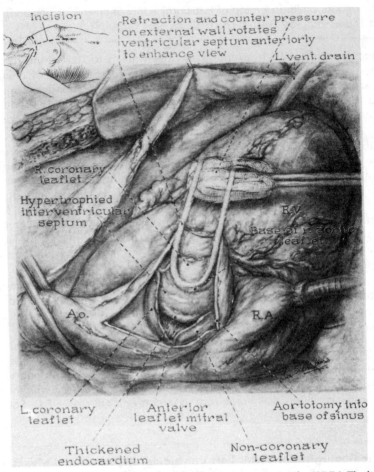

Fig 14–3.—Operative exposure of interventricular septum in preparation for LVMM. The bulging hypertrophied septum is visible below the right coronary leaflet, which is retracted anteriorly and to the left by the cloth-covered retractor. Ao indicates aorta; R.A., right atrium; R.V., right ventricle. (From Brown PS Jr, Roberts CS, McIntosh CL, et al: *Ann Thorac Surg* 51:585–592, 1991.) (Courtesy of Morrow AG: *J Thorac Cardiovasc Surg* 76:423–430, 1978.)

verse between them. All were continued for at least 4 cm toward the apex in an attempt to incorporate the fibrous plaque of mitral-septal contact (Fig 14–4). In later operations, incisions were begun 5–10 mm below the annulus (Fig 14–5).

Patients.—Of 525 patients with hypertrophic cardiomyopathy treated by LVMM, 496 had nonregurgitant trileaflet aortic valves preoperatively. Follow-up in this group was 99% complete; patients were seen routinely in the outpatient clinic every year or so. After LVMM, aortic regurgitation developed in 19 patients (12 women, 7 men; mean age, 35 years). In 5 patients, LVMM was followed immediately by aortic valve replacement

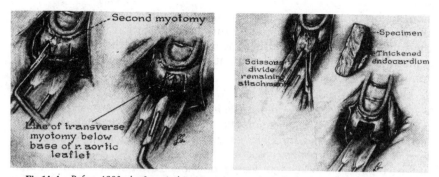

Fig 14–4.—Before 1982, the 2 vertical incisions were made at the aortic annulus and carried down toward the ventricular apex. (From Brown PS Jr, Roberts CS, McIntosh CL, et al: *Ann Thorac Surg* 51:585–592, 1991. Courtesy of Morrow AG: *J Thorac Cardiovasc Surg* 76:423–430, 1978.)

or valvuloplasty. In 7, aortic regurgitation developed 6 months or less postoperatively, and 3 patients required surgical repair. In the 7 remaining patients, aortic regurgitation developed 3 or more years after LVMM; 3 patients required repair. Those who had aortic regurgitation before 6 months had either a very small aortic annulus (21 mm or less), a low mitral-septal contact lesion (35 mm or more below the aortic annulus), or both. None of the patients with late aortic regurgitation had an aortic annulus of this size, and only 1 had a low mitral-septal contact point. When these problems were present, they made the operation much more difficult and necessitated increased retraction of the aortic valve and annulus to expose the interventricular septum.

Conclusions.—A 3.8% incidence of aortic regurgitation occurred after LVMM. When a very small aortic annulus, low mitral-septal contact le-

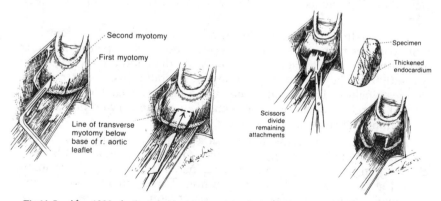

Fig 14–5.—After 1982, the 2 vertical incisions were made 5–10 mm below the aortic annulus. After completion of the resection, a rectangular channel 1 × 1.5 cm extends from the valve annulus toward the apex for about 4.5 cm. (From Brown PS Jr, Roberts CS, McIntosh CL, et al: *Ann Thorac Surg* 51:585–592, 1991. Courtesy of McIntosh CL: *Current Therapy in Cardiothoracic Surgery*, Grillo HC, ed. Toronto, B.C. Decker, 1989.)

sion, or both, are present in a patient undergoing LVMM, the surgeon should use great care in operating through the aortic valve and evaluate the valve postoperatively. Other means of exposing the interventricular septum, or mitral valve replacement, should be considered if LVMM cannot be done easily.

▶ This elegant report from the National Heart Institute well analyzes the uncommon but serious complication of aortic insufficiency after left ventricular myomectomy for hypertrophic cardiomyopathy. Among 496 patients treated in a 30-year period, aortic regurgitation developed in 19 (4%). In 14 of the 19 patients, aortic regurgitation developed after operation, in 7 within 6 months and in 7 after 3 years. About half of the patients required operative repair.

The authors suggest that development of this complication after 3 years may represent a separate disease entity, not preventable by known techniques. The classic Schlossberg illustrations are excellent.—F.C. Spencer, M.D.

Repair of Aortic Coarctation in Infants

Brouwer MHJ, Kuntze CEE, Ebels T, Talsma MD, Eijgelaar A (Univ of Groningen, The Netherlands)
J Thorac Cardiovasc Surg 101:1093–1098, 1991   14–8

Background.—There is still a considerable risk of recoarctation in infants younger than age 2 years who undergo repair of aortic coarctation. In addition to young age, risk factors are reported to include the morphology of the coarctation and the suture material used. Data were reviewed on 53 patients to determine any further risk factors for recoarctation.

Patients.—In a 13½-year period, 35 male infants and 18 female infants younger than age 2 years underwent operative repair of aortic coarctation. The median age of the 53 was 83 days and the median weight was 4,000 g. The main clinical finding at operation were severe congestive heart failure. Thirty-four infants had a discrete juxtaductal lesion and 19 had a preductal isthmic narrowing. Ten of the 20 who had a left-to-right shunt had an atrial septal defect.

Treatment.—All patients underwent a left posterolateral thoracotomy. Sixty percent had resection and end-to-end anastomosis, 36% had subclavian flap angioplasty, and 4% had patch angioplasty. Four infants died, 1 as late as 3 months after operation. Three patients had postoperative hypertension with no signs of recoarctation.

Outcome.—At a mean follow-up of 5.6 years, 11 patients had recoarctation, a rate of 21%. This included 13% of patients who had resection and end-to-end anastomosis compared to 33% of those who had subclavian flap or patch angioplasty. On multivariate stepwise logistic regression analysis the risk factors for recoarctation were patient weight, rather than age, and the residual gradient after operation. When expressed as a ratio of systolic arm pressure, the latter factor was even more significant, because this takes background hemodynamics into account.

Conclusions.—Patient weight at operation and gradient ratio appear to be the only incremental risk factors for recoarctation. Weight is more important than age; thus the operation should be deferred only in infants who are gaining weight. The gradient ratio should be as low as possible, because even small gradients have a strong incremental effect in low weight infants. Currently, resection and end-to-end anastomosis is the preferred technique, although the current study does not suggest that it decreases the risk of recoarctation.

▶ This report from The Netherlands describes results in 53 consecutive infants undergoing repair of a coarctation. Resection and end-to-end anastomosis was performed in 32 patients and subclavian flap angioplasty in 19. Recoarctation occurred in 13% of the patients undergoing resection and direct anastomosis, but in 33% of 21 patients undergoing subclavian flap angioplasty or patch angioplasty. The authors clearly emphasize that the problem remains unsolved. Statistical analysis found that the weight at the time of operation, rather than age, was a stronger predictor of late recurrence. When clinically possible, deferment of operation until the child is larger is suggested.—F.C. Spencer, M.D.

End-to-End Repair of Aortic Coarctation Using Absorbable Polydioxanone Suture

Arenas JD, Myers JL, Gleason MM, Vennos A, Baylen BG, Waldhausen JA (Pennsylvania State Univ)

Ann Thorac Surg 51:413–417, 1991   14–9

Introduction.—Various suture materials have been tried in attempts to avoid residual and recurrent coarctation of the aorta. Polydioxanone, an absorbable monofilament suture, is useful in various cardiovascular procedures because it allows vascular anastomoses to grow.

Methods.—Fifteen patients aged 2 months to 9 years underwent repair of aortic coarctation by resection and end-to-end anastomosis. Polydioxanone monofilament absorbable suture was used. The mean preoperative catheterization gradient was 43 mm Hg.

Results.—Thirteen patients were followed for a mean of 23 months after repair. Doppler and color echocardiography and MRI demonstrated good anatomical repair with no anastomotic aneurysms. No patient had residual coarctation. Color flow mapping of the aortic arch demonstrated virtually normal laminar flow in the descending aorta with minimal turbulence.

Conclusion.—No vascular complications were related to repair of aortic coarctation with absorbable polydioxanone suture material.

▶ A crucial question about vascular anastomoses in children, especially infants, is the ability of the area of the anastomosis to grow with increasing age. Absorbable sutures, if safe, would seem to be the ideal solution. Hence the data in this report are of particular importance. In a period of 6 years, absorbable sutures were used in the operative repair of coarctation in 15 patients between 3 months and 9 years of age. Evaluation in 13 of these patients, after 11–49 months, found no signs of aneurysm formation. Although not conclusive, it seems unlikely that aneurysms would develop later if they are not evident at this time. This report thus seems particularly significant.—F.C. Spencer, M.D.

Hypoplastic Transverse Arch and Coarctation in Neonates: Surgical Reconstruction of the Aortic Arch—A Study of Sixty-Six Patients
Lacour-Gayet F, Bruniaux J, Serraf A, Chambran P, Blaysat G, Losay J, Petit J, Kachaner J, Planché C (Paris-Sud Univ, Le Plessis Robinson, France)
J Thorac Cardiovasc Surg 100:808–816, 1990   14–10

Patients.—From 1983 to 1988, 66 consecutive neonates with coarctation of the aorta and marked hypoplasia of the transverse aortic arch underwent resection of the coarctation and arch reconstruction. The mean age at operation was 2 weeks. Associated lesions were present in 80% of the patients; 25 infants had complex intracardiac lesions. More than 80% of the infants had hypoplasia of the distal transverse aortic arch.

Technique.—The ductus often is divided to gain a better approach to the terminal end of the ascending aorta. The incision of the transverse arch is extended well proximal to the left carotid origin. An extended oblique anastomosis is performed over the entire aortic arch using 6–0 polypropylene suture material. Pulmonary artery banding was performed in 19 infants.

Results.—The postoperative mortality was 14%; for 25 infants with complex lesions it was 28%. There were 6 late deaths, none among infants having simple coarctation. In 4 surviving infants, there was prolonged left ventricular dysfunction. Actuarial survival at 5 years was 75%. Recurrent coarctation was diagnosed in 7 patients, 5 of whom underwent reoperation.

Conclusion.—This procedure relieves obstruction at the level of the transverse arch. Wide resection of ductus tissue might prevent recurrent coarctation. Preoperative prostaglandin administration is helpful.

▶ This report from France describes a significant experience with operations on 66 infants with hypoplastic transverse arch. The mean age at operation was 14 days. The coarctation was an isolated abnormality in only 25% of the patients.

The operative technique is well described, employing wide mobilization of the entire aortic arch and descending aorta through a left thoracotomy in the third interspace. A radical resection was then performed, placing the proximal occlusion clamp proximal to the left carotid artery. Early mortality was 14%, including that from repair of an associated anomaly. There were only 4 recurrences, all of which were successfully operated on.

Hypoplastic transverse arch was defined as a 50% reduction in the diameter of the transverse arch in comparison with the diameter of the ascending aorta. As the authors indicate, the significance of this degree of obstruction is not clearly known.

No complications from temporary occlusion of the left carotid occurred. The operative approach has the attractiveness of a wide anastomosis with complete excision of abnormal tissue, without the use of prosthetic material.—F.C. Spencer, M.D.

Coarctation and Hypoplasia of the Aortic Arch: Will the Arch Grow?
Siewers RD, Ettedgui J, Pahl E, Tallman R, del Nido PJ (Univ of Pittsburgh; Children's Hosp of Pittsburgh)
Ann Thorac Surg 52:608–614, 1991   14–11

Introduction.—Infants with coarctation of the aorta commonly have various degrees of hypoplasia of the transverse aortic arch. It is questionable whether operations designed to correct these stenoses will relieve pressure gradients between the ascending and descending aorta. In addition, more infants with complex coarctation are being treated surgically, partly because of the ability to stabilize their condition with prostaglandin E_1. Isolated coarctation with hypoplasia appears to be related as much to the presence of ductal tissue in the wall of the aortic isthmus as to fetal blood flow patterns. Based on study of autopsy specimens, the diameter of the normal distal aortic arch is at least half that of the ascending aorta. An arch index (transverse aortic arch to ascending aorta diameter ratio) of less than .5 can therefore define transverse aortic arch hypoplasia (Fig 14–6). To determine whether the arch can grow after correction of discrete coarctation stenosis, arch indices were studied in a group of conventionally treated infants.

Patients and Methods.—Coarctation repair was performed in 229 patients during a 10-year period. Fifty-six percent of the patients were less than 12 months old; of these, 102 had preoperative cineangiograms suitable for use in determining transverse arch hypoplasia and arch index. Most had subclavian flap arthroplasty, but others had classic resection and end-to-end anastomosis. The mean follow-up in 92 survivors was 50 months.

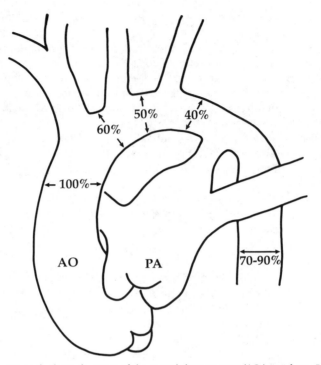

Fig 14–6.—Minimal relative diameters of the normal thoracic aorta (AO) in infancy. PA indicates pulmonary artery. (Adapted from Moulaert AJ, Bruins CC, Oppenheimer-Dekker A: *Circulation* 53:1101–1105, 1976. From Siewers RD, Ettedgui J, Pahl E, et al: *Ann Thorac Surg* 52:608–614, 1991.)

Findings.—A hypoplastic aortic arch was present in 33 infants; 27 of these had major associated cardiac anomalies. For 18 patients, data on the preoperative and postoperative arch index were available. The mean preoperative index was .40, and the mean postoperative index was .69 within an average of 39 months postoperatively. Change in the arch index was unrelated to type of operation or age at the time of repair.

Conclusions.—In children with hypoplasia of the aortic arch and coarctation of the aorta, growth of the arch can occur after surgical repair. Recurrent coarctation does not appear to result from the persistently hypoplastic and flow-restrictive transverse aortic arch. It is recommended that extended arch repair be reserved for infants with arch indices of less than .25.

▶ This important paper addresses the major question of the growth potential of a hypoplastic transverse aortic arch. This question is especially pertinent, with the recommendation by some groups of performing extensive resection of the transverse hypoplastic arch at the time of repair of coarctation.

In this retrospective analysis of 120 children younger than 12 months at the time of operation, 32% had a hypoplastic arch, defined as an aortic arch index of less than .5. Also, 82% of this group had major associated cardiac anomalies, perhaps constituting a major contributing factor to underdevelopment of the aortic arch. Nonetheless, on late follow-up, satisfactory growth of the aortic arch was found in all 18 patients available for study, with a mean postrepair index of .7. The authors further emphasize that not a single patient was seen in whom moderate hypoplasia of the transverse aortic arch was associated with a significant postoperative arm-leg pressure gradient. The recommendation was made that extensive resection of the aortic arch be confined to a severe degree of hypoplasia, i.e., a ratio of .25 or less.—F.C. Spencer, M.D.

15 Valvular Heart Disease

The Pericardial Valve in the Aortic Position Ten Years Later

Gonzalez-Lavin L, Gonzalez-Lavin J, Chi S, Lewis B, Amini S, Graf D (Robert Wood Johnson Univ Hosp, New Brunswick, NJ; Ingham Med Ctr, East Lansing, Mich)
J Thorac Cardiovasc Surg 101:75–80, 1991
15–1

Introduction.—The Ionescu-Shiley bovine pericardial valve (ISBPV) was the initial prototype of its kind. It was removed from the market, but experience gained in the past decade might provide important information now that second-generation pericardial valves are available.

Methods.—Aortic valve replacement was performed with the standard ISBPV in 240 patients (mean age, 62.5 years) in 1977–1983. Aortic stenosis was the predominant aortic valve defect. Nearly half of the patients had concomitant procedures, most often for ischemic heart disease. The mean follow-up was 5 years 2 months.

Results.—Late mortality in the 224 hospital survivors was 28%, and the rate of cardiac-related death was 16.5%; 9 deaths (4%) were valve related, 7 of which deaths were caused by infective valve dysfunction. Risk factors for late death included age older than 60 years, more severe cardiac dysfunction, infective endocarditis, and concomitant surgery. The rate of thrombotic events was 1.2% per patient-year of follow-up, and that of intrinsic tissue failure, 2.4% per patient-year. Thirteen patients had prosthetic valve endocarditis, and paravalvular leaks developed in 2. The rate of death and/or reoperation attributable to valve-related events was 3.6% per patient-year, the risk increasing markedly after 80 months.

Conclusion.—The ISBPV provides good hemodynamics and only infrequently causes thromboembolism, but its durability is limited. Elimination of calcific degeneration is the most important goal in developing new pericardial valves for use in the aortic position.

▶ This short report well documents the importance of a 10-year follow-up of new valve prostheses. Pericardial valves are similar to the fascia lata valves of years ago in that early results were encouraging and led to wide use of the prosthesis. This report well documents the poor results in 240 patients 10 years after insertion of a pericardial aortic prosthesis. Although thromboembolism was rare, there was an exponential rise in the frequency of valve deterioration more than 7 years after operation.—F.C. Spencer, M.D.

Management of Aortic Insufficiency in Chronic Aortic Dissection

Pêgo-Fernandes PM, Stolf NAG, Moreira LFP, Pereira Barreto AC, Bittencourt D, Jatene AD (Univ of São Paulo Med School, Brazil)
Ann Thorac Surg 51:438–442, 1991   15–2

Background.—In chronic aortic dissection with valvular insufficiency there has been a tendency to replace the valve, but in recent years aortic valve preservation has been preferred.

Patients.—Aortic insufficiency was present in 44 of 62 patients with chronic aortic dissection who were treated surgically between 1980 and 1988. Seventy percent of the patients had a type I dissection. In 41 patients the proximal aorta was substituted, whereas in 3 patients aortoplasty with a patch was performed. In 48% of the patients the aortic valve was preserved by commissural resuspension. Twenty-three patients underwent valve replacement.

Results.—The 37 operative survivors were followed for a mean of 18 months. Only 2 patients with a preserved aortic valve had mild aortic insufficiency. Two had persistent dissection at the descending aorta without clinical sequelae. Those patients who had valvoplastic surgery had higher survival rates than those who underwent valve replacement; however, the difference was not significant. All 7 patients with Marfan's syndrome had valve replacement.

Conclusions.—Valve resuspension is a satisfactory procedure in patients with chronic aortic dissection who have evidence of aortic insufficiency. Autoplastic surgery should be avoided because of the high risk of redissection.

▶ In most centers attempts are made to preserve the aortic valve with acute dissection, but usually the aortic valve is replaced in chronic aortic dissections with aortic insufficiency—hence the importance of this report from the Heart Institute in São Paolo, Brazil, by Jatene and associates. Among 44 patients with chronic aortic dissection and aortic insufficiency who were operated on, it was possible to preserve the aortic valve in nearly half (48%). The valve was removed routinely in patients with Marfan's syndrome or annuloaortic ectasia.

The authors emphasize that determining the mechanism of aortic insufficiency is important in reaching a decision. Techniques of valvular reconstruction are only briefly described but included primarily resuspension of the leaflets, similar to that used with acute dissection. Let's hope that this encouraging trend to lessen the frequency of prosthetic replacement can be duplicated by others.—F.C. Spencer, M.D.

Reoperation for Persistent Outflow Obstruction in Hypertrophic Cardiomyopathy

Roberts CS, McIntosh CL, Brown PS Jr, Cannon RO III, Gertz SD, Clark RE

(Natl Heart, Lung, and Blood Inst, Bethesda, Md)

Ann Thorac Surg 51:455–460, 1991   15–3

Background.—Hypertrophic cardiomyopathy has been treated operatively since 1958. Of 535 patients so treated at the National Heart, Lung, and Blood Institute, 23 required reoperation for persistent left ventricular outflow obstruction. Twelve had a second left ventricular myotomy and myectomy (M+M) and 11 had mitral valve replacement (MVR). Results of these 2 procedures at reoperation were compared.

Methods.—The clinical records of patients were reviewed, and patients were contacted by telephone to update the records. Seven of the M+M patients had the initial procedure performed at another institution.

Outcome.—The M+M group was significantly younger at the initial operation, had a longer interval between operations, and remained significantly younger at reoperation. At 6 months, the 2 groups had similar improvements in mean functional class, cardiac index, and left ventricular outflow gradient at rest. Outflow gradients with provocation, however, were 57 mm Hg in the M+M group and 14 mm Hg in the MVR group. The average follow-up periods were 5.9 years in the M+M group and 3.4 years in the MVR group. The 3-year actuarial survival was 83% in the M+M group and 92% in the MVR group. Five-year survivals were 76% and 77%, respectively.

Conclusions.—Both procedures effectively relieve hemodynamic obstruction and reduce symptoms; however, because it avoids the complications of anticoagulation and substitute valves, M+M is preferred. Inadequate length or depth of the M+M trough may result in persistent left ventricular outflow obstruction.

▶ This significant report from the National Institutes of Health analyzes 23 patients undergoing reoperation for left ventricular outflow obstruction. At this institution, more than 500 operations have been performed since 1959 for hypertrophic cardiomyopathy. Of the 23 patients undergoing a repeat operation, 11 had mitral valve replacement and 12 had a second myocardial resection. Seven of the latter 12 had their initial operation performed elsewhere.

The follow-up averaged 4–6 years after the second operation. Results were quite similar, indicating that a second myocardial resection is preferable to avoid the complications of anticoagulation with prosthetic valves.

The authors briefly mention the current use of intraoperative echocardiography to confirm the adequacy of the myocardial resection. Key characteristics of an adequate resection are the length, depth, and location. Extending the trough of the resection far enough apically is especially crucial.—F.C. Spencer, M.D.

Mitral Valve Repair in the Extensively Calcified Mitral Valve Annulus
El Asmar B, Acker M, Couetil JP, Perier P, Dervanian P, Chauvaud S, Carpentier A (Hôpital Broussais, Paris)
Ann Thorac Surg 52:66–69, 1991   15–4

Background.—Mitral valve repair is not performed on patients with a heavily calcified mitral annulus because of the increased risk of ventricular rupture. However, mitral valve replacement is also a risky procedure. Extensive decalcification of the annulus was performed before mitral valve repair in 12 patients. All patients had a calcified bloc in the posterior of the mitral annulus, which extended further in some of them.

Technique.—The type of mitral disease and the degree and location of the calcification are analyzed. Decalcification of the annulus is initiated by incision of the ventricular endothelium around the borders of the calcified bar. Scissors are used to excise the calcium (Fig 15–1). After removal of the calcium, interrupted mattress sutures are used to close the trench created by the decalcification. The posterior leaflet is then reattached (Fig 15–2). After annular reconstruction, other lesions are repaired.

Results.—There were no thromboembolic events, need for reoperations, or deaths. All patients are currently in New York Heart Association class I or II.

Conclusion.—Mitral valve repair can be performed successfully on patients with an extensively calcified mitral annulus, avoiding the risks associated with mitral valve replacement.

▶ The key basis for mitral valve reconstruction is the ability to excise more than 50% of the annulus of the mural leaflet, followed by annuloplasty and valve reconstruction. The valve resection-annuloplasty technique is dependent on a pliable annulus in the mural leaflet. Hence extensive calcification is

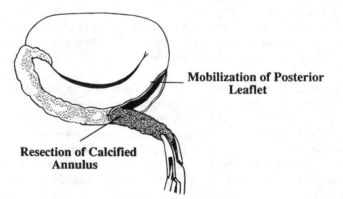

Fig 15–1.—Mobilization of posterior leaflet and decalcification of annulus. (Courtesy of El Asmar B, Acker M, Couetil JP, et al: *Ann Thorac Surg* 52:66–69, 1991.)

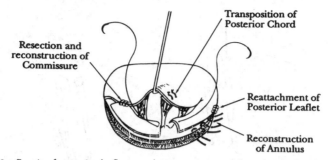

Fig 15–2.—Repair of posterior leaflet, annulus, commissure, and anterior leaflet. (Courtesy of El Asmar B, Acker M, Couetil JP, et al: *Ann Thorac Surg* 52:66–69, 1991.)

often considered a contraindication to reconstruction. This short report from Carpentier's group in Paris, where many of the techniques for mitral valve reconstruction originated, describes successful results with radical calcium débridement of the annulus of the mural leaflet in 12 patients. At my institution, selective excision of calcium has been performed in a number of patients, after which reconstruction was possible, although the extensive decalcification method described by Carpentier has not been utilized. Knowing that such extensive débridement is possible and safe will, we hope, encourage others to evaluate this novel approach.—F.C. Spencer, M.D.

Mitral Valve Repair by Replacement of Chordae Tendineae With Polytetrafluoroethylene Sutures

David TE, Bos J, Rakowski H (Univ of Toronto; Toronto Hosp)
J Thorac Cardiovasc Surg 101:495–501, 1991   15–5

Background.—Mitral valve incompetence resulting from prolapse of the anterior leaflet or of both leaflets may be difficult or impossible to repair because of inadequate chordal tissue. Thickened and calcified chordae may cause a similar problem in patients with advanced rheumatic mitral valve disease. A 5-year experience in the use of chordal replacement with expanded polytetrafluoroethylene (PTFE) sutures was reviewed.

Patients.—The series included 43 patients (28 men and 15 women) whose mean age was 55 years. Thirty patients had degenerative and 11 had rheumatic mitral valve disease; 2 had ischemic mitral regurgitation. Most patients were in New York Heart Association (NYHA) class III or IV.

Technique.—The technique involves passing a double-armed PTFE suture twice through the fibrous part of the papillary muscle and tying it down. Suture arms are then brought up to the free margin of the leaflet and passed through the attachment of the native chorda, the lengths of the 2 arms are adjusted, and the ends tied together on the ventricular side of the leaflet. A 5-0 suture is used

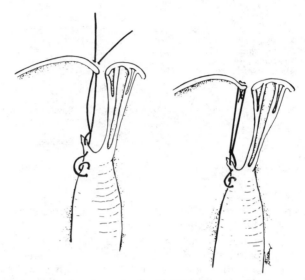

Fig 15–3.—Replacement of a primary chorda with 5-0 PTFE suture. The 2 arms of the suture are placed in the same area of the leaflet. (Courtesy of David TE, Bos J, Rakowski H: *J Thorac Cardiovasc Surg* 101:495–501, 1991.)

for replacement of a single chorda (Fig 15–3) and a 4-0 suture for prolapse of a wider segment of anterior leaflet or for replacement of 2 adjacent chordae (Fig 15–4).

Results.—No patient died perioperatively. At a mean follow-up of 13 months, most patients had normal mitral valve function, as shown by Doppler echocardiography. The operation failed in 2 patients, 1 with acute mitral regurgitation and 1 with hemolysis. Two patients with degenerative disease died 14 months and 22 months postoperatively, 1 of myocardial infarction and the other of a ruptured cerebral aneurysm. Thirty-one of 39 survivors were in NYHA class I and 8 were in class II.

Conclusions.—Suture replacement of chordae tendineae is a simple procedure that allows reconstruction rather than replacement of the mitral valve. It is especially valuable for patients with degenerative disease and prolapse of both the anterior and posterior leaflets. Long-term follow-up studies are needed.

▶ Reconstruction, rather than replacement, of mitral valves with ruptured chordae tendineae is now frequently performed—in more than 90% of cases in my institution. Repair can be particularly complicated with rupture of chordae to the anterior leaflet. Hence long-term results with this preliminary technique reported by Dr. David and associates will be especially significant. The short-term data are excellent. Forty-three patients have been operated on, with reconstruction of the chordae using 4-0 or 5-0 PTFE sutures (Gortex).

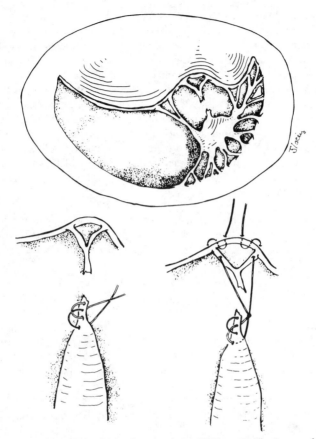

Fig 15–4.—Replacement of chordae tendineae with 4-0 PTFE suture. The 2 arms of the suture are placed in separate but adjacent areas of the leaflet. (Courtesy of David TE, Bos J, Rakowski H: *J Thorac Cardiovasc Surg* 101:495–501, 1991.)

There were no operative deaths and only 2 failures requiring mitral valve replacement.—F.C. Spencer, M.D.

Repair of Flail Anterior Leaflets of Tricuspid and Mitral Valves by Cusp Remodeling
Sutlic Z, Schmid C, Borst HG (Hannover Med School, Germany)
Ann Thorac Surg 50:927–930, 1990   15–6

Background.—Several pathologic conditions may result in chordae tendineae rupture. An alternative approach to this problem was used in 2 patients, 1 with tricuspid trauma and 1 with mitral valve bacterial endocarditis.

Case Report.—Man, 30, had several attacks of leg edema and dyspnea in a 3-year period. Exercise tolerance had progressively decreased, and he could walk up only 10 stairs. As a child he had sustained minor thoracic trauma after falling out a window. He had a grade 3/6 systolic murmur over the left sternal border in the fifth intercostal space, massive enlargement of the right atrium and ventricle was seen on chest radiographs. Severe tricuspid insufficiency was noted on 2-dimensional echocardiography. At total cardiopulmonary bypass, a greatly enlarged tricuspid annulus was seen with tearing of the caudal two thirds of the chordae of the anterior leaflet and rupture of the chordae of the posterior leaflet. Flail portions of both leaflets were resected, the cut edges were united by a running 5-0 suture, and the annulus segment without leaflets was plicated. A tricuspid valve orifice measuring 3 cm² was achieved. The patient regained full exercise tolerance.

Conclusions.—An alternative treatment method was used for extensive chordae tendineae rupture with flail anterior leaflets. Maximal use of the remaining leaflets and their chordal support provided an adequate valve orifice.

▶ This short report from Germany describes significant experiences in 4 patients who had unusual defects in the mitral or tricuspid valves resulting from either endocarditis or trauma. An alternative form of resection of the diseased cusp tissue, followed by mobilization of the remaining leaflets with subsequent suture repair, was used. These techniques produced a competent valve, avoiding prosthetic replacement.—F.C. Spencer, M.D.

Tricuspid Valve Repair for Tricuspid Valve Endocarditis: Tricuspid Valve "Recycling"
Allen MD, Slachman F, Eddy AC, Cohen D, Otto CM, Pearlman AS (Univ of Washington)
Ann Thorac Surg 51:593–598, 1991   15–7

Background.—The traditional operations for tricuspid valve endocarditis are excision or replacement of the diseased valve. Many patients who have excision ultimately need replacement, which necessitates implantation of foreign material in an infected field. To avoid this problem, a program of tricuspid valve repair, applying the principles of mitral valve repair, was initiated.

Patients and Methods.—Four patients were treated—2 intravenous drug abusers and 2 patients with recent dental abscesses. All had recurrent septic emboli. Preoperative echocardioghoraphy showed 3 to 4+ tricuspid regurgitation with evidence of progressive right ventricular enlargement and mobile vegetations. Intraoperatively, all patients had involvement of the anterior leaflet, free margin, and associated chordae and papillary muscles extending up to the annulus. The surgeons used monofilament sutures and pledgets constructed of pericardium. After

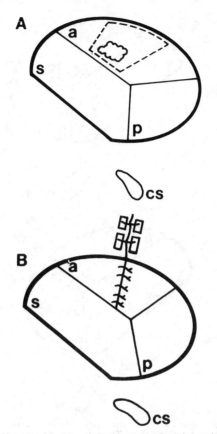

Fig 15–5.—A, one half to three fourths of the anterior leaflet of the tricuspid valve and attached chordae were excised with a quadrangular resection. **B,** an annuloplasty was performed with pericardial pledgets. The leaflet margins were approximated with 5-0 Prolene suture. *a* indicates anterior leaflet; *cs,* coronary sinus; *p,* posterior leaflet; *s,* septal leaflet. (Courtesy of Allen MD, Slachman F, Eddy AC, et al: *Ann Thorac Surg* 51:593–598, 1991.)

excision of leaflet and chordae, leaflet margins were approximated with 5-0 Prolene suture (Fig 15–5). In 1 patient, the leaflet could not be closed, and the anterior and posterior halves had to be sutured after annular plication, resulting in a bicuspid valve (Fig 15–6). In the most recent patient, a new anterior leaflet was constructed of pericardium, and basilar chordae were mobilized to form new papillary muscles.

Outcome.—Postoperative echocardiography showed reduction of tricuspid regurgitation and right ventricular dimensions in 2 patients despite the loss of leaflet tissue. The other 2 patients were left with only mild dilation. Valve tissue specimens all showed bacteria on Gram stain or culture, but all of the repaired valves were successfully sterilized. There were no recurrent infections.

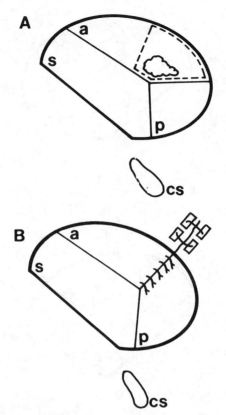

Fig 15–6.—A, the posterior half of the anterior leaflet of the tricuspid valve was excised with involved chordae. **B,** annuloplasty was performed. The remaining anterior leaflet was sutured to the intact posterior leaflet. (Abbreviations as in previous figure.) (Courtesy of Allen MD, Slachman F, Eddy AC, et al: *Ann Thorac Surg* 51:593–598, 1991.)

Conclusions.—In patients with complicated tricuspid valve endocarditis, the valves can be repaired to allow eradication of the infection and possible improvement in valve function. Excision of vegetations alone may be successful in most patients if performed early. Other reported procedures have included chordal transposition, reconstructive valvuloplasty, and Carpentier ring annuloplasty.

▶ This intriguing paper describes reasonably good results in 4 patients with tricuspid valve endocarditis limited to the anterior leaflet. Different combinations of anterior leaflet resection and reconstruction were performed. Significant regurgitation remained in 3 of the 4 patients.

Selected reports by others are described in the paper. The cumulative data seem clear that some method of tricuspid valve reconstruction may be applied safely in patients with endocarditis limited to the leaflet. Probably, the concomitant use of a Carpentier ring to stabilize the annulus would minimize late recurrence. This was avoided by the authors because of the risk of infection, but long-term data following standard Carpentier ring reconstructions uniformly show that the risk of endocarditis is very small—less than 1%.—F.C. Spencer, M.D.

16 Coronary Artery Disease

Ten-Year Follow-Up of Quality of Life in Patients Randomized to Receive Medical Therapy or Coronary Artery Bypass Graft Surgery: The Coronary Artery Surgery Study (CASS)
Rogers WJ, Coggin CJ, Gersh BJ, Fisher LD, Myers WO, Oberman A, Sheffield LT, for the CASS Investigators (Davis K, Univ of Washington)
Circulation 82:1647–1658, 1990   16–1

Introduction.—Little information is available about long-term effects of coronary artery bypass graft surgery in terms of patient quality of life.

Methods.—Data on quality of life for 780 patients in the Coronary Artery Surgery Study were examined 10 years after the patients were randomized to medical or operative management. Ten-year mortalities were 22% in the medical group and 19% in the surgical group. Thirty-seven percent of patients randomized to medical care had undergone operation because of progressive chest pain. The mean follow-up was 11 years.

Outcome.—After 1 year, 66% of surgical patients and 30% of the medical group were asymptomatic. The respective figures at 5 years were 63% and 38%. At 10 years, 47% of surgical patients and 42% of the medical group were free of angina. Surgical patients were less limited in their activities and used less β-blocker and nitrate medication than did medical patients at 1 year and 5 years. The groups did not differ significantly with respect to employment or recreational status, the frequency of nonprotocol hospitalization, or heart failure.

Discussion.—The marked improvement in quality of life for surgical patients observed in the first 5 years is much less evident after 10 years. Patients with normal left ventricular function can be managed medically at the outset if bypass is offered when angina worsens. More than one third of such patients will require revascularization in the first decade of follow-up.

▶ A 10-year follow-up in the Coronary Artery Surgery Study of 780 patients initially randomized to medical or surgical therapy was done. Initially, quality of life was substantially better in the surgical group, but 10 years later the differences were less. Forty-seven percent of the surgical patients were free of angina as opposed to 42% of the medical group. Use of antianginal medications was similar. Other indices of quality of life (e.g., increase in activity) also were similar. These similarities reflect the return of symptoms in the surgical group to some extent, but also the performance of late surgery in a significant portion of those initially assigned to medical therapy.—F.C. Spencer, M.D.

Ten-Year Follow-Up of Survival and Myocardial Infarction in the Randomized Coronary Artery Surgery Study
Alderman EL, Bourassa MG, Cohen LS, Davis KB, Kaiser GG, Killip T, Mock MB, Pettinger M, Robertson TL, for the CASS Investigators (Davis K, Univ of Washington)
Circulation 82:1629–1646, 1990   16–2

Introduction.—The Coronary Artery Surgery Study is designed to assess the effect of coronary bypass surgery on mortality and selected nonfatal end points.

Methods.—A total of 780 patients in the study were randomized to coronary artery surgery or medical management. Nearly all of the patients randomized to coronary surgery received vein grafts, and 16% received internal mammary artery grafts.

Results.—Of the patients randomized to medical care, 6% were operated on within 6 months and 40% by 10 years. Cumulative survival at 10 years was 79% in the medical group and 82% in the surgical group, not a significant difference. There also was no significant difference in the rates of nonfatal myocardial infarction. Patients with an ejection fraction of less than .5 did better with initial operative treatment, whereas the others appeared to do better if randomized to medical treatment with respect to the proportion free of death and the risk of infarction. Adjusting for heart failure, age, hypertension, and extent of coronary disease failed to reveal significant differences in survival or freedom from myocardial infarction.

Conclusion.—Patients with mild stable angina and normal left ventricular function have a comparable course whether treated medically, with an option for surgery if symptoms progress, or by initial surgery.

▶ This is a 10-year follow-up of the Coronary Artery Surgical Study that initially randomized 780 patients to either coronary surgery or medical therapy. Ten years later there is no significant difference in survival—82% vs. 79%. As the authors indicate, however, patients who were initially treated medically promptly had surgery if symptoms developed. Forty percent of the group had surgery within 10 years.

The data also reaffirm that patients with an ejection fraction of less than .50 did substantially better with initial surgical therapy. Long-term survival was 79% with surgery and 61% with medical therapy.—F.C. Spencer, M.D.

Bilateral Internal Mammary Artery Grafts in Reoperative and Primary Coronary Bypass Surgery
Galbut DL, Traad EA, Dorman MJ, DeWitt PL, Larsen PB, Kurlansky PA, Button JH, Ally JM, Gentsch TO (Miami Heart Inst)
Ann Thorac Surg 52:20–28, 1991   16–3

Background.—The established technique for myocardial revascularization is bilateral internal mammary artery (IMA) grafting. There are few data, however, on the use of bilateral IMA grafts in coronary bypass reoperation. Data were reviewed on 88 such patients, to assess the operative risk and long-term benefits.

Patients and Methods.—The 77 men and 11 women, (mean age, 62 years) had reoperation for myocardial revascularization with bilateral IMA and supplemental vein grafts over a 7½-year period. For comparative purposes, the results of a subset of 88 patients who had primary revascularization with bilateral IMA grafts were also analyzed. These groups were matched for age, sex, left ventricular function, angina, and left main coronary artery disease. There was unstable angina in 62.5% and reduced ejection fraction in 43.2% of each group. Left main coronary artery disease was present in 21% of the reoperation group and 20.5% of the primary operation group. Twenty-five percent of patients reoperated on required preoperative intra-aortic balloon support.

Findings.—Hospital mortality was 6.8% in the reoperation group and 3.4% in the primary operation group. In each group the intra-aortic balloon pump was used after operation in 1.1%. The 2 groups showed no difference in the incidence of sternal infection or perioperative myocardial infarction. However, 13.6% of the reoperation group had respiratory insufficiency vs. 3.4% of the reference group (table). Approximately

	Comparison of Operative Results by Patient Group		
Variable	Reoperation group	Reference group	*p* Value
Reoperation for bleeding	5 (5.7)	4 (4.5)	NS
Sternal infection	3 (3.4)	2 (2.3)	NS
Respiratory failure	12 (13.6)	3 (3.4)	<0.015
Perioperative myocardial infarction	7 (8.0)	2 (2.3)	NS
Stroke	3 (3.4)	1 (1.1)	NS
Mechanical support (IABP)	31 (35.2)	13 (14.8)	<0.001
Mean hospitalization (days)	16.9 ± 18.5	12.5 ± 5.6	<0.038

Abbreviations: IABP, intra-aortic balloon pump; NS, not significant.
NOTE: Numbers in parentheses are percentages.
(Courtesy of Galbut DL, Traad EA, Dorman MJ, et al: *Ann Thorac Surg* 52:20–28, 1991.)

13.5% of the patients in each group had recurrent angina. The reoperation group had a long-term survival (5 years) of 85.3% vs. 91.6% for the reference group. Equality of survival distribution was not significantly different for the 2 groups.

Conclusions.—Bilateral IMA grafting carries an acceptable operative risk in patients who undergo reoperation. Long-term survival and functional improvement are similar to those in patients who have their first revascularization. This appears to be the technique of choice for patients who have reoperation and may help to avoid the need for a third operation.

▶ This interesting report is from the Miami group who have had extensive experience with bilateral IMA grafting for more than a decade. Performing bilateral IMA grafts as a repeat operation would seem surely to increase operative morbidity because of the number of complications associated with re-operation, however it is performed. This report described experiences with 88 patients operated on in a period of 7 years, clearly a select group of about 1 patient per month. It is significant that the intra-aortic balloon pump was used before operation in more than 20% of patients and only 1% post-operatively. There was a higher frequency of respiratory failure, 13%, as well as perioperative infarction, 8%, with an overall mortality of 7%. Hence it seems that undertaking bilateral IMA grafting at the time of reoperation should be done only with careful assessment of the frequency of associated complications.—F.C. Spencer, M.D.

Clinical Outcome of Single Versus Sequential Grafts in Coronary Bypass Operations at Ten Years' Follow-Up
Meeter K, Veldkamp R, Tijssen JGP, van Herwerden LL, Bos E (Erasmus Univ, Rotterdam)
J Thorac Cardiovasc Surg 101:1076–1081, 1991   16–4

Background.—The internal mammary artery implant is generally thought to be a better bypass conduit than the saphenous vein, but the vein is still often used for various reasons. The long-term results in patients treated with sequential and single vein grafts were investigated.

Patients.—The outcome of 234 patients with single venous grafts (group I) was compared with that of 234 patients who had predominantly sequential grafts (group II). All patients had angina pectoris before surgery and had 3-vessel or left main stem coronary artery disease. The patients underwent their operations from 1975 to 1980. The mean follow-up was 10.5 years, ranging from 8.5 to 13.6 years.

Outcomes.—Perioperative mortalities were 3% in group I and 1% in group II; the difference was not significant. The 5-year survival probabilities were 90% for group I and 88% for group II. At 10 years they were 71% and 72%, respectively. Multivariate analysis identified no risk difference related to graft type. The group II vs. group I hazard ratio was .82. An increased risk with depressed left ventricular function was observed. An age of 60 years or more also carried an increased risk.

Conclusions.—The technique of sequential grafting with the reversed saphenous vein is easier than the single grafting technique and produces comparable long-term results. If mammary artery implantation is not possible, or if an addition to the arterial bypass is needed, the sequential venous graft with 1 anastomosis on the aorta and peripheral anastomoses on the remaining graftable coronary arteries may be useful.

▶ This report from The Netherlands compares clinical results 10 years after operation between 234 patients with single grafts vs. 234 with sequential grafts. Both early and long-term results are strikingly similar with a 5-year survival of 90% vs. 88% and a 10-year survival of 71% vs. 72%. Late angiograms were not performed. However, the clinical data indicate that the sequential technique is certainly not inferior to the single graft technique and may be particularly valuable when multiple anastomoses are necessary or satisfactory venous conduits are limited.—F.C. Spencer, M.D.

Does Use of Gastroepiploic Artery Graft Increase Surgical Risk?
Suma H, Wanibuchi Y, Furuta S, Takeuchi A (Mitsui Mem Hosp, Tokyo; Osaka Med College, Japan)
J Thorac Cardiovasc Surg 101:121–125, 1991   16–5

Introduction.—The right gastroepiploic artery (GEA) is a viable alternative graft to the internal mammary artery in coronary artery bypass grafting (CABG). However, there is still some concern about the additional risk associated with laparotomy. Whether use of the GEA graft increases the perioperative risk in patients undergoing CABG was determined.

Patients and Methods.—During a 3-year period, 10 women and 60 men (mean age, 56.8 years) underwent nonurgent CABG with the GEA graft; 15 women and 55 men (mean age, 61.8 years) had nonurgent CABG without the GEA graft. All patients were operated on by the same surgeon, who used essentially the same technique in all of them. Sixty-eight patients (97%) having GEA grafts and 61 patients (87%) not having a GEA graft also received an internal mammary artery graft. A saphenous vein graft was also used in 39 patients (56%) having a GEA graft and in 66 of the others (94%). The patients treated with the GEA graft were significantly younger than the other patients, but all other preoperative parameters were similar. In 5 patients, gastric mucosal blood flow was measured before and after division of the GEA by endoscopic laser Doppler velocimetry. Forty-six patients having a GEA graft and 42 patients not having this graft underwent postoperative angiography within 6 months after operation.

Results.—There were 2 early deaths (2.9%) and 1 late death (1.4%) among patients treated with a GEA graft and 2 early deaths (2.9%) and 2 late deaths (2.9%) in the other group. Two patients in each group had new Q-wave infarction. Five patients with a GEA graft and 3 without the GEA graft required intra-aortic balloon pumping. Major postoperative complications were similar and rare. Postoperative angiography showed similar patency rates. Gastric mucosal blood flow as measured intraoperatively by laser Doppler velocimetry in 5 patients with a GEA graft showed no reduction of blood flow after division of the GEA. Previous cholecystectomy was not a contraindication to GEA grafting.

Conclusion.—Use of the GEA graft is safe and does not increase the perioperative risk. The right GEA graft also can be used safely in patients with associated disease requiring a combined operation.

▶ This short report compares mortality and morbidity in 70 patients in whom the GEA was used with 70 other patients undergoing bypass. There were no significant differences in outcome. This report reflects the continuing search for alternative arterial conduits. It is encouraging that the increased surgical dissection, combined with opening the abdomen, did not significantly influence operative complications.—F.C. Spencer, M.D.

Technique for Use of the Inferior Epigastric Artery as a Coronary Bypass Graft
Mills NL, Everson CT (Cardiology Ctr, New Orleans)
Ann Thorac Surg 51:208–214, 1991   16–6

Background.—Late patency of the saphenous vein graft is less than that of arterial grafts, prompting use of the inferior epigastric artery (IEA) as a coronary arterial bypass graft.

Technique.—A paramedian incision is made to harvest the IEA, stopping about 5 cm above the level of the inguinal ligament (Fig 16–1). The posterior peritoneal branches are ligated adjacent to the IEA; electrocautery serves to free interdigitations of the rectus muscle from its sheath (Fig 16–2). The IEA is harvested as a pedicle with its 2 accompanying veins (Figs 16–3 and 16–4). Finally, the vessel is dissected to its origin and suture-ligated. If the artery follows a lateral path, exposure is facilitated by dissecting the lateral border of the rectus muscle (Fig 16–5). Distal anastomoses are sutured using a S-1 to 6-mm coronary arteriotomy and 8-0 polypropylene suture material, starting at the heel of the graft and proceeding circumferentially around the toe; both ends end in the midportion of the arteriotomy. The proximal anastomoses are made either to the ascending aorta, or end-to-side to an internal mammary artery or saphenous vein graft. The IEA-internal mammary proximal anastomoses may be made before cardiopulmonary bypass is instituted.

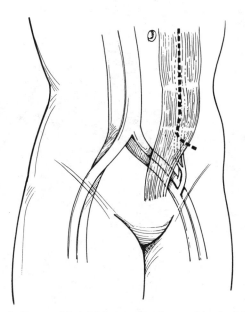

Fig 16–1.—Incision for harvest of the left inferior epigastric artery is made slightly lateral to the midline of the rectus muscle and is angled toward the femoral vessels. The incision stops well above the femoral crease. (Courtesy of Mills NL, Everson CT: *Ann Thorac Surg* 51:208–214, 1991.)

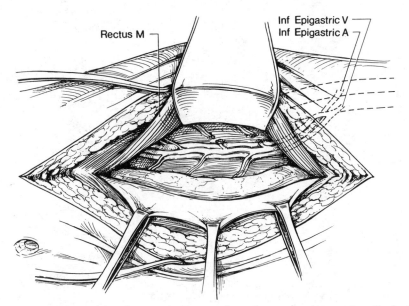

Fig 16–2.—Harvest of the inferior epigastric artery is begun by retracting the rectus laterally after its fascia is opened directly anterior for the length of the incision. Undue traction on the rectus muscle (M) at this point can avulse penetrating branches. *Abbreviations: A,* artery; *Inf,* inferior; V, vein. (Courtesy of Mills NL, Everson CT: *Ann Thorac Surg* 51:208–214, 1991.)

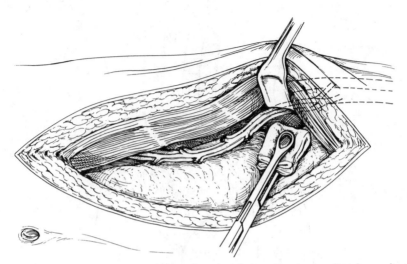

Fig 16–3.—Dissection is first carried inferiorly as the inferior epigastric artery branches are ligated and divided. Traction with a sponge-stick on the peritoneal tissues enhances exposure. (Courtesy of Mills NL, Everson CT: *Ann Thorac Surg* 51:208–214, 1991.)

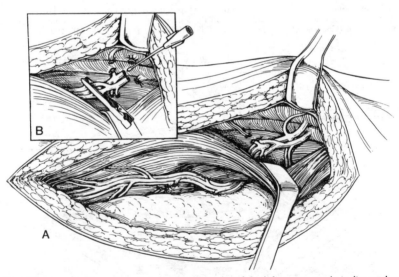

Fig 16–4.—**A,** to facilitate dissection, the lateral border of the left rectus muscle is dissected away from its fascia for 4–5 cm. The origin of the inferior epigastric artery is exposed through this approach. **B,** the external spermatic artery and the pubic branch of the inferior epigastric artery are ligated as well as the inferior epigastric vein. The inferior epigastric artery itself is ligated at its origin, and after a 2-mm soft, plastic olive-tip needle is tied in place, the graft is withdrawn from under the rectus muscle. (Courtesy of Mills NL, Everson CT: *Ann Thorac Surg* 51:208–214, 1991.)

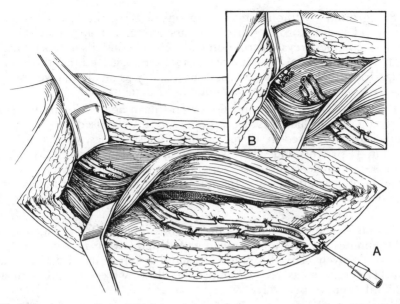

Fig 16–5.—**A,** in some instances, it is necessary to enhance exposure superiorly by separating the rectus muscle from its lateral attachment for a 4 to 5-cm distance. It is then retracted medially. **B,** the upper end of the inferior epigastric artery is divided and ligated to complete harvest of the graft. (Courtesy of Mills NL, Everson CT: *Ann Thorac Surg* 51:208-214, 1991.)

Clinical Experience.—Eighteen patients had IEA grafts made to 19 coronary arteries. Graft length ranged from 11.5 cm to 17 cm. No deaths occurred during follow-up for 1–18 months. There was 1 late wound infection before the routine use of Jackson-Pratt drains. No hernias resulted from the dissection, and there was no evidence of rectus muscle necrosis. Three postoperative angiograms demonstrated widely patent IEA grafts within 10 days of surgery.

▶ The fact that the patency rate in internal mammary grafts is well over 90% 10 years after operation, with no signs of late deterioration, has intensified the search for other arterial conduits. This preliminary report describes the use of the inferior epigastric artery in 18 patients. The illustrations of the technique are excellent. Short-term results are good, but as with all new conduits, the key question is the patency rate at 1–5 years after operation.—F.C. Spencer, M.D.

Use of the Inferior Epigastric Artery as a Free Graft for Myocardial Revascularization
Barner HB, Naunheim KS, Fiore AC, Fischer VW, Harris HH (St. Louis Univ)
Ann Thorac Surg 52:429–437, 1991   16–7

Background.—Although many surgeons now use the internal thoracic artery (ITA) for coronary artery bypass grafting, it is not possible to achieve complete revascularization with arterial conduits in most patients with 3-vessel disease. Preliminary reports have suggested that the internal epigastric artery (IEA) can be used successfully as an alternative conduit. The IEA was used as a bypass conduit in 47 patients.

Patients.—The 41 men and 6 women (mean age, 59 years) were undergoing myocardial revascularization. One IEA was used in 37 cases and both IEAs were used in 10 for 62 distal anastomoses. Both ITAs were used in 41 patients and 1 ITA was used in 6 patients for 100 distal anastomoses. A single saphenous vein graft was used in 5 patients. The total number of anastomoses was 167, or 3.55 per patient. A paramedian incision was used to harvest single IEA grafts and a midline incision for bilateral grafts.

Results.—The mean harvest time was 36.5 minutes for IEA grafts, and 29.6 minutes for ITA grafts; mean graft lengths were 11.9 cm and 16.5 cm, respectively. The IEA grafts measured 2 mm in distal diameter and the ITA grafts measured 2.1 mm; graft flows were 49.7 mL/min and 48.7 mL/min, respectively.

Segments of both types of grafts were examined microscopically in 14 patients. The internal elastic laminae were similar and fenestrations were equal in number. The 2 conduits had comparable combined intimal and medial thickness. The ITA grafts had more prominent medial elastic tissue, however, and this tissue was missing in 8 of 14 IEA grafts. Half of the IEA grafts contained gross plaque in the proximal 1–3 cm, but there was no luminal compromise and only minimal microscopic thickening. Surprisingly, medial calcifications without atherosclerosis were found in 2 of 14 IEAs. One patient died while hospitalized, another had an abdominal wound infection, and another had fat necrosis superficial to the sternum.

Conclusions.—The IEA appears to be a satisfactory conduit for myocardial revascularization. Operative morbidity is limited, and there have been no ischemic events after discharge; however, follow-up has been short. The durability of IEA grafts has yet to be established.

▶ This report from St Louis University describes experiences with inferior epigastric grafts in 47 patients; 10 were double grafts. Short-term results seem satisfactory, although no postoperative angiograms were done. Clearly, the technique can be applied when adequate venous conduits are not present. Until postoperative angiographic data are available, however, the approach should be considered an interesting experimental one, yet unproved.—F.C. Spencer, M.D.

Reduction of Myocardial Infarction After Emergency Coronary Artery Bypass Grafting for Failed Coronary Angioplasty With Use of a Normothermic Reperfusion Cardioplegia Protocol

Bottner RK, Wallace RB, Visner MS, Stark KS, Recientes E, Katz NM, Hopkins RA, Patrissi GA, Kent KM (Georgetown Univ Hosp)

J Thorac Cardiovasc Surg 101:1069–1075, 1991   16–8

Background.—Up to 13.5% of patients who have elective percutaneous transluminal coronary angioplasty require emergency coronary artery bypass grafting. Many of these patients sustain a myocardial infarction, and 18% to 46% of which result in new Q waves. A revised protocol based on research suggesting the use of normothermic cardioplegia to limit myocardial injury and necrosis was used for myocardial preservation in 19 patients.

Technique.—Patients who undergo emergency bypass grafting for failed angioplasty have induction of cardioplegia with a normothermic cardioplegia solution. Then, a 4° C blood cardioplegic solution is administered for 5 minutes, followed by additional doses into the aortic root every 20 minutes. After completion of each distal anastomosis, additional doses of cold solution are infused through the vein grafts. Rewarming is begun during completion of the last anastomosis.

Observations.—The 19 patients treated by the revised protocol were compared to 45 patients treated previously by induction and maintenance with cold solution and no reperfusion. Sixty-five percent of the group treated with cold cardioplegia had myocardial infarction, compared to 26% of the group that received normothermic cardioplegia. Patients who received cold cardioplegia had a median peak creatine kinase myocardial band level of 57 IU/L vs. 10 IU/L in the normothermic cardioplegia group; this suggests that the latter group had not only fewer but also smaller infarcts. Factors independently associated with the absence of infarction included use of the revised protocol, nontotal occlusion of the angioplasty vessel, and presence of collateral flow to the angioplasty vessel.

Conclusions.—In patients who undergo emergency coronary bypass grafting for failed angioplasty, normothermic induction, cold maintenance, and normothermic reperfusion of blood cardioplegia may reduce the incidence of myocardial infarction. Because of the nonrandomized and noncurrent nature of this study, however, a prospective, randomized trial should be done.

▶ The editor has long been intrigued by the uniformly high frequency of myocardial infarction after emergency bypass for failed angioplasty; the rates range from 10% to 50% in different reports. The possibility exists that some such infarctions are caused by embolization at the time of angioplasty and hence are irreversible.

The approach described in this report is based on the theory developed by Buckberg and associates who proposed normothermic induction of cardioplegia to restore substrait before proceeding with the operation, followed by normothermic reperfusion afterward. In this report the frequency of infarction decreased from 65% to 26%, but the authors emphasize that the study was both nonrandomized and nonconcurrent. Whatever the explanation, the data strongly suggest that the techniques of myocardial preservation may significantly influence the frequency of perioperative infarction. In the future, the new technique of continuous cardioplegia, now being evaluated in several centers, may be applicable to this type of clinical problem.—F.C. Spencer, M.D.

Starting Aspirin Therapy After Operation: Effects on Early Graft Patency

Goldman S, Copeland J, Moritz T, Henderson W, Zadina K, Ovitt T, Kern KB, Sethi G, Sharma GVRK, Khuri S, Richards K, Grover F, Morrison D, Whitman G, Chesler E, Sako Y, Pacold I, Montoya A, DeMots H, Floten S, Doherty J, Read R, Scott S, Spooner T, Masud Z, Haakenson C, Harker LA, and the Dept of Veterans Affairs Cooperative Study Group (VA Med Ctr, Tucson)
Circulation 84:520–526, 1991   16–9

Background.—Aspirin treatment before surgery improves vein graft patency after coronary artery bypass grafting. However, it also causes bleeding. The effects on early graft patency of aspirin therapy started before surgery were compared with those of aspirin therapy started 6 hours after surgery. The prospective, centrally directed, randomized, double-blind, placebo-controlled trial enrolled 489 men.

Methods.—Patients were assigned to receive aspirin, 325 mg, or placebo the night before surgery. After surgery, all patients received aspirin, 325 mg daily, the first dose being administered through the nasogastric tube 6 hours postoperatively. Angiography was done in 72% of patients a mean 8 days after surgery. The primary end point was saphenous vein graft patency in 351 patients. Internal mammary artery graft patency was assessed in 246 patients because many received both internal mammary artery and vein grafts.

Results.—Patients given aspirin before surgery had a vein graft occlusion rate of 7.4%, compared with 7.8% in those given placebo. Patients receiving Y grafts who were given aspirin preoperatively had no occlusions, compared with 7% of this subgroup given placebo. The internal mammary artery occlusion rate in the aspirin-treated group was 0% and in the placebo-treated group, 2.4%. Patients given aspirin needed more transfusions than those given placebo. The reoperation rate for bleeding was 6.3% in the aspirin-treated group and 2.4% in the group given placebo. The median chest tube drainage within the first 6 hours of operation in the 2 groups was 5 mL and 448 mL, respectively.

Conclusions.—Preoperative aspirin increases bleeding complications without improving early vein graft patency when compared with aspirin therapy begun 6 hours after surgery. A nonsignificant trend was noted toward improved early patency for Y grafts and internal mammary artery grafts when aspirin therapy was given before surgery.

▶ This extensive report describes the results of a multi-institutional study developed by the Veterans Administration. It addresses the significant question of whether preoperative aspirin, which admittedly increases the risk of bleeding during bypass, would significantly improve graft patency as compared to starting aspirin therapy 6 hours after operation, which is the standard approach.

As demonstrated in the original Mayo Clinic studies, there was a significant increase in the frequency of transfusions and reoperation rate for bleeding (6% vs. 2.4%) when aspirin was used. There was no major improvement in early vein graft patency, however, indicating that the benefit from preoperative aspirin is negligible and it clearly increases the frequency of bleeding.—F.C. Spencer, M.D.

Combined Myocardial Revascularization and Abdominal Aortic Aneurysm Repair
Hinkamp TJ, Pifarre R, Bakhos M, Blakeman B (Loyola Univ Med Ctr, Maywood, Ill)
Ann Thorac Surg 51:470–472, 1991   16–10

Introduction.—Late survival after repair of abdominal aortic aneurysm (AAA) appears to be affected directly by coronary artery disease. The myocardial stress of aneurysm repair may be heightened by coronary artery disease. The results of combined myocardial revascularization and AAA repair performed in hemodynamically stable patients during a 5-year period were reviewed.

Methods.—Of 128 patients who underwent elective or urgent AAA repair, 17 had a combined procedure after undergoing coronary angiography for coronary artery disease. Coronary artery disease was found at catheterization in 14 patients undergoing elective AAA repair, and 3 had increasing angina. Cardiopulmonary bypass with myocardial revascularization was performed through a median sternotomy, which was then extended for AAA repair. All patients were considered to be hemodynamically stable before abdominal surgery.

Results.—Complications included mediastinal bleeding, tension pneumothorax, and a small subendocardial myocardial infarction. Within 30 days, 1 patient died; the others were well at follow-up. Average transfusion requirements were 4 units of packed red blood cells and 1.7 units of fresh-frozen plasma; however, routine use of the Cell Saver significantly reduced the need for blood in the latter patients.

Conclusions.—In patients with serious coronary artery disease and AAA, both conditions can be treated safely in a single operation. The mortality of this procedure is 5.9%, and costs and hospitalization are decreased.

▶ This short report describes a seemingly radical approach to the problem of patients who have both significant coronary disease and AAA. It is well known that the major cause of death after AAA resection, both initially and in the next 5 years after operation, is myocardial infarction. At the editor's institution, such patients usually undergo myocardial revascularization, followed in 6–8 weeks by excision of the AAA. There are several reports, however, of fatal rupture of an AAA after different types of operative procedures. Hence this report describing combined coronary bypass grafting with excision of the AAA in 17 patients, only 1 of whom died, is of particular interest. The authors state that this combined procedure has been used frequently in the past 6 years. Perhaps other institutions can duplicate these impressive results.—F.C. Spencer, M.D.

Meralgia Paresthetica After Coronary Bypass Surgery
Parsonnet V, Karasakalides A, Gielchinsky I, Hochberg M, Hussain SM (Univ of Medicine and Dentristry of New Jersey; Newark Beth Israel Med Ctr; St Barnabas Med Ctr, Livingston, NJ)
J Thorac Cardiovasc Surg 101:219–221, 1991   16–11

Introduction.—Meralgia paresthetica is characterized by paresthesia and numbness of the anterolateral aspect of the thigh, and it involves the lateral femoral cutaneous nerve. In addition, meralgia paresthetica has been associated with hematoma and scar tissue formation in the inguinal canal, femoral catheterization, obesity, pregnancy, trauma, retroperitoneal tumors, and surgery that is remote from the lateral femoral cutaneous nerve. Three patients who experienced meralgia paresthetica after cardiac surgery were assessed.

Case Reports.—Man, 57, had symptoms of meralgia paresthetica in both thighs after 5-vessel coronary bypass surgery. The "frog-leg" position was not used in harvesting the grafts. Paresthesia persisted at follow-up 4 years later, however, it did not impede daily activities.

Man, 64, underwent triple bypass surgery using veins harvested from both thighs. The patient was in a modified frog-leg position. Full sensation returned 3 years later.

Man, 71, whose total pump time was 140 minutes, also had meralgia paresthetica, but normal sensation returned 30 months later.

Discussion.—Meralgia paresthetica is a rare complication of cardiac surgery that may be related to positioning of the lower extremities during graft harvesting. The disorder is benign and self-limited. Extreme and protracted positioning should be avoided unless absolutely necessary.

▶ This short report describes the unusual neurologic complication of meralgia paresthetica, which was observed in 3 patients. The report is particularly valuable for its follow-up; 1 patient had persistent numbness 4 years later, and the other 2 recovered within 2–3 years. The occurrence of this disorder in the 3 patients could not be related to any variation in surgical technique. This unusual problem may not be preventable; its development varies with the anatomical relationship of the lateral femoral cutaneous nerve and the size of the foramen through which it passes below the fascia lata. The editor has personally observed a similar complication in a few patients.

As the authors indicate, reassurance is all that is necessary, explaining the benign nature of the condition, but with the caution that in a few patients the numbness may be permanent.—F.C. Spencer, M.D.

17 Miscellaneous Cardiac Conditions and the Great Vessels

Discriminate Use of Electrocautery on the Median Sternotomy Incision: A 0.16% Wound Infection Rate
Nishida H, Grooters RK, Soltanzadeh H, Thieman KC, Schneider RF, Kim W-P
(Iowa Methodist Med Ctr, Des Moines)
J Thorac Cardiovasc Surg 101:488–494, 1991   17–1

Background.—Sternotomy infection and mediastinitis have been reported in up to 5% of patients who have undergone cardiac surgery. Studies in dogs suggest that extensive electrocautery of the presternal soft tissues may predispose to sternotomy infection.

Study Design.—The value of limiting electrocautery to pinpoint hemostasis in the sternotomy soft tissues was examined in 3,118 consecutive patients who underwent median sternotomy for cardiac surgery during a 2-year period. All of the patients lived for more than a week after surgery. The presternal soft tissues were divided with a scalpel, and electrocautery was reserved for pinpoint hemostasis.

Results.—Five patients (.16%) had mediastinal wound infection, and the incidence of deep mediastinitis was .13%. No patient required major sternal débridement or muscle flap reconstruction. The only factor related to sternotomy infection was an operating time exceeding 3 hours.

Conclusion.—The selective use of electrocautery during median sternotomy appears to limit the occurrence of wound infection in patients who undergo cardiac surgery.

▶ This report describes an astonishingly low frequency of mediastinitis in a series of 3,118 patients undergoing sternotomy in a period of 12 years. Only 5 patients, 0.16%, acquired an infection. The authors emphasize that this low infection rate is lower than those reported in 28 previously published studies. The electrocautery was used for pinpoint hemostasis only, the presternal tissues being divided with a scalpel.

An infection rate of 0.16% is clearly far lower than normally reported. The authors' hypothesis that this may reflect better preservation of the vascularity of the soft tissues is interesting, especially as the technique described on the sternum seems to be a standard one. The electrocautery was used as needed on the periosteum. Bone wax also was used. With widespread demonstration of the efficacy of muscle flaps for control of infection, the authors' technique of minimal use of the cautery in the anterior chest wall merits serious consideration.—F.C. Spencer, M.D.

Long-Term Results of Pectoralis Major Muscle Transposition for Infected Sternotomy Wounds

Pairolero PC, Arnold PG, Harris JB (Mayo Clinics and Found, Rochester, Minn)
Ann Surg 213:583–590, 1991   17–2

Introduction.—Wound infection after sternotomy is a rare, but potentially lethal, complication of thoracic surgery. The short-term results of treating infected sternotomy wounds by aggressive débridement and muscle transposition were reported previously. The same group of patients were followed to assess long-term results.

Patients and Methods.—During an 11.5-year period, 79 males and 21 females aged 5–85 years underwent surgical repair of a recalcitrant infected median sternotomy wound. Sternal drainage occurred a median of 3 weeks after sternotomy. The median time interval between onset of sternal drainage and sternal repair was 7.5 weeks. Sixty-five patients had undergone unsuccessful attempts at closure. Initial treatment involved débridement of the manubrium and sternum in each patient. In addition, the manubrium and sternum were resected completely in 43 patients and partially in 33. All 76 patients had associated costochondral arches resected from the back to the ribs. The wound was closed at initial débridement in 11 patients; in the others, wound closure was performed a median of 14 days after initial débridement. The median number of operations in these 100 patients was 4. Hospitalization ranged from 7 to 210 days. The median follow-up period was 4.2 years.

Outcome.—Forty-two patients had 59 complications, including 8 with prolonged wound infections. One of the 2 perioperative deaths was related to sepsis. Reconstruction was entirely with muscle transposition in 79 patients, omental transposition in 4, and both in 15. In all, 175 muscles were transposed. Thirty patients required mechanical ventilation beyond the second postoperative day. Twenty-six patients had a recurrent sternal infection. The median time from surgical closure to recurrence was 5.5 months. The cause of recurrence was inadequate removal of cartilage in 16 patients and bone in 6, and a retained foreign body in 4. There were 30 late deaths, but only 1 was related to recurrent infection. At the time of death or at the last follow-up visit, 92 patients had a healed chest wall.

Conclusion.—Vigorous sternal débridement and obliteration of dead space by muscle transposition remains an excellent method for managing infected sternotomy wounds.

▶ The editor read this spectacular report with particular interest for it has been a subject of individual research for many years.

This impressive paper merits careful study by any surgeon dealing with the complicated problem of an infected sternotomy incision. Experiences with 100 patients treated in a period of 11 years are described. It is quite important to realize that the data are somewhat skewed, because the initial sternotomy operations were not performed by the authors; 44 of the 100 patients had their sternotomies performed at another institution. Hence the overall time for treatment, 7½ weeks after onset of sternal drainage, is far later than that reported by many groups.

The pectoral muscle was used in 79 patients, and omentum with or without the rectus abdominus in 19. The preferred approach was radical débridement, followed in an average of 14 days by muscle flap closure. Mechanical ventilation was required in 30 patients. Only 2 perioperative deaths occurred. Nonetheless, 26 patients had recurrent infection, which developed within an average of 5 months after closure. Among the 26 patients, recurrence was almost always the result of inadequate débridement, including inadequate removal of cartilage in 16 instances and bone in 6. The majority of these 26 recurrences were treated successfully at another operation.

The authors' classification of sternal wound infection is excellent, describing 3 types. Type I is an early infection without extensive mediastinitis. Type II is a fulminant mediastinitis within a few weeks, involving sternal osteomyelitis and areas of bone necrosis. The degree of rigidity of the mediastinum varies widely, which, in turn, influences the capacity of suction drainage to obliterate the mediastinal space after sternal closure. Type III infections are those occurring months to years later with chronic draining sinuses.

The discussion of the paper by Dr. Jurkiewicz from Atlanta described experiences with 246 patients, but the majority were treated much earlier as most came from the same institution. The rectus abdominus had been used with increasing frequency, and a single-stage closure was performed in 139 patients.

In summary, the available data indicate the paramount influence of early diagnosis in determining the type of effective therapy. Prompt recognition of a sternal infection, often by needle aspiration, within 7–10 days after operation, permits early débridement and wound closure with irrigation therapy, because suction at this time would obliterate the mediastinal space. If the diagnosis is not made for 2 or 3 weeks or longer, the development of osteomyelitis, as well as the rigidity of the mediastinum, indicates that more radical therapy (e.g., radical resection and muscle flap transposition) is necessary.—F.C. Spencer, M.D.

Delayed Chest Wall Pain Due to Sternal Wire Sutures
Eastridge CE, Mahfood SS, Walker WA, Cole FH Jr (Univ of Tennessee; VA Med Ctr, Memphis)
Ann Thorac Surg 51:56–59, 1991   17–3

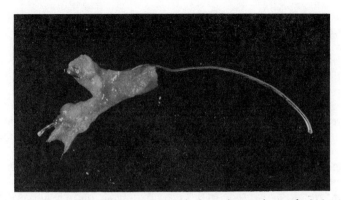

Fig 17–1.—Exaggerated fibrous reaction at the anodic (twisted portion) area of a 316 stainless steel wire used to reapproximate the sternum. (Courtesy of Eastridge CE, Mahfood SS, Walker WA, et al: *Ann Thorac Surg* 51:56–59, 1991.)

Introduction.—The appearance or persistence of anterior chest wall pain weeks after median sternotomy usually is ascribed to incisional trauma, anxiety, or a musculoskeletal disorder. Other possible causes are a scar-entrapped neuroma and a hypersensitivity reaction to nickel in stainless steel suture material.

Methods.—Eighteen patients (mean age, 55 years) were seen 2–84 months after median sternotomy with disabling chest wall pain apparently caused by sternal wire sutures. The patients had mostly undergone coronary bypass surgery. Pain developed within an average of 21 months postoperatively. Either sharp, stabbing pain or an ill-defined deep-seated aching was described.

Results.—A total of 64 wires were removed. All patients were totally relieved of pain and tenderness. Wires from areas that were tender to palpation exhibited a thick fibrous tissue reaction about the twisted part of the wire (Fig 17–1). Electrical potential measurements revealed a mean of 200 mV in wires causing pain and values of 5–30 mV for those not associated with pain or tenderness. Ferroxyl testing of wires with increased potential values showed ionization of iron at the twisted portion.

Conclusion.—If the protective chromic oxide coating on stainless steel wire is damaged, the area becomes relatively anodic, producing a voltaic cell, and current flows to the cathodic (undamaged) part of the wire through body fluids. Appreciable corrosion leads to the accumulation of metal particles in tissue near the anode; eventually, the area is invested by fibrous tissue. Treatment consists of removing the wires and adjacent scar tissue.

▶ This short intriguing paper describes 18 patients with persistent chest wall pain from sternal wire sutures that developed 2–84 months after operation. Pain was relieved by removal of the wires.

In 6 patients the electrical potential of the wires removed was studied, with the finding of an average potential in the painful wires of 200 mV as compared to 5–30 mV in other wires and 10 mV in unused 316 stainless steel wire.

The authors describe the stainless steel as an alloy of carbon and iron with resistance to corrosion achieved by adding various amounts of either chromium, nickel, or molybdenum. Resistance to corrosion from body fluids is provided by a thin continuous film of chromium oxide on the surface. If this protective chromium oxide coat is broken, the change in the electrical potential results in this area becoming anodic to the rest of the wire, constructing a simple voltaic cell; body fluids and electric current thus flow from the anodic portion to the cathodic portion. This flow of electric current may result in the accumulation of iron ions in the area adjacent to the anode, stimulating an inflammatory response.

To the editor's knowledge, this elegant analysis well defines what is the most plausible cause of painful stainless steel wires—simply an inadvertent break in the chromium oxide coat, producing a voltaic cell. Clearly, with this concept in mind, a persistent painful wire should be removed, rather than attempts made to treat by injection or other forms of therapy. The authors are to be congratulated for this significant study.—F.C. Spencer, M.D.

Overdose Reperfusion of Blood Cardioplegic Solution: A Preventable Cause of Postischemic Myocardial Depression
Kofsky ER, Julia PL, Buckberg GD (Univ of California, Los Angeles)
J Thorac Cardiovasc Surg 101:275–283, 1991   17–4

Introduction.—Reperfusion of warm blood cardioplegic solution is helpful to minimize reperfusion damage after myocardial ischemia. It is possible, however, that overzealous administration of blood cardioplegia at the time of reperfusion can depress ventricular performance.

Methods.—Of 31 dogs having 45 minutes of normothermic global ischemia on vented bypass, 6 received normal blood reperfusion and 25 were reperfused with a warm aspartate/glutamate-enriched blood cardioplegic solution. The mean dosage was 3,600 mL in 8 of the latter animals and 1,180 mL in the other 17 animals. Cardioplegia was administered for 10–20 minutes. An average of 5,100 mL of blood cardioplegic perfusion was administered to 5 other dogs without ischemia previously.

Results.—Ventricular function remained intact in animals not subjected to ischemia. After ischemia, normal blood reperfusion was associated with marked left ventricular dysfunction and a mortality of 33%. High-dose cardioplegic perfusion provided for marginal recovery of ventricular function; mortality was 25%. Reperfusion with a limited dose of blood cardioplegic solution permitted 100% survival and restored the stroke work index to 90% of control.

Conclusion.—Reperfusion injury may be avoided by the initial administration of limited doses of substrate-enriched blood cardioplegic solution. In reperfusion, more of a good treatment is not necessarily better.

▶ This experimental study clearly defines the harmful effects of high-dose cardioplegia reperfusion. The ischemic injury, 45 minutes of aortic clamping at 37°C, is a severe one. Without mechanical support, mortality is very high; with 24 hours of mechanical support, survival is near 70%.

Somewhat paradoxically, this study documents that reperfusion with a limited dose of cardioplegia (approximately 1,200 mL in 10–20 minutes) was valuable, whereas infusion of 5 L in a similar period of time was harmful. The exact mechanism is unclear. This harmful effect was seen only in ischemic hearts, as infusion of high doses without ischemia did not cause significant harm.—F.C. Spencer, M.D.

Superiority of Retrograde Cardioplegia After Acute Coronary Occlusion

Haan C, Lazar HL, Bernard S, Rivers S, Zallnick J, Shemin RJ (Boston Univ)
Ann Thorac Surg 51:408–412, 1991   17–5

Background.—Antegrade cardioplegia may limit the distribution of cardioplegia beyond a coronary occlusion. Retrograde coronary sinus cardioplegia was investigated to determine whether it provides better myocardial protection during revascularization of an acute coronary occlusion.

Methods.—The second and third diagonal branches in 20 adult pigs were occluded with a snare for 1.5 hours. The pigs were then placed on cardiopulmonary bypass. Thirty minutes of ischemic arrest with multidose, potassium, crystalloid cardioplegia was begun. The cardioplegia was administered antegrade through the aortic root in 10 pigs and retrograde through the coronary sinus in the other 10. After arrest, the coronary snares were released and the hearts reperfused for 3 hours.

Results.—Hearts protected with retrograde coronary sinus cardioplegia had less tissue acidosis than those protected with antegrade cardioplegia. The change in pH was .08 in the former and .41 in the latter group. The retrograde group also had higher wall motion scores—2 compared with 1.3—although this difference was nonsignificant. Myocardial necrosis occurred in 43.4% of the group having retrograde cardioplegia and in 73.3% of those having antegrade cardioplegia.

Conclusions.—In emergent revascularization for acute coronary occlusion, retrograde coronary sinus cardioplegia results in significantly less myocardial necrosis than antegrade cardioplegia does despite the absence of significant improvement in wall motion scores in the area of risk between the techniques. This persistent depression in systolic shortening is probably the result of a "stunned" myocardium, providing further evidence that depressed wall motion just after reperfusion is not a valid index of myocardial necrosis.

▶ This experimental method compared antegrade vs. retrograde cardioplegia in 20 adult pigs with temporary occlusion of regional coronary arteries for 90 minutes. Animals treated with retrograde cardioplegia had significantly less myocardial necrosis in the ischemic zone than did those with antegrade cardioplegia. These studies support the concept that retrograde cardioplegia may be a superior method of delivery of cardioplegic solutions in patients treated after an acute infarction.—F.C. Spencer, M.D.

Retrograde Continuous Warm Blood Cardioplegia: A New Concept in Myocardial Protection
Salerno TA, Houck JP, Barrozo CAM, Panos A, Christakis GT, Abel JG, Lichtenstein SV (St Michael's Hosp, Toronto; Univ of Toronto)
Ann Thorac Surg 51:245–247, 1991   17–6

Background.—Retrograde coronary sinus cardioplegia is a safe and effective procedure. Use of a coronary sinus catheter with a self-inflating balloon has simplified the technique, eliminating the need for bicaval cannulation and snaring in most cases. A series of 113 patients scheduled for cardiac surgery received continuous warm blood cardioplegia through the coronary sinus with warm body perfusion during cardiopulmonary bypass.

Patients and Methods.—The most common preoperative diagnosis was stable angina, followed by unstable angina and aortic valve disease. The series included 85 men and 28 women (mean age, 61 years). Twenty-two percent of the patients were older than 70 years, and 39% were in New York Heart Association class IV. Mean coronary sinus flow of cardioplegia was 122 mL/min, and the total administered volume ranged from 300 to 5,200 mL.

Results.—Three patients died, 2 of them in the early postoperative period because of graft failure after urgent coronary artery bypass grafting. Transient intra-aortic balloon pump support was needed in 8 patients, and 7 had evidence of perioperative myocardial infarction with no clinical sequelae. Spontaneous return of rhythm occurred in 96% of the patients. The coronary sinus was not injured.

Conclusions.—The new technique of retrograde continuous warm blood cardioplegia appears to be simple, safe, and reliable. This may be a promising technique for high-risk operations.

▶ This short report describes the use of continuous warm blood cardioplegia, a concept originating with one of the authors. His technique was a sequel to the use of continuous cold cardioplegia for about 7 years.

The report is primarily of significance for the technique described. The results in 113 patients are not impressive and certainly do not demonstrate superiority of the technique. There were 3 deaths, 8 patients required a balloon pump for a short time, and 6 had signs of an infarction. The duration of aortic clamping was not reported, but it must have been short because the mean coronary sinus infusion rate was 122 mL/min, but the total administered volume ranged between 300 mL and 5,200 mL. This is a preliminary report, but the concept is interesting. Further data are awaited with interest.—F.C. Spencer, M.D.

Technique and Pitfalls of Retrograde Continuous Warm Blood Cardioplegia

Salerno TA, Christakis GT, Abel J, Houck J, Barrozo CAM, Fremes SE, Cusimano RJ, Lichtenstein SV (St Michael's Hosp, Toronto; Sunnybrook Health Service Ctr, Toronto)

Ann Thorac Surg 51:1023–1025, 1991   17–7

Background.—With the advent of normothermic myocardial preservation and systemic perfusion during cardiopulmonary bypass, the necessity of hypothermia during cardiac surgery has come into question. The technique of continuous normothermic blood cardioplegia through the coronary sinus was used in nearly 300 patients during a 4-month period.

Technique.—Retrograde continuous warm blood cardioplegia begins with cannulation of the coronary sinus, usually transatrially. Arrest is achieved with 4 portions of blood to 1 of high-potassium Fremes solution. The retrograde cannula is used for perfusion as soon as diastolic arrest occurs. Low-potassium Fremes solution is given at a mean maximum pressure of 40 mm Hg, with cardioplegic delivery not to exceed 250 mL/min. Pressures and flows are monitored constantly, with additional high-potassium cardioplegia given retrogradely if electric activity occurs. Cardioplegia is stopped and the cannula withdrawn before the aortic clamp is removed.

Special Considerations.—Initial antegrade cardioplegia is given to achieve arrest, even in patients with severe aortic insufficiency. The cannula is advanced into the coronary sinus as far as it will go; otherwise it may be displaced into the coronary sinus. Proper position can be assessed by careful insertion and placement of the atrial pursestring suture. The most reliable method, however, is pressure monitoring on the side port of the cannula. Blood in the operative field is managed by local irrigation with warm saline, placing a probe into the coronary artery, and snaring the artery, or brief discontinuation of cardioplegia. Flow rates generally range from 40 mL/min to 150 mL/min in coronary artery disease and 250 mL/min in hypertrophied hearts. The technique is useful for combined valvar and coronary procedures. Potassium at the end of the procedure is usually not a problem. In nearly 300 patients treated, no coronary sinus injuries occurred. Questions remain, however, about the extent of right ventricular preservation during retrograde continuous warm blood cardioplegia.

Discussion.—This new concept of myocardial protection offers many advantages over the antegrade method. However, the surgeon must exercise caution during its use and follow the principles of cardioplegic delivery. More research is necessary to establish the superiority of this method.

▶ This short technique paper describes current guidelines and experiences with continuous retrograde warm cardioplegia, a method adopted by this Canadian group who have popularized continuous warm cardioplegia by the antegrade technique in the past few years. The technique described is quite recent and was used in about 300 patients in the past few months. The uncertain questions include how much cardioplegia should be given—the range is 40–250 mL/min—and whether excess potassium becomes a problem. The authors use transatrial cannulation of the coronary sinus, advancing the coronary sinus catheter as far into the coronary sinus as possible. Because this is well beyond the entry of right ventricular veins; the efficacy of the technique is presumably based on wide distribution through the coronary venous system, regardless of the position of the cannula. A pressure up to 40 mm is considered safe.—F.C. Spencer, M.D.

Warm Heart Surgery

Lichtenstein SV, Ashe KA, El Dalati H, Cusimano RJ, Panos A, Slutsky AS (St Michael's Hosp; Mt Sinai Hosp, Toronto)
J Thorac Cardiovasc Surg 101:269–274, 1991   17–8

Introduction.—The use of cold blood cardioplegia remains controversial. Hypothermia can influence enzyme function, membrane stability, glucose utilization, adenosine triphosphate generation and utilization, and tissue oxygen uptake. Because electromechanical work is the chief determinant of myocardial oxygen consumption, the heart might ideally be electromechanically arrested and perfused with blood.

Methods.—A new approach that allows for aerobic arrest during cardiac surgery overcomes many of the disadvantages of ischemic hypothermia. The heart is maintained at 37° C with continuous warm blood cardioplegia. This approach was used in 121 consecutive coronary bypass operations and compared with a historical group of 133 consecutive patients given hypothermic cardioplegia.

Results.—Mortality was 2.2% in patients with cold cardioplegia and .9% in those with warm cardioplegia. Perioperative infarction, low output syndrome, and the need for intra-aortic balloon pumping all were significantly less in the group given warm blood cardioplegia. Nearly all of these patients had a spontaneous return of normal sinus rhythm compared with only 10% of the cold cardioplegia recipients. Reperfusion was required for a significantly shorter time in the warm cardioplegia group. Only in this group was the cardiac output after discontinuing bypass significantly greater than the prebypass output.

Conclusion.—Warm blood cardioplegia is a safe and effective means of preserving myocardial function during cardiac surgery.

▶ This interesting paper compares 121 coronary bypass procedures with a historical cohort of 133 consecutive patients operated on previously. Results were clearly much better in the group with warm cardioplegia, although, as the authors indicate, the significance of the difference is limited by the absence of properly matched controls.

The paper is particularly significant because it challenges several concepts of myocardial protection, especially the importance of hypothermia. Normothermic arrest was used, initially arresting the heart with 1,500 mL of warm blood having a potassium concentration of 20 mEq. Subsequent low potassium infusions were carried out—6 mEq/L at a rate of 50–150 mL/min. It is quite disappointing that, for unknown reasons, neither the cross-clamp times nor the total amount of potassium given were provided. This significantly limits the objective significance of the data.

The authors state that the method can be used either in the aortic root or the coronary sinus. However, there is no mention of the pressure in the aortic root during infusion of a small amount of blood, 50–150 mL/min. With a mild degree of aortic insufficiency, such blood would simply run into the ventricular cavity. Unless aortic root pressures are measured, it is difficult to imagine where the infused blood was going.

Obviously, however, no harm resulted. The editor has long commented that an unknown defect must exist with techniques of hypothermic myocardial preservation because of the high mortality from acute operations such as mitral valve replacement for ruptured papillary muscle. Hence this new approach is clearly welcome and may be a very significant one. Obviously, further data are needed.—F.C. Spencer, M.D.

Warm Heart Surgery and Results of Operation for Recent Myocardial Infarction
Lichtenstein SV, Abel JG, Salerno TA (St Michael's Hosp; Univ of Toronto)
Ann Thorac Surg 52:455–460, 1991   17–9

Background.—Compared with elective coronary artery bypass grafting, revascularization procedures after recent myocardial infarction have a higher mortality and morbidity. Traditional myocardial protection methods further insult ischemically the already compromised myocardium. Although continuous cold blood cardioplegia may eliminate ischemia, it still may leave the heart anaerobic. Warm aerobic arrest is theoretically an attractive alternative to standard hypothermic ischemic arrest in these cases.

Methods.—Within 6 hours to 7 days of acute myocardial infarction, 115 patients underwent coronary artery bypass grafting. Continuous cold or continuous warm blood cardioplegia was used for myocardial protection. The 51 patients treated after 1988 with warm blood cardioplegia were compared with a historical control group of 64 patients treated before 1988 with cold blood cardioplegia.

Results.—No patient undergoing warm cardioplegia died, compared with 10.9% of patients undergoing cold cardioplegia. The former group had a myocardial infarction rate of 2%, compared with 9.3% in the latter group. The use of an intra-aortic balloon pump in the 2 groups was 0% and 12.5%, respectively.

Conclusions.—Continuous warm aerobic arrest may minimize ischemia and anaerobic metabolism during surgery. It may be beneficial to patients with a limited tolerance of ischemic insult.

▶ In this interesting report the authors describe experiences in 115 patients treated in the past few years with bypass grafting after an infarction sustained 6 hours to 7 days previously. Before 1988, 64 patients were treated with continuous cold cardioplegia; since that time, patients have been treated with continuous warm blood cardioplegia. The group having warm cardioplegia had no mortality, but 11% of those having cold cardioplegia died. The myocardial infarction rate was 2% in the group having warm cardioplegia and 9% in the group having cold cardioplegia, although in the discussion the authors stated that this was not statistically significant. In both groups it was necessary to interrupt the cardioplegia for short periods of time during performance of an anastomosis. The aortic clamp time was near 60 minutes in both groups.

It is difficult to believe that the lower mortality resulted from using warm cardioplegia rather than cold. On a theoretical basis, one can argue that the reverse could be predicted, because a period of cold should protect from ischemia during the short period of interruption of circulation. Most likely the differences are attributable to a change in technique or referral patterns over this period of time. It is impressive, however, that more than 60 patients could be operated on with no mortality, even though an infarction had occurred in the previous week. Future reports from others using this interesting technique will be enlightening.—F.C. Spencer, M.D.

The Dynamics of Antegrade Cardioplegia With Simultaneous Coronary Sinus Occlusion: Effects on Aortic Root Infusion Pressure, Coronary Sinus Pressure, and Myocardial Cooling

Sun S-C, Diaco M, Laurence RD, DiSesa VJ, Cohn LH (Brigham and Women's Hosp, Boston)

J Thoracic Cardiovasc Surg 101:517–525, 1991　　　　　　　　17–10

Background.—Some physicians have proposed that antegrade cardioplegia with the coronary sinus occluded improves myocardial cooling and limits myocardial injury in the presence of coronary artery occlusion. Little is known, however, of the exact relationships among the rate of infusion, aortic root pressure, degree of coronary sinus occlusion, coronary sinus pressure, and myocardial cooling.

Methods.—These relationships were examined in sheep placed on cardiopulmonary bypass. The distal left anterior descending coronary artery was occluded, and the proximal coronary sinus was snared. Various infusion rates (3–9 mL/kg/min) and no, partial, or full coronary sinus occlusion was imposed for 2-minute periods of antegrade cardioplegia.

Observations.—The infusion rate was related linearly to the aortic root infusion pressure under all test conditions. Coronary sinus occlusion had a positive effect on the aortic root infusion pressure, and increasing infusion rates with various degrees of coronary sinus occlusion produced elevated coronary sinus pressures. The myocardial temperature in the area of coronary occlusion remained lower when the coronary sinus was occluded. In other myocardial regions, temperature declined as the infusion rate increased.

Recommendations.—A coronary sinus pressure of 25–35 mm Hg appears to be safe. Further studies should assess an infusion rate of 5 mL/kg/min with subtotal or total coronary sinus occlusion.

▶ This experimental study in 22 sheep evaluates a different approach to cardioplegia, combining antegrade cardioplegia with constriction of the coronary sinus. Similar experimental studies have been reported by Lazar et al. (1). The studies analyze the combinations of rate of infusion of cardioplegic solution with the degree of occlusion of the coronary sinus, determining the myocardial temperature with each technique. The authors concluded that a degree of coronary sinus occlusion that produces a coronary sinus pressure between 25 mm and 35 mm is probably ideal; this corresponds to an infusion rate of cardioplegic solution of 5 mL/kg/min. Theoretically, this combined approach could obviate the maldistribution that occurs with the traditional method of antegrade cardioplegia.—F.C. Spencer, M.D.

Reference

1. Lazar HL, et al: *Ann Thorac Surg* 46:202–207, 1988.

Role of Potassium Concentration in Cardioplegic Solutions in Mediating Endothelial Damage

Mankad PS, Chester AH, Yacoub MH (Natl Heart and Lung Inst, London; Harefield Hosp, England)
Ann Thorac Surg 51:89–93, 1991   17–11

Background.—Potassium, a vascular irritant, has been used to denude vessels of endothelium. Hyperkalemic crystalloid cardioplegic solution is demonstrably toxic to cultured endothelial cells.

Methods.—The dose-dependent rise in coronary flow caused by 5-hydroxytryptamine (5-HT) in the isolated perfused rat heart depends on an intact endothelium. This model was used in examination of the effect of potassium in different cardioplegic solutions on the coronary vascular endothelium. After induction of increased coronary flow by 5-HT or nitroglycerin, hearts were perfused for 30 minutes or 60 minutes with St Thomas' solution or Bretschneider solution containing 20 mM of potassium per liter, or for 30 minutes with either solution containing 30 mM of potassium per liter.

Observations.—Infusion of solution containing potassium, 20 mM/L, for 60 minutes maintained the basal vasodilatory response of the coronary vessels. In contrast, infusion of a higher-potassium solution for 30 minutes abolished the 5-HT-induced rise in coronary flow. Nitroglycerin-induced vasodilation was unaffected.

Conclusion.—The potassium concentration of the cardioplegic solution is a critical factor in whether endothelial damage will occur.

▶ This short report assessed the influence of the potassium concentration on endothelial cell function in hearts perfused for 30–60 minutes with either 20 or 30 mM of potassium solution (St Thomas or Bretschneider). With either of the 2 solutions, a potassium concentration of 20 mM routinely preserved function, whereas a higher concentration of 30 mM abolished such function. With increasing interest in methods of continuous cardioplegia requiring the use of potassium in smaller amounts, such studies are of particular relevance.—F.C. Spencer, M.D.

When Do Cerebral Emboli Appear During Open Heart Operations? A Transcranial Doppler Study

van der Linden J, Casimir-Ahn H (Univ of Uppsala, Sweden)
Ann Thorac Surg 51:237–241, 1991   17–12

Background.—Embolization of air to the brain is always a risk in open-heart surgery. The ultrasonic Doppler method now allows intraoperative imaging of both cardiac function and blood flow, and it has demonstrated air embolization often, even after standard procedures for deairing.

Methods.—Emboli were monitored in the middle cerebral artery using the transcranial Doppler method in 10 patients having electric aortic or mitral valve replacement. Only flat membrane oxygenators without arterial filters were used during these operations.

Findings.—A transient change in the Doppler record indicated scattered emboli in all but 1 of the 10 patients studied during insertion of the aortic cannula. Four patients had emboli at the start of cardiopulmonary bypass. Small amounts of emboli were seen just after release of the aortic clamp, and scattered emboli were observed during reperfusion with the heart beating empty. When extensive deairing maneuvers were performed before declamping in 2 patients, only small amounts of emboli were evident. One patient had partial anopsia at discharge, with CT showing hypodensity in the area supplied by the left cerebellar artery.

Recommendations.—Cerebral air emboli are especially likely to occur during filling of the beating heart, even after meticulous deairing is carried out. Careful deairing should be done before declamping the aorta. In addition, brief filling of the beating heart may be helpful before final closure of the aortic incision or vent. Reduced cerebral blood flow from hyperventilation or anesthesia during filling of the empty beating heart also might lower the risk of cerebral embolism.

▶ The transcranial Doppler technique detected air emboli in all 10 patients during open-heart operations; the emboli occurs primarily when the heart began to beat and eject into the aorta. Emboli were not recorded during the operation during cross-clamping. Membrane oxygenators were used. The clinical significance is uncertain, because detailed neuropsychological studies were not done. One small neurologic defect was recognized.

The surgical technique used for removal of air from the heart before unclamping would be considered seriously inadequate by this editor, especially as the left ventricle was not vented in the majority of patients. Nonetheless, the occurrence of what was apparently air emboli despite their absence of recognition clinically is alarming, especially in view of their possible relationship to the frequency of neurologic injury of unknown cause after bypass. We hope that further use of this non-invasive technique will be attempted in other centers.

This study has considerable potential significance, because the primary morbidity from open-heart operations is neurologic injury. The frequency is small, but the disability can be severe.—F.C. Spencer, M.D.

Role of Perfusion Pressure and Flow in Major Organ Dysfunction After Cardiopulmonary Bypass

Slogoff S, Reul GJ, Keats AS, Curry GR, Crum ME, Elmquist BA, Giesecke NM, Jistel JR, Rogers LK, Soderberg JD, Edelman SK (Texas Heart Inst, Hous-

ton: St Luke's Episcopal Hosp, Houston)
Ann Thorac Surg 50:911–918, 1990   17–13

Introduction.—A clear association between low perfusion pressure during cardiac operations requiring cardiopulmonary bypass (CPB) and new postoperative cerebral or renal adverse events has been established in some studies. Others, however, have failed to support this association. The relationship between perfusion pressure and flow with moderate hypothermia and hemodilution and new postoperative CNS or renal dysfunction was examined.

Patients.—During a 7-month period, 511 patients aged 19–89 years (mean age, 61 years) underwent elective operations requiring CPB. All were studied during 5 observation periods. The CPB flow was targeted at more than 40 mL/kg^{-1}/min^{-1}, and perfusion pressure at more than 50 mm Hg.

Results.—During onset CPB, perfusion flows less than target occurred in 21.6% of patients and perfusion pressures less than target occurred in 97.1%. Of 504 evaluable patients, 15 (3%) experienced new perioperative renal events and 13 (2.6%) new CNS dysfunction. Two patients had both new renal and new CNS dysfunction. Patients with new renal dysfunction had significantly higher incidences of preoperative renal and CNS dysfunction, peripheral vascular disease, and diabetes than did those who had no new postoperative renal events. New CNS events were significantly associated only with preoperative renal and left ventricular dysfunction. However, neither perfusion pressure nor perfusion flow less than target during CPB were predictors of new renal or CNS dysfunction. Multivariate analysis identified intra-aortic balloon counterpulsation, excessive blood loss in the intensive care unit (ICU), vasopressor drug therapy before CPB, postoperative myocardial infaction, emergency reoperation, excessive postoperative transfusion, and chronic renal disease as independent predictors of new postoperative renal events. Cardiopulmonary resuscitation in the ICU, intracardiac thrombus or valve calcification, and chronic renal disease were independent predictors of new postoperative CNS events.

Conclusion.—Perfusion pressure and flow during hypothermic CPB with hemodilution are not related to new postoperative CNS or renal dysfunction. Rather, both adverse outcomes are strongly related to hypoperfusion during failure of the native circulation immediately after CPB or in the early postoperative period.

▶ This extensive report examined the frequency of postoperative renal or cerebral dysfunction after bypass in 504 patients. Particular scrutiny was given to those who had a perfusion pressure above or below 50 mm Hg or a flow less than 40 mL/kg/min. Renal problems developed in 3% of the patients and neurologic problems in 2.6%.

A detailed analysis of various hemodynamic factors did not detect either defective flow or hypotension as a major cause. The authors conclude that other factors must exist. This report well emphasizes the important basic fact that the small but significant frequency of renal and cerebral injury after bypass is often of unknown origin and hence not preventable by present techniques.—F.C. Spencer, M.D.

Risk Factors for Pancreatic Cellular Injury After Cardiopulmonary Bypass

Fernández-del Castillo C, Harringer W, Warshaw AL, Vlahakes GJ, Koski G, Zaslavsky AM, Rattner DW (Massachusetts Gen Hosp, Boston; Harvard Univ, Cambridge)
N Engl J Med 325:382–387, 1991   17–14

Introduction.—Cardiac complications after heart surgery have been reduced in recent years, but certain noncardiac complications continue to result in postoperative morbidity and mortality. The cause of one such complication, pancreatitis, remains unknown. Three hundred patients undergoing cardiac surgery with cardiopulmonary bypass were evaluated to determine variables associated with pancreatitis.

Patients.—The 300 patients consecutively underwent surgery from December 1989 to March 1990. Criteria for pancreatic cellular injury were hyperamylasemia (> 123 units per liter) and either elevated serum lipase activity (> 24 units per liter) or a disproportionate increase in the pancreatic isoamylase peak, or both. Serum amylase, pancreatic isoamylase, and serum lipase levels were measured on postoperative days 1, 2, 3, 7,

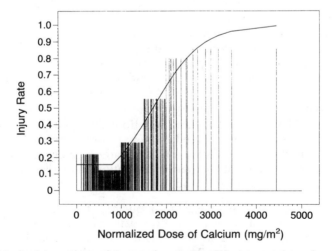

Fig 17–2.—Logistic regression of the rate of pancreatic cellular injury on the total normalized calcium dose (the amount of calcium chloride administered during surgery and 24 hours postoperatively per square meter of body-surface area). The curve represents predicted probabilities. (Courtesy of Fernández-del Castillo C, Harringer W, Warshaw AL, et al: N Engl J Med 325:382–387, 1991.)

and 10. In the last 101 patients studied, trypsinogen-activation peptides, an indication of intrapancreatic enzyme activation, were determined.

Results.—Three patients died within the first 24 hours after surgery. Hyperamylasemia developed postoperatively in 120 (40%) of the remaining patients. Pancreatic cellular injury occurred in 80 patients (27%), 23 of whom had postoperative signs or symptoms suggestive of pancreatitis. The incidence of severe pancreatitis was 1% (3 of 297 patients). Multivariate analyses yielded 4 variables significantly associated with the development of pancreatitis: preoperative renal insufficiency, valve surgery, postoperative hypotension, and perioperative administration of calcium chloride. The level of trypsinogen-activation peptides did not differentiate between patients who had pancreatic cellular injury and those who did not.

Conclusion.—The administration of large doses of calcium chloride (> 800 mg/m²) is an independent predictor of pancreatic cellular injury (Fig 17-2). Although calcium chloride is often used routinely, the dose should be limited or other drugs substituted.

▶ This paper found a surprisingly high frequency of pancreatic cellular injury after bypass in 300 consecutive patients. In all, 27% of the patients had signs of pancreatic injury; either pancreatic abscess or necrotizing pancreatitis developed in 3, with 2 deaths. This high frequency is far greater than that encountered in the editor's institution. The finding that the frequency of pancreatitis correlated markedly with the amount of calcium given, starting with a calcium dose of 800 mg/m², seems quite significant (Fig 17–2). The authors are to be complimented on this perceptive and significant report.—F.C. Spencer, M.D.

Cerebral Blood Flow Response to Changes in Arterial Carbon Dioxide Tension During Hypothermic Cardiopulmonary Bypass in Children

Kern FH, Ungerleider RM, Quill TJ, Baldwin B, White WD, Reves JG, Greeley WJ (Duke Univ)

J Thorac Cardiovasc Surg 101:618–622, 1991   17–15

Background.—Loss of pressure-flow autoregulation occurs during deep hypothermic cardiopulmonary bypass in infants and children and leads to pressure-dependent cerebral blood flow (CBF). The different physiologic milieu endured by children during bypass may therefore have different effects on the CBF compared with those in adults. Infants and children are exposed to greater physiologic extremes during bypass, and carbon dioxide management methods are divergent; therefore, the effect of arterial carbon dioxide tension ($PaCO_2$) on CBF was studied.

Methods.—The relationship of changes in $PaCO_2$ on CBF responsiveness was examined in 20 children undergoing hypothermic cardiopulmonary bypass. Xenon-133 clearance methodology at 2 different arterial tensions was used to measure CBF during steady-state hyopthermic by-pass.

Results.—There was no significant change in mean arterial pressure, nasopharyngeal temperature, pump flow rate, or hematocrit value. Cerebral blood flow was significantly higher at greater arterial CO_2 tensions; for every millimeter of mercury rise in a $PaCO_2$, there was a 1.2 mL · 100 g^{-1} · min^{-1} rise in CBF. Deep hypothermia and age less than 1 year reduced the effect of CO_2 on CBF responsiveness but did not eliminate it.

Conclusions.—Cerebral blood flow remains responsive to $PaCO_2$ in children undergoing hypothermic CPB. Although temperature and age affected the degree of CO_2 reactivity during extracorporeal circulation, adding CO_2 produces a potent stimulus that increases cerebral perfusion. Still unknown is the effect of increased CBF in response to elevated $PaCO_2$ on cerebral metabolism and flow-metabolism coupling.

▶ Adequacy of the CBF, of course, is a major consideration during cardiac operations in infants and small children, especially with hypothermia and circulatory arrest. This elegant study in 20 patients undergoing operation clearly documents that the cerebral vascular bed remains reactive to changes in $PaCO_2$, even with severe hypothermia. These data support the policy of maintaining CO_2 with the "alpha-stat" technique during bypass. The paper supplements an earlier publication from the same group demonstrating that, with deep hypothermia, pressure flow autoregulation did not function, thus flow was pressure dependent.—F.C. Spencer, M.D.

Current Treatment for Wolff-Parkinson-White Syndrome: Results and Surgical Implications
Bolling SF, Morady F, Calkins H, Kadish A, de Buitleir M, Langberg J, Dick M, Lupinetti FM, Bove EL (Univ of Michigan)
Ann Thorac Surg 52:461–468, 1991   17–16

Background.—Surgical division of an accessory atrioventricular (AV) pathway in management of Wolff-Parkinson-White (WPW) syndrome has become the primary treatment for many of these young and otherwise healthy patients. Preliminary studies have suggested that catheter ablation of accessory AV connections with radiofrequency current is also successful. In a retrospective study, the results of surgical treatment were compared with results in a group who had radiofrequency catheter ablation of accessory AV connections.

Patients.—During a 4½-year period, surgical ablation of aberrant conduction pathways was conducted in 123 patients with WPW syndrome. The 85 male and 38 female patients had a mean age of 26 years. Thirteen patients had associated anomalies, including Ebstein's anomaly, sudden death syndrome, coronary artery disease, cardiomyopathy, abdominal aortic aneurysm, neurofibromatosis, and other arrhythmias, as well as congenital heart diseases. Multiple accessory pathways were present in 41 patients. Between March 1990 and January 1991, a total of 124 WPW patients had catheter ablation with radiofrequency current. Five of these patients had other abnormalities, and 9 had multiple accessory pathways.

Outcome.—The mean follow-up in the surgical group was 26 months. The initial failure rate in this group was 7%, dropping to 3% with repeat operations. Six patients had concomitant valve repair or replacement; other concurrent procedures included right ventricular conduit replacement, subaortic resection, Fontan repair, corrected transposition repair, coronary artery bypass, and placement of an automatic defibrillator. There were no operative deaths; complications included mitral regurgitation and myocardial infarction. The mean follow-up in the catheter group was 7 months. All accessory AV connections were ablated in 90% of patients; these patients remained symptom free. In 12 patients the procedure failed; 5 then had surgery and 7 were treated medically. Complications in this group included circumflex coronary artery occlusion, excessive bleeding, perforated valve, and a cerebral vascular accident.

Conclusions.—Surgical ablation and catheter ablation of aberrant conduction pathways both give good results in patients with WPW syndrome. Longer follow-up is needed, however, to establish the success of the latter technique. Surgery may be indicated when catheter ablation fails, or multiple pathways are present, or when additional procedures are needed.

▶ The changing method of treatment of WPW syndrome is clearly described in this report from the University of Michigan.

Initially, most patients were treated surgically, with 123 patients operated on in a period of 5 years with a 90% success rate. However, in 1990, 124 patients underwent catheter ablation with radiofrequency current; again, the success rate was 90%. If the early results with radiofrequency ablation are durable, operation will probably be used in the future only for the patients who do not respond to radiofrequency techniques.—F.C. Spencer, M.D.

Catheter Ablation of Accessory Atrioventricular Pathways (Wolff-Parkinson-White Syndrome) by Radiofrequency Current
Jackman WM, Wang X, Friday KJ, Roman CA, Moulton KP, Beckman KJ, McClelland JH, Twidale N, Hazlitt HA, Prior MI, Margolis PD, Calame JD, Overholt ED, Lazzara R (Univ of Oklahoma; VA Med Ctr, Oklahoma City)
N Engl J Med 324:1605–1611, 1991
17–17

Background.—Surgical or catheter ablation of the accessory pathway has been used therapeutically for more than 20 years in patients with the Wolff-Parkinson-White syndrome. The high morbidity and mortality associated with accessory pathway ablation led to exploration of high-energy shock and nonsurgical alternatives for ablation. Radiofrequency current delivered via catheter provides an alternative energy source for ablation with less morbidity and mortality. Catheter techniques for applying radiofrequency ablation were tested and evaluated in 166 patients with 177 accessory pathways.

Method.—Radiofrequency current was delivered through a catheter electrode positioned against the mitral or tricuspid annulus or a branch of the coronary sinus. The placement ensured that the radiofrequency current produced lesions potentially effective for accessory pathway ablation. Accessory pathways were localized by recording accessory pathway activation potentials.

Results.—Ventricular preexcitation and atrioventricular reentrant tachycardia were eliminated in 164 of 166 patients. A single procedure was required in 148 patients; in 16 others, 2 procedures were required. There was no mortality in this series and only 6 complications. The recurrence of preexcitation or atrioventricular reentrant tachycardia in 15 patients was treated successfully by a second ablation.

Conclusion.—Catheter delivery of a radiofrequency current guided by direct recording of accessory pathway activation was a highly effective method of ablation. There was no mortality and less morbidity in patients treated with a radiofrequency current compared to surgical or catheter ablation with high-energy shocks.

▶ This dramatic report clearly documents the safety and efficacy of radiofrequency catheter ablation of accessory atrioventricular pathways. Initially, 164 of 166 patients (99%) were treated successfully. Recurrences developed in 9%, in all of whom a second radiofrequency ablation was successful. Complications occurred in only 1.8% of patients. There was no mortality. Hence the radiofrequency technique developed in recent years, in contrast to earlier techniques that used higher electrical energy with direct current, seems highly effective with minimal morbidity.—F.C. Spencer, M.D.

Current Indications, Risks, and Outcome After Pericardiectomy

DeValeria PA, Baumgartner WA, Casale AS, Greene PS, Cameron DE, Gardner TJ, Gott VL, Watkins L Jr, Reitz BA (Johns Hopkins Med Insts)
Ann Thorac Surg 52:219–224, 1991   17–18

Background.—Surgeons disagree as to the optimal surgical approach to effusive and constrictive pericarditis. Ten years of experience with pericardiectomy were reviewed to determine long-term survival and any improvement in function after surgery.

Patients.—A total of 38 male and 22 female patients (median age, 49.5 years) underwent pericardiectomy during the study period. Thirty-six had restrictive and 24 had effusive disease; in 6 cases pain was the primary reason for intervention. The cause of disease was idiopathic in 45% of patients and a previous cardiac operation in 16.7%. A median sternotomy was performed in 52 patients, 4 of whom required cardiopulmonary bypass; a left anterior thoracotomy was carried out in 8. A previous, limited pericardial procedure in 9 patients necessitated a formal pericardiectomy. Operative mortality was 4.2% among patients with effusive disease and 5.6% among those with constrictive disease.

Outcome.—Fifty-three patients were followed for a median of 57 months. The mean actuarial survivals were 82% at 1 year, 72% at 5 years, and 60% at 10 years. Cox proportional hazards regression analysis demonstrated that a history of malignancy, previous pericardial operation, and preoperative New York Heart Association class IV were predictors of poor survival. The most common causes of late death were complications of malignancy, myocardial infarction, and noncardiac-related sepsis. All patients who had surgery primarily for effusion and associated pain were alive at follow-up, with improved functional capacity and no need for steroids.

Conclusions.—Complete pericardiectomy is a safe procedure that can lead to long-term survival and good functional results. A complete rather than limited procedure should be done in patients with effusive disease resistant to conservative treatment. For those with refractory chest pain, complete pericardiectomy is usually safe and effective.

▶ Experiences with 60 patients undergoing pericardiectomy in a period of 10 years at the John Hopkins Hospital were reviewed. It is significant that almost half of the patients were operated on for recurrent pericardial effusion, rather than for pericardial constriction. Radical excision of the pericardium was uniformly effective in management of recurrent effusion refractory to simpler measures. Refractory pain was the primary indication for operation in 6 patients. Results were excellent, clearly indicating that operation perhaps should be carried out more frequently, rather than accepting the morbidity caused by the continued use of steroids over a period of months or longer.—F.C. Spencer, M.D.

Endothelial Cell Toxicity of Solid-Organ Preservation Solutions
von Oppell UO, Pfeiffer S, Preiss P, Dunne T, Zilla P, Reichart B (Univ of Cape Town, South Africa)
Ann Thorac Surg 50:902–910, 1990   17–19

Introduction.—Solutions used to preserve kidneys and livers in cold storage are formulated primarily to abolish energy-consuming transmembranous electrolyte gradients. Cardioplegic solutions are formulated primarily to produce diastolic arrest because the myocardium has a high rate of energy consumption. Although the endothelium may be even more vulnerable to ischemia than is myocardium, few studies have examined to what extent preservation solutions affect the endothelium. The endothelial cell damage caused by standard renal, hepatic, and cardiac preservation solutions was examined.

Methods.—Endothelial cells were harvested from human saphenous vein segments obtained during coronary artery bypass grafting and organ transplantation. Monolayer cell cultures were exposed to St Thomas' Hospital No. 2 (ST) and Bretschneider-HTK (B-HTK) cardioplegic solutions, modified Collins kidney preservation solution, and to University of Wisconsin cold storage solution. All solutions were gassed with 95% oxygen and 5% carbon dioxide 30 minutes before use to ensure pH stability and uniform oxygen content. The normothermic experiments were performed at 37° C and the hypothermic experiments were performed at 4–10°C. Endothelial cells were exposed to preservation solution for 12 hours, after which the cell morphology was examined by light microscopy. After removal of the solution, the cells were rinsed and reincubated to assess cell survival.

Results.—Hypothermic exposure for 12 hours to ST cardioplegic solution caused the cells to contract. Endothelial cell survival 24 hours after exposure was 51%. Exposure to B-HTK cardioplegic solution yielded a 24-hour postexposure cell survival of 80%. Exposure to University of Wisconsin cold storage solution did not alter the cells' appearance and best preserved cell morphology, but postexposure cell survival was only 70%. Postexposure cell survival with modified Collins kidney preservation solution was 62%. The superior cell survival after exposure to B-HTK cardioplegic solution was attributed to its additives histidine, tryptophan, and KH-2-oxygluterate, and its low chloride content. When ST was modified by decreasing its chloride content, cell survival improved to 71%. Normothermic exposure to B-HTK, modified Collins kidney preservation solution, and University of Wisconsin cold storage solutions was cytotoxic, whereas normothermic exposure to ST solution was not.

Conclusion.—Bretschneider-HTK cardioplegic solution is the least cytotoxic to endothelial cells at hypothermia, and ST cardioplegic solution is the least harmful at normothermia.

▶ The search for the ideal solution for solid organ preservation has recently focused on endothelial cell viability. This report from South Africa compared 4 commonly used preservation solutions—the Bretschneider, the St. Thomas', the Collins, and the University of Wisconsin. The Bretschneider solution with the addition of histidine, tryptophan, and KH-2-oxygluterate provided the best results when combined with hypothermia.

We hope that this type of study will make it increasingly possible to achieve long-term organ preservation with excellent preservation of the critical endothelial layer.—F.C. Spencer, M.D.

Perioperative Myocardial Ischemia in Patients Undergoing Noncardiac Surgery: II. Incidence and Severity During the 1st Week After Surgery

Mangano DT, Wong MG, London MJ, Tubau JF, Rapp JA, and the Study of Perioperative Ischemia (SPI) Research Group (Univ of California, San Francisco; VA Med Ctr, San Francisco)
J Am Coll Cardiol 17:851–857, 1991   17–20

Introduction.—Part I of this study showed that postoperative myocardial ischemia is a major predictor of adverse cardiac outcome in patients at risk for coronary artery disease (CAD) who undergo major noncardiac operations under general anesthesia. The incidence and characteristics of myocardial ischemia during the late postoperative period were determined in the same 100 at-risk patients studied in part I.

Methods.—Continuous postoperative monitoring with an ambulatory single-channel ECG monitor was initiated in the first hour after operation and continued for up to 7 days afterward. The total ECG monitoring time in this part of the study was 10,445 hours.

Results.—During the first week after operation, 27 patients had 437 episodes of ST segment changes suggestive of myocardial ischemia. Of the 437 episodes, 284 occurred on days zero–3 and 153 occurred on days 4–7. The total duration of myocardial ischemia in all patients during the first postoperative week was 18,658 minutes, or 1.8 minute of ischemia per 1 hour of monitoring. Thus ischemia was most severe during the early postoperative period. However, 8% of patients had late severe episodes. Tachycardia was associated with 58% of ischemic episodes, and 84% of episodes were clinically silent. More than half of the ischemic episodes were associated with tachycardia, which was most fre-

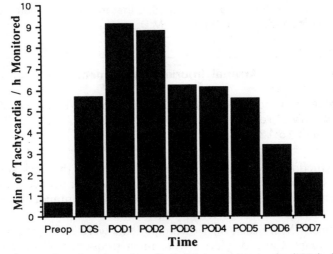

Fig 17–3.—Pattern of postoperative tachycardia. For each postoperative day (*POD*), the average number of tachycardic (heart rate $\geq$ 100 beats per minute) min/h monitored was calculated by dividing total minutes of tachycardia by total hours monitored. *Preop* indicates preoperative. (Courtesy of Mangano DT, Wong MG, London MJ, et al: *J Am Coll Cardiol* 17:851–857, 1991.)

quent on the first 2 postoperative days (Fig 17–3). Patients undergoing vascular procedures had the highest incidence of ischemia. There were 13 adverse cardiac outcomes, 5 of which were severe and included 1 death. All 5 were preceded by postoperative ischemia occurring 1 day or later before the adverse cardiac event.

Conclusion.—Postoperative ECG ST changes consistent with myocardial ischemia in at-risk patients undergoing major noncardiac operations are most common during the first 3 days after operation. Changes persist for 1 week or longer.

▶ One hundred high-risk patients had continuous ECG monitoring for 1 week after major noncardiac surgery. Reversible ST abnormalities consistent with ischemia were identified in 27% of the patients. These occurred most frequently in the first 3 days, but in 8% they occurred after 4 or 5 days. Further, 84% of the episodes were silent, unaccompanied by symptoms of angina or syncope, and 57% were associated with tachycardia, a heart rate of more than 100 per minute. All 5 adverse cardiac outcomes—unstable angina, myocardial infarction, or cardiac death—were preceded by an episode of postoperative ischemia in the previous 24 hours.

No difference was found in the frequency of ischemia in patients receiving preoperative antianginal medication and those who did not. Presumably, this medication was not continued postoperatively during the period of monitoring.

These studies are particularly important, because a cardiovascular event is the principal cause of mortality and morbidity after major surgery. Because the cost implications of such extensive monitoring for 1 week afterward are large, however, future studies are needed that may define even more clearly those patients at risk.—F.C. Spencer, M.D.

Cerviocothoracic Arterial Injuries: Recommendations for Diagnosis and Management
George SM Jr, Croce MA, Fabian TC, Mangiante EC, Kudsk KA, Voeller GR, Pate JW (Univ of Tennessee)
World J Surg 15:134–140, 1991   17–21

Introduction.—Mortality from arterial injuries in the neck and thoracic outlet is reported to be as high as 30%. Data were reviewed on 118 patients treated for such injuries in 1974–1988 by immediate exploration or selective care at the attending surgeon's discretion.

Patients.—More than 80% of the patients were males; the average age was 33 years. Carotid injuries were most frequent, followed by axillary and subclavian artery injuries. Penetrating wounds were present in 78% of the patients, one third of whom underwent angiography. Also, all but 2 of the 26 patients with blunt injuries were evaluated primarily by angiography.

Morbidity and Mortality of Cervicothoracic Trauma

Artery (N)	Amputation	Death
Innominate (6)	–	1
Carotid (57)	–	11
Subclavian (24)	1	4
Axillary (31)	1	1
Total 118	2 (2%)	17 (14%)

(Courtesy of George SM Jr, Croce MA, Fabian TC, et al: *World J Surg* 15:134–140, 1991.)

Treatment.—Interposition grafts were used to repair 29% of carotid artery injuries and 47% of subclavian injuries. Half of the axillary injuries also were treated by interposition grafting. The carotid artery was ligated in 12% of patients. Nearly half of the patients with carotid injury were treated by anticoagulation.

Results.—The overall mortality was 14% (table). Nearly one fourth of patients with blunt carotid injuries died; all of the other deaths followed penetrating trauma. Of 12 patients with hemiplegia, 10 survived.

Conclusion.—Angiography should be used liberally in stable patients with nonspecific physical findings. Proximal and distal control remains the key to operative management. If primary repair is not feasible, an interpositon graft may be placed or ligation performed. Patients with multiple injuries and blunt carotid dissection may safely be treated with anticoagulants. Hemiplegic patients with penetrating carotid injury usually survive after revascularization but seldom improve appreciably.

▶ Experiences with 118 patients with cervicothoracic arterial injuries seen in a period of 13 years are briefly described in this report. Diagnosis was greatly facilitated by the liberal use of angiography. Adequate exposure was clearly essential, as is well illustrated in the paper. The authors quite properly indicate the value of the 1973 monograph by Henry as a classic anatomical reference for surgical exposure (1).

The overall rate of mortality was 14%; 5% of deaths were attributed to shock and 7% to ischemia. The gravity of injury to the carotid artery is clear, as 11 of 57 patients who sustained such injuries died. The results are even worse in those patients who had neurologic defects. Among 20 patients who had either hemiplegia or coma before operation, only 5 were improved afterward; 8 remained unchanged and 7 died.—F.C. Spencer, M.D.

Reference

1. Henry AK: *Extensive Exposure,* ed 2. Edinburgh, Churchill Livingston, 1973.

Composite Graft Repair of Marfan Aneurysm of the Ascending Aorta: Results in 100 Patients

Gott VL, Pyeritz RE, Cameron DE, Greene PS, McKusick VA (Johns Hopkins Med Insts)

Ann Thorac Surg 52:38–45, 1991   17–22

Background.—A composite graft technique for the repair of ascending aortic aneurysms in Marfan's syndrome has greatly improved operative and long-term survival. The long-term results of 100 such procedures performed consecutively between 1976 and 1989 were reviewed.

Technique.—Standard hypothermic bypass is carried out with crystalloid potassium cardioplegic arrest. Direct anastomosis of the coronary ostia to the graft is used (Fig 17–4). Originally, a Cabrol interposition graft was used for patients whose coronary ostia had not migrated sufficiently for direct anastomosis (Fig 17–5), but it was found later that direct anastomosis could be achieved by placing pledgeted valve sutures below the annulus. Currently, if either ostium is extremely low, it is excised with a collar of aortic wall, mobilized, and the anastomosis performed slightly more distally. The aneurysm wall is tacked loosely over the composite graft, rather than being wrapped.

Patients and Outcome.—The 74 male and 26 female patients had a mean age of 31 years. The average aortic diameter was 7 cm. Ascending aortic dissection was done at the time of graft repair in 22 cases, and 18 patients had a mitral valve operation. Operative procedures were done on an elective basis in 92 patients, none of whom died. There was 1 operative death among the 8 who had emergency procedures. The overall in-hospital mortality was 1%, and late mortality was 10%. Five deaths occurred in the first 11 patients in the series and 5 in the last 88. The cause of death was graft endocarditis in 3 cases. Endocarditis occurred in 3 other patients as well, but they were treated by aortic root replacement with cryopreserved homografts. One patient died of late coronary dehiscence, but another had successful repair of dehiscence. At 5 years the actuarial survival was 92.6% and at 10 years, 75.8%.

Conclusions.—Patients with Marfan's syndrome and aneurysm of the ascending aorta can be treated successfully with composite graft repairs. The Bentall procedure should be used in those with an aneurysmal diameter of 6 cm or more, even if they are asymptomatic.

▶ This elegant report from Johns Hopkins describes experiences with 100 consecutive patients with Marfan's syndrome undergoing composite graft repair in a period of 13 years. There were no hospital deaths among 92 patients undergoing elective repair. Ten late deaths occurred, however; 3 were caused by composite graft endocarditis and 2 by late coronary dehiscence. The actuarial survival rate at 5 years was 92%. These data clearly document the recommendation for elective operation in patients with Marfan's syn-

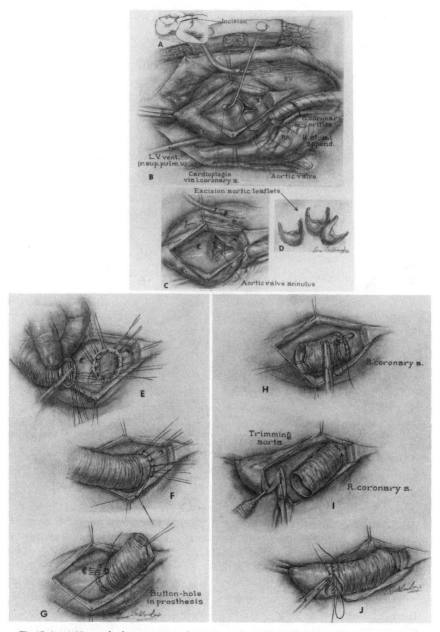

Fig 17–4.—**A-H,** standard composite graft repair as adapted from Bentall and DeBono. **E,** mattress sutures are placed below annulus if coronary ostia are low. **I,** aorta is completely transsected to facilitate distal end-to-end anastomosis. **J,** no-wrap technique is used; redundant aneurysm wall is tacked loosely over composite graft. *Abbreviations: LV,* left ventricular; *RA,* right atrium; *RV,* right ventricle. (Courtesy of Gott VL, Pyeritz RE, Cameron DE, et al: *Ann Thorac Surg* 52:38–45, 1991.)

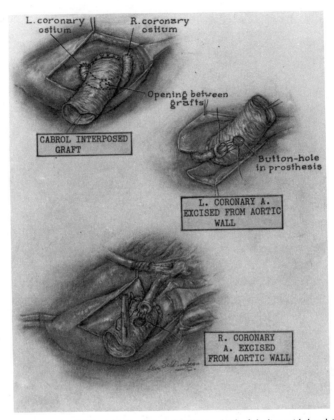

Fig 17–5.—Technique of Cabrol interposed graft. This method of dealing with low-lying coronary ostia has been replaced by mobilization of coronary ostia as depicted. (Courtesy of Gott VL, Pyeritz RE, Cameron DE, et al: *Ann Thorac Surg* 52:38–45, 1991.)

drome when the diameter of the aortic root reaches 6 cm.—F.C. Spencer, M.D.

Sixteen-Year Experience with Aortic Root Replacement: Results of 172 Operations
Kouchoukos NT, Wareing TH, Murphy SF, Perrillo JB (Wash Univ, St Louis)
Ann Surg 214:308–320, 1991   17–23

Introduction.—The results of 172 aortic root replacements in 168 patients treated in a 16-year interval were evaluated. The follow-up concluded in 1990. In 1981 an open technique replaced the inclusion/wrap technique used in the first 105 procedures in this series.

Technique.—In the open procedure, after excision of the aortic valve and completion of the sutures between the annulus and the prosthetic valve, buttons of graft opposite the coronary ostia are excised. The aortic wall next to the coronary ostia is sutured to these openings.

Results.—The hospital mortality rate was 5%. The only significant independent predictor of early death was the duration of cardiopulmonary bypass. The mean duration of follow-up was 81 months. Actuarial survival was 61% at 7 years and 48% at 12 years. There was no significant difference in survival rate between the inclusion/wrap and open technique; however, the frequency of reoperation was significantly less with the open procedure. Actuarial freedom from thromboembolism for 152 patients with prosthetic valves was 82% at 12 years.

Conclusion.—These results support continued use of composite graft replacement of the aortic root for annuloaortic ectasia and persistent aneurysm of the sinuses of Valsalva, and for patients with ascending aortic dissection. The open technique was associated with fewer reoperations and is the method of choice. The use of aortic allografts and pulmonary autografts has broadened the indications for aortic root replacement.

▶ This detailed report describes experiences with 168 patients undergoing aortic root replacement during a period of 16 years. Basic causes were either Marfan's syndrome, annuloaortic ectasia, or aortic dissection. Operative mortality was 5% but 4 of the 9 deaths in the series occurred among patients operated on for acute dissection.

Actuarial survival was 61% at 7 years. Hence the data clearly demonstrate the safety and reliability of aortic root replacement for these complex problems.—F.C. Spencer, M.D.

Management and Long-Term Outcome of Aortic Dissection
Glower DD, Speier RH, White WD, Smith LR, Rankin JS, Wolfe WG (Duke Univ)
Ann Surg 214:31–41, 1991   17–24

Background.—Operative treatment for types I and II aortic dissection is standard, but there is disagreement about aortic valve replacement vs. resuspension, management of aortic arch involvement, aortic repair vs. grafting, and the use of inclusion vs. exclusion grafting techniques. Data were reviewed on 163 patients treated in a 14-year period with aortic dissection.

Patients and Methods.—Most of the patients (74%) were men. The mean age was 56 years. There were 68 type I, 23 type II, and 72 type III dissections. The diagnosis was confirmed by aortography or CT in most cases. Surgically treated patients had a woven Dacron graft sutured proximally just above the coronary ostia, and the distal suture line was completed with 3-0 polypropylene. Intraoperative mortality was 11% for type I and 14% for type II patients; 30-day mortality was 26% and 14%,

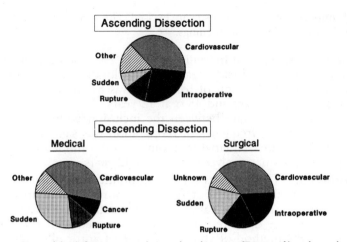

Fig 17–6.—Cause of death for patients with ascending dissection (*Top panel*) or descending dissection with medical or surgical therapy (*bottom panel*). (*Courtesy of Glower DD, Speier RH, White WD, et al: Ann Surg* 214:1 31–41, 1991.)

respectively. The 5-year survival was 56% and 87%, respectively. Thirty-three percent of types I and II patients had aortic valve resuspension and 14% had valve replacement. Of type III patients, 53 had medical management and 19 required operation for aortic rupture or expansion.

Results.—Among patients treated surgically, the intraoperative mortality was 11%. Thirty-day mortality in medically treated patients was 18%. At 9 or 10 years, 29% of type I, 46% of type II, and 29% of type III patients were still alive. Thirteen percent of patients with primary aortic dissection needed subsequent aortic surgery. Among late deaths, 38% resulted from other cardiovascular disease, 24% from sudden death, 21% from other medical conditions, and 18% from rupture of another segment of the aorta (Fig 17–6).

Conclusions.—Operative therapy remains the technique of choice in patients with types I and II aortic dissection, but it should be reserved for selected type III dissections. Although the long-term survival rate is acceptable, patients must be followed carefully to control any concurrent cardiovascular or residual aortic disease. This should include chest films, CT, or angiography.

▶ This report from Duke University describes experiences with dissection in 163 patients seen during a 13-year period. Type I and type II dissections were promptly operated on, with an intraoperative mortality of 11%; type III dissections were managed medically in 53, reserving operation for 19 with threatened rupture or expansion. Aortic valve resuspension was performed in 22 patients with acute dissection involving a normal valve; whereas 9 patients with intrinsic aortic valve disease required aortic valve replacement.

The 9- to 10-year survival rates were 29%, 46%, and 29% for types I, II, and III, respectively. This high late fatality rate, especially with dissection involving the aorta distal to the left subclavian artery, clearly indicates the importance of continuing long-term follow-up.—F.C. Spencer, M.D.

Treatment of Postoperative Infection of Ascending Aorta and Transverse Aortic Arch, Including Use of Viable Omentum and Muscle Flaps

Coselli JS, Crawford ES, Williams TW Jr, Bradshaw MW, Wiemer DR, Harris RL, Safi HJ (Baylor College of Medicine; Methodist Hosp, Houston)
Ann Thorac Surg 50:868–881, 1990   17–25

Background.—Because wounds created by reconstruction of the ascending aorta (AA) or the transverse aortic arch (TAA) communicate directly with the skin, complications that would be trivial at other sites have grave consequences. In the 1% to 6% of patients in whom abdominal aortic and peripheral arterial operative sites become infected, an external bypass graft, resection of the infected graft, and 1–6 months of antibiotic therapy produce survival rates of 50% to 90%. This approach is not suitable for most infections of the AA and TAA. The results of in situ surgery and lifelong antibiotic therapy were studied in patients with such infections.

Methods.—In 40 patients (average age, 55 years), postsurgical infections developed 1 week to 5.5 years after graft replacement of the AA, TAA, or both. Infections resulted in complications such as aortic-right ventricular, aortobronchial, or aortocutaneous fistulas (Fig 17-7), periaortic abscess; infection of a false aneurysm (Figs 17-8 and 17-9); suture line rupture; insufficiency of the aortic valve; and chest wall problems. Complications were treated medically or by surgical methods including resuturing, débridement, graft or valve and graft replacement, and patch-graft closure of false aneurysm. An important feature was the use of local tissue, distant muscle flaps, and omentum to fill dead space in the mediastinum. All surgical patients had intravenous antibiotic therapy for 4–6 weeks followed by lifelong oral suppressive antibiotics. Patients were followed for 3 months to 6.5 years.

Results.—Although 5 patients died of complications during surgery and 2 died in the subsequent 2 months, 29 surgically treated and 4 medically treated patients (83% overall) survived the early postoperative period. At last follow-up, 70% were alive and well. None of the late deaths resulted from recurrent infection, a hazard avoided by all surgically treated patients.

Conclusions.—The lifelong postoperative use of suppressive antibiotics permitted conservative treatment of infected grafts. In situ operations with lifelong suppressive antibiotic therapy appear to be an appropriate, if not the only possible, surgical intervention for graft infection of AA and TAA grafts.

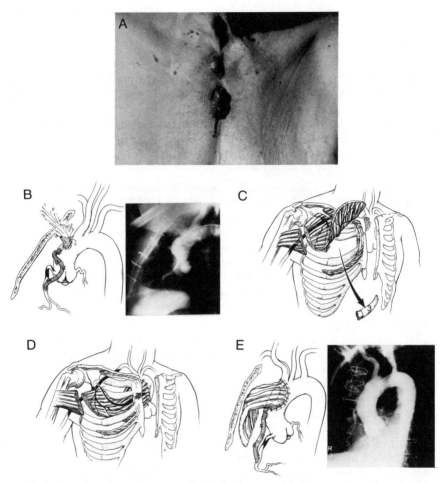

Fig 17-7.—Patient with aortocutaneous fistula after coronary artery bypass grafting. **A,** anterior chest wall has a healing external aortocutaneous fistula in the upper end of the old scar and a fresh external opening with protruding granulation tissue just below it. **B,** false aneurysm arising from the site of previous patch-graft repair of infected false aneurysm. **C,** a large segment of the right pectoralis major was completely mobilized. **D,** the mobilized muscle was transferred into the chest through a window created by removing the medial end of the third rib and costal cartilage. **E,** the mobilized muscle was sutured around the ascending aorta, which was repaired by débridement and reinsertion of a new Dacron patch (*drawing*), thus producing a satisfactory aortic reconstruction (*aortogram*). (Courtesy of Coselli JS, Crawford ES, Williams TW Jr, et al: *Ann Thorac Surg* 50:868–881, 1990.)

▶ This classic paper describes a large experience with the dread complication of postoperative infection of the aorta and aortic arch. Because the 40 patients varied widely in complexity, generalized conclusions are limited by the amount of comparable data. Twenty-one patients contracted infection between 1 week and 2 years after operation at the authors' institution, representing a 3% infection rate following 652 operations. Nineteen patients were referred for well-established chronic infections. Quite significant is the fact that 9 of the 40 patients became infected between 1 and 6 years after operation. Long-term survival was about 70%. Several general comments can be made, but the paper should be studied in detail by anyone treating a patient with this serious complication.

The authors previously introduced the novel concept of lifelong antibiotics. This is based on the fact that a few patients stopped taking antibiotics even after 1 year and promptly had recurrence of the infection. The basis for this concept is probably analogous to long-term prophylaxis with penicillin for rheumatic fever, but it is probably applicable only to organisms that do not develop resistant strains. In this series, 57% of the organisms were gram positive, 23% were gram negative, only 3% were fungi.

Muscle flaps or omentum were used effectively in some patients, but no data are given. Some of the illustrations dramatically illustrate impressive results. Figure 17–8 shows a large muscle flap used after 11 previous operations were ineffective.

Table 3 in the full-length article documents different methods of treatment. The concept of not removing the entire infected prosthesis was employed. However, simple suture of the origin of a false aneurysm in 8 patients resulted in eventual death in 5 of them. A composite valve graft replacement was done in 9 patients, only 4 of whom survived, whereas graft replacement was successful in 7 others.

The most important concept to be derived from the paper is that most patients can be treated successfully by a variety of the current techniques available, including circulatory arrest, widespread débridement and removal of

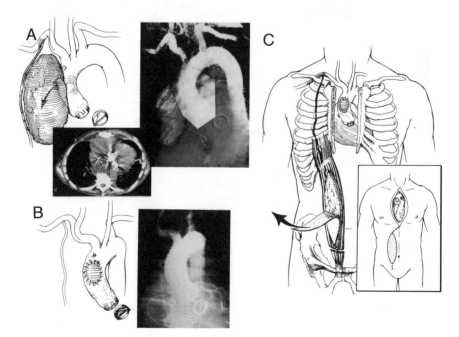

(continued)

Fig 17–8 (cont).

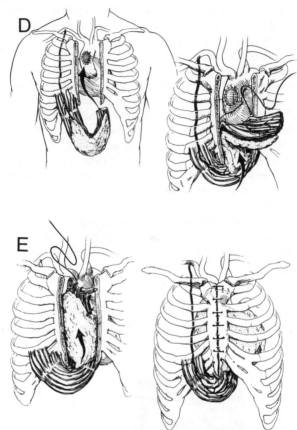

Fig 17–8.—Patient with large retrosternal false aneurysm after replacement of aortic and mitral valves. **A**, drawing, CT scan, and aortogram showing aneurysm. **B**, with circulation arrested, the chest was opened and the aneurysm site was débrided and closed with a large Dacron patch. **C**, a musculocutaneous flap was created to cover the aorta and fill the mediastinal dead space. **D**, the flap was introduced into the mediastinum, thus covering the reconstructed aorta. **E**, the bulky segment of flap filled the dead space, and the wound was closed. (Courtesy of Coselli JS, Crawford ES, Williams TW Jr, et al: *Ann Thorac Surg* 50:868–881, 1990.)

infected tissue, and application of muscle or omental grafts. The authors are to be congratulated for this important contribution.—F.C. Spencer, M.D.

Reappraisal of Surgical Treatment of Traumatic Transection of the Thoracic Aorta
Zeiger MA, Clark DE, Morton JR (Maine Med Ctr, Portland)
J Cardiovasc Surg 31:607–610, 1990   17–26

Introduction.—Repair of traumatic transection of the thoracic aorta without shunt or bypass, as introduced by Crawford in the mid-1970s, is

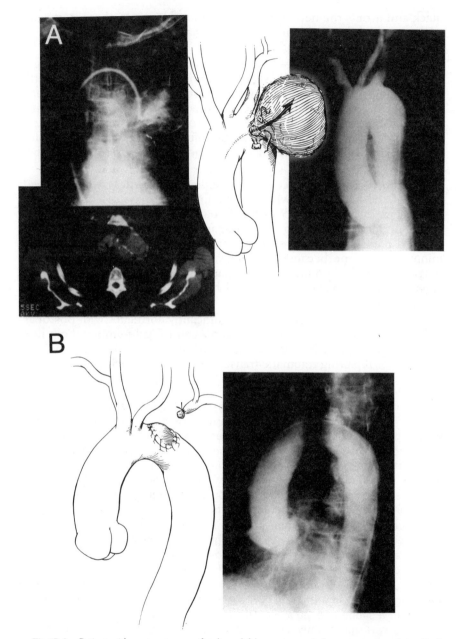

Fig 17–9.—Patient with aortocutaneous fistula and false aneurysm in lesser curvature of the distal aortic arch after aortic injury during a Chamberlain procedure. **A,** percutaneous angiogram (*upper left*) performed through the chronic aortocutaneous sinus tract, CT scan (*bottom left*), and drawing show the false aneurysm and route of the aortocutaneous fistula. Preoperative aortogram (*right*) was nondiagnostic. **B,** drawing and postoperative aortogram show satisfactory aortic reconstruction using the left subclavian artery for repair of coarctation. (Courtesy of Coselli JS, Crawford ES, Williams TW Jr, et al: *Ann Thorac Surg* 50:868–881, 1990.)

quick and avoids the need for heparinization. However, there is growing evidence that the incidence of paraplegia with this method may be greater than is justified by its advantages.

Patients and Methods.—Between 1975 and 1988, 54 patients aged 15–70 years (mean age, 28 years) sustained traumatic thoracic aortic transection. Most patients had multiple associated injuries. Nine patients could not be resuscitated. Another 5 patients who were alive on admission died before operation could be performed. The remaining 40 patients underwent repair of their aortic injury. Fourteen patients underwent repair with some type of bypass and shunt, and 26 patients had repair without a shunt.

Outcome.—All 40 patients who underwent aortic repair survived. None of the 14 patients who had repair with bypass or shunt became paraplegic. In contrast, in 9 of the 26 patients who had repair without a shunt, permanent paraplegia or paraparesis developed. Of the 26 non-shunted patients, 11 had repair with aortic clamp times of less than 28 minutes and none became paraplegic. Of 8 patients with clamp times ranging from 28–35 minutes, 1 had paraparesis and 1 had complete paraplegia. The remaining 7 patients all had clamp times of more than 35 minutes and all became paraplegic.

Conclusion.—Aortic clamp time significantly correlates with postoperative paraplegia. Left heart bypass using a centrifugal pump without heparin combined with a separate blood salvage system may be the best method for repairing traumatic transection of the thoracic aorta.

▶ For more than 20 years the debate has continued about the best approach in management of traumatic rupture of the aorta: use of a bypass with heparin or no-bypass or shunt. Operation is shorter and simpler by the latter method because heparinization increases bleeding significantly. However, virtually all data show an unacceptable frequency of paraplegia if the aorta is occluded for more than 30 minutes. Paraplegia, in all likelihood, is simply ischemic infarction of the spinal cord, although undoubtedly a number of factors influence the collateral circulation.

This review from the Maine Medical Center of experiences with 40 patients found a zero frequency of paraplegia in 14 repaired with a shunt and a 35% frequency in those repaired without a shunt. All cases of paraplegia occurred with occlusion times of more than 28 minutes.

A tabulation of 16 published reports found a similar variation in the rate of paraplegia, 2.9% in a total of 136 cases operated on with a pump, 7.9% in 165 with a shunt, and 20% in 108 operated on without a shunt. Mortality, however, was significantly higher with heparinization, 26% vs. about 14%.

These data are similar to those summarized in the important report by Pate in 1985, which should have been cited in the Bibliography (1).

As the authors indicate, the availability of the Bio-medicus centrifugal pump, permitting bypass without heparinization, may well be the best approach to this problem.—F.C. Spencer, M.D.

Reference

1. Pate JW: *Ann Thorac Surg* 39:531, 1985.

Traumatic Rupture of the Descending Thoracic Aorta
Von Oppell UO, Thierfelder CF, Beningfield SJ, Brink JG, Odell JA (Univ of Cape Town, South Africa; Groote Schuur Hosp, Cape Town)
S Afr Med J 79:595–598, 1991   17–27

Background.—Controversy remains about the management of acute traumatic rupture of the thoracic aorta, especially regarding the prevention of perioperative paraplegia. A 6-year review was made of the management of this problem.

Patients.—In all, 150 patients underwent aortography for suspected acute traumatic rupture of the descending thoracic aorta. The diagnosis was made in 18, 3 of whom had other findings on thoracotomy. Another patient had operation without aortography, giving a total of 16 patients. There were 13 males and 4 females (mean age, 29.4 years). All had been involved in motor vehicle accidents. Radiographically, all patients had mediastinal widening, and most had obliteration of the aortopulmonary window and left apical pleural cap. Multiple injuries were present in all patients, resulting in 5 missed diagnoses. Four patients successfully underwent other surgical procedures before aortic surgery was done.

Management.—One patient with a circumferential tear died as the operation was begun. Eight patients had simple aortic cross-clamping without augmentation; 1 died intraoperatively of cardiac arrhythmia and 2 died postoperatively of major bleeding. Three patients had postoperative paraplegia (table). Five patients were treated by partial heparinless bypass with a centrifugal vortex pump. None of these patients died or had hemorrhagic or new paraplegic complications after surgery.

Conclusions.—Partial heparinless bypass appears to be a better procedure for management of traumatic rupture of the descending thoracic aorta than simple aortic cross-clamping, which is often complicated by paraplegia. The bypass provides partial neutralization and extends the time for the operative procedure. Clinicians who treat victims of severe trauma must maintain a high index of suspicion for these injuries.

▶ This short report from the University of Cape Town in South Africa was selected because it clearly shows in a small series the utility of the Bio-Medicus pump in protecting from cardioplegia. Eight patients were treated early in the series with simple aortic cross-clamping; 3 deaths and 2 instances of paraplegia resulted. Since September 1988, the Bio-Medicus pump has

---

Outcomes of 16 Patients With Traumatic Rupture of
the Descending Thoracic Aorta and Surgical
Techniques Used

Initial deaths (_N_ = 3)
  Severe cerebral trauma 1
  Exsanguination after aortography
  (diagnosis missed for 46 h) 1
  Exsanguination at commencement of
  surgery (inability to obtain proximal
  aortic control) 1
Simple aortic cross-clamping (_N_ = 8)
  Deaths
    Intra-operative cardiac arrest on cross-
    clamping 1
    Postoperative, consequential to major
    secondary haemorrhages requiring
    re-operation 2
  Pre-operative paraplegia 1
  Postoperative

Paraplegia	No paralysis
3	4
Cross-clamp time (min)	
35 - 70	19 - 25
(mean 46,7)	(mean 21,75)
Interposition grafts	
2	2

Partial heparin-less bypass (_N_ = 5)
  Pre-operative paraplegia 1
  Postoperative

Paraplegia	No paralysis
1	4
Cross-clamp time (min)	
26	17 - 37
	(mean 24,5)
Interposition grafts	
1	3

(Courtesy of Von Oppell UO, Thierfelder CF, Beningfield SJ, et al: _S Afr Med J_ 79:595–598, 1991.)

---

been used in 5 patients with no fatalities and no postoperative paraplegia. As reported by others, paraplegia particularly occurs if clamp time exceeds 30 minutes. If the aortic tear is circumferential, an occlusion time longer than 30 minutes is often necessary.

The Bio-Medicus pump has the attractiveness of avoiding the use of heparin in a patient with multiple injuries, especially head injury, but permits perfusion of the distal aorta; the frequency of paraplegia should thus be greatly decreased without a corresponding increase in morbidity from hemorrhage.—F.C. Spencer, M.D.

The Value of Pulmonary Artery and Central Venous Monitoring in Patients Undergoing Abdominal Aortic Reconstructive Surgery: A Comparative Study of Two Selected, Randomized Groups

Isaacson IJ, Lowdon JD, Berry AJ, Smith RB III, Knos GB, Weitz FI, Ryan K (Emory Univ Hosp)
J Vasc Surg 12:754–760, 1990   17–28

Introduction.—Cardiac complications are the chief cause of morbidity and death after reconstruction of the abdominal aorta. It is important to define the extent of coronary disease and of myocardial reserve before surgery.

Methods.—To determine whether the choice between the central venous catheter (CVC) and pulmonary artery catheter (PAC) for hemodynamic monitoring influences the outcome, 102 patients undergoing abdominal aortic reconstruction were assigned prospectively to monitoring with a CVC or a PAC. None of the patients had uncompensated cardiopulmonary or renal disease.

Results.—There were no differences in morbidity between the 2 groups. On the second postoperative day, 1 patient in the PAC group died in cardiogenic shock. Dysrhythmias occurred in 3 patients in the CVC group and 5 in the PAC group. Hospital costs did not differ significantly, but anesthesia charges were significantly lower in the CVC group.

Conclusion.—Hemodynamic monitoring using a CVC seems adequate during abdominal aortic reconstructive surgery in most patients, but large-scale, multicenter studies are desirable.

▶ The 102 patients undergoing abdominal aortic reconstructive surgery were prospectively allocated randomly to 2 groups, monitoring either with a CVC or PAC. There was no significant difference in the results between the 2 groups. One death occurred in the pulmonary-artery-monitored group, and 1 myocardial infarction occurred in each group. The major difference between the 2 techniques was that there was a slight decrease in cost by avoiding pulmonary artery monitoring.

An important point is that patients were carefully screened for coronary artery disease, frequently using the dipyridamole-thallium scan. Patients with severe coronary artery disease were treated beforehand or were not operated on. This approach may be the major explanation for the low frequency of cardiovascular complications in either group.—F.C. Spencer, M.D.

18 The Arteries, the Veins, and the Lymphatics

Natural History of Patients With Abdominal Aortic Aneurysm
Glimåker H, Holmberg L, Elvin A, Nybacka O, Almgren B, Björck C-G, Eriksson I (Univ Hosp, Uppsala, Sweden; Central Hosp, Falun, Sweden)
Eur J Vasc Surg 5:125–130, 1991   18–1

Objective.—The factors determining the outcome of abdominal aortic aneurysm were examined retrospectively in a series of 187 consecutive patients seen at a single hospital in a 9-year period. All of the aneurysms were diagnosed ultrsonically, and the study was repeated in patients not having primary operative treatment.

Course.—Overall, 27% of the aneurysms expanded more rapidly than .4 cm/yr. Larger lesions tended to expand more rapidly. The cumulative rate of aneurysmal rupture was 12% at 5 years. The rate in patients with aneurysms less than 5 cm in size was 2.5% at 7 years, and no lesion was documented as being smaller than this at the time of rupture. Among 9 aneurysms 5 cm or larger in size, 28% ruptured within 3 years. The overall patient survival was 51% at 5 years. The proportion of deaths caused by aneurysmal rupture in patients with small lesions was 5.5%, compared with 53% in patients with large anerurysms. Life-tables were similar for large and small aneurysms when deaths from aneurysmal rupture were excluded.

Conclusions.—Abdominal aortic aneurysms expand at highly individual rates. The initial diameter of the lesion is the only recognized predictor of rupture.

▶ This represents an extremely low rate of rupture for aneurysms less than 5 cm in size and certainly suggests that patients with aneurysms smaller than 5 cm can be followed with sequential ultrasonogoraphy. Interestingly, the authors noted that a majority of aneurysms did not expand at all. Demonstration by Ellis et al. (1) that the accuracy of measurement with ultrasound is ± 0.47 because of observer variability makes this method of surveillance a reasonable one.—S.I. Schwartz, M.D.

Reference

1.   Ellis M, Greenhalgh RM, Mannick JA (eds), et al: *in The Cause and Management of Aneurysms.* London, WB Saunders, 1990, pp 117–121.

Surgery for Abdominal Aortic Aneurysms: A Survey of 656 Patients
Olsen PS, Schroeder T, Agerskov K, Røder O, Sørensen S, Perko M, Lorentzen JE (Rigshospitalet, Copenhagen)
J Cardiovasc Surg 32:636–642, 1991   18–2

Introduction.—Epidemiologic studies have shown that the incidence and mortality from abdominal aortic aneurysms (AAAs) have been steadily increasing in the past 2 decades. Elective surgery for AAAs can now be performed with a mortality of less than 5%. However, most aneurysmectomies are still performed acutely in the Scandinavian countries.

Methods.—Data were reviewed on 543 men and 113 women (median age, 69 years) who were operated on for AAA from 1979 to 1988. Of these 656 patients, 287 (44%) had elective procedures and 369 were operated on acutely; 218 patients had a ruptured AAA. The records of all patients were reviewed for associated diseases, preoperative clinical status, postoperative complications, and mortality.

Results.—Patients with symptomatic AAA had an increased incidence of arteriosclerotic heart disease and impaired renal function compared with patients operated on electively. Patients with arteriosclerotic heart disease, hypertension, impaired renal funtion, or chronic pulmonary disease had increased perioperative mortality compared with patients who did not have any of these risk factors. All patients with ruptured AAA and 80% of patients with symptomatic AAA had abdominal or back pain and a palpable pulsatile abdominal mass as the main features. Of the patients with a ruptured AAA, 51% were admitted in shock and had a systolic blood pressure below 100 mm Hg. There were ischemic symptoms in 28% of the patients without and in 14% of the patients with AAA rupture. Postoperative failure of 1 or more organs occurred in 153 patients (23%). The mortality rate among patients with multiorgan failure was 68%. In 93 patients, (14%) there were complications that required reoperation.

Conclusions.—The overall perioperative mortality was 18.8%. The perioperative mortality was 4.8% for patients operated on electively, 17.2% for symptomatic patients, and 37% for patients with AAA rupture. The 5-year survival rate was 48% after ruptured AAA, 70% after symptomatic AAA, and 75% after electively treated AAA. However, after 6 months the life expectancy in all 3 groups was identical and comparable to that in a sex- and age-matched control population. The overall survival rate after aneurysmectomy of an AAA could be improved by substantially increasing the proportion of patients operated on electively.

▶ The article reports the current state of the art of surgery for AAA. I would make a plea that the article subdivide the category of ruptured aneurysms. The operative mortality for retroperitoneal rupture without hypertension is obviously significantly better than that associated with free ruptures of the peritoneal cavity with portal hypertension. The 2 lesions are distinct and should be considered as such in providing statistical analysis of the operative procedures.—S.I. Schwartz, M.D.

Treatment of Patients with Aortic Dissection Presenting with Peripheral Vascular Complications
Fann JI, Sarris GE, Mitchell RS, Shumway NE, Stinson EB, Oyer PE, Miller DC
(Stanford Univ)
Ann Surg 212:705–713, 1990   18–3

Introduction.—Controversy exists over the optimal therapeutic approach in patients with aortic dissection complicated by peripheral vascular problems. A review was made of a 25-year experience with such patients, in whom an aggressive approach directed primarily at repair of the dissected thoracic aorta was followed.

Patients.—Between 1963 and 1987, 272 consecutive patients underwent surgery after spontaneous aortic dissection. Two types of dissection were distinguished: type A involved the ascending aorta and type B did not. Acute dissections were those in which symptoms occurred less than 14 days earlier; dissections in which symptoms appeared more than 14 days earlier were defined as chronic. The frequency of specific complications by acuity and type of dissection is shown in figure 18–1. The

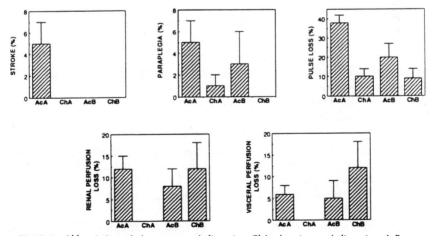

Fig 18–1.—*Abbreviations: AcA*, acute type A dissection; *ChA*, chronic type A dissection; *AcB*, acute type B dissection; *ChB*, chronic type B dissection. The frequency of specific individual peripheral vascular complications subdivided according to acuity and type of aortic dissection. (Courtesy of Fann JI, Sarris GE, Mitchell RS, et al: *Ann Surg* 212:705–713, 1990.)

patient group was predominantly male (196 patients) and had a mean age of 57 years. Eighty-five patients had sustained 1 or more peripheral vascular complications.

Operative Technique and Outcome.—Patients with type A dissections were approached by a median sternotomy. Those in the type B group underwent a left posterolateral thoracotomy. The overall hospital mortality rate was 25%. The rate in patients with acute type A dissections (25%) was not significantly different from that in patients with chronic type A dissections (20%). In the type B group, however, acute dissections resulted in a significantly higher operative mortality rate than chronic dissections, 40% vs. 18%.

Implications.—The presence of peripheral vascular complications did not significantly affect overall operative mortality, although multivariate analysis revealed that impaired renal perfusion was a significant independent predictor of increased operative mortality risk. After repair of the thoracic aorta, the outcome was less favorable in patients with paraplegia and impaired visceral perfusion. Prompt surgical repair of the aorta will obviate the need for most peripheral revascularization procedures.

▶ The current knowledge about aortic dissecting aneurysm was well reviewed by DeSanctis et al. (1). The importance of long-term follow-up has been emphasized by several reports demonstrating that nearly 30% of deaths result from the development and rupture of another aneurysm. The long-term survival rate for patients with this disease has improved, the overall actuarial 10-year survival now being approximately 40%.—S.I. Schwartz, M.D.

Reference

1. DeSanctis RW, et al: *N Engl J Med* 317: 1060, 1987.

Spontaneous Abdominal Arteriovenous Fistulae: Report of Eight Cases and Review of the Literature
Gilling-Smith GL, Mansfield AO (St Mary's Hosp, London)
Br J Surg 78:421–426, 1991   18–4

Background.—The hemodynamic disturbance resulting from the spontaneous rupture of an abdominal aneurysm into an adjacent major vein is profound and worsens rapidly. The diagnosis must be made promptly and the fistula surgically closed if the patient is to survive. Eight cases and the literature on this subject were reviewed.

Diagnosis.—The condition is always fatal if operation is not done. Usually, the diagnosis is made clinically, because most patients have at least some signs of fistula. The "full house" presentation of palpable abdominal aneurysm, machinery murmur, high-output cardiac failure, and

TABLE 1.—Symptoms, Signs, and Operative Findings in 8 Cases of Spontaneous Abdominal Arteriovenous Fistula

Case	Sex	Age (years)	Symptoms/duration	Signs	Operative findings	Procedure	Outcome
1	F	72	Low back pain, 2 weeks; dyspnoea, 4 days	Palpable AAA – machinery bruit; BP 120/50 mmHg; CVP+30 cmH$_2$O	Infrarenal AAA (12 cm); fistula into IVC (2 cm)	Fistula sutured; bifurcation graft	Well, 2 years
2	M	67	Low back pain, 2 days	Palpable AAA; BP 70/– mmHg	Infrarenal AAA (11 cm); retroperitoneal rupture; fistula into IVC (3 cm); (CVP+32 cmH$_2$O)	Fistula sutured; bifurcation graft	Well, 4 years
3	M	80	Low back pain, 4 days	Palpable AAA; BP 80/– mmHg	Infrarenal AAA (12 cm); retroperitoneal rupture; fistula into IVC (4 cm) (machinery thrill)	Fistula sutured; straight graft	Well, 1 year
4	M	81	Back pain, 10 days; abdominal pain, 2 days	Palpable AAA – tender; BP 100/60 mmHg	Infrarenal AAA (10 cm); retroperitoneal rupture; fistula into IVC (2 cm); (CVP+24 cmH$_2$O)	Fistula sutured; bifurcation graft	Well, 1 year

(continued)

regional venous hypertension is uncommon. A spontaneous abdominal arteriovenous fistula should be considered in any patient with an atypical-appearing abdominal aneurysm or chronic congestive cardiac failure refractory to medical treatment. In patients whose condition is stable,

Table 1 (continued)

5	M	65	Back pain, 2 weeks; haematuria, 2 days	Palpable AAA – machinery bruit; BP 110/20 mmHg; cyanotic legs; priapism and pulsating varicose veins	Aorto right iliac aneurysm; fistula: right CIA into IVC (3 cm)	Fistula sutured; bifurcation graft	Well, 6 months
6	F	73	LIF pain, weakness and lethargy, 10 weeks; vomiting, 1 week	Palpable aortoiliac aneurysm; systolic bruit; BP 150/70 mmHg; acute renal failure	Aorto left iliac aneurysm; fistula: left CIA into left CIV (machinery thrill, CVP+20 cmH$_2$O)	Fistula sutured; bifurcation graft	Well, 3 months
7	M	66	Dyspnoea, 3 years; swollen legs, 2 years	Pulsating RIF mass – machinery bruit; BP 140/40 mmHg; CVP+28 cmH$_2$O; gross pulmonary oedema; cyanotic legs	Right CIA aneurysm; fistulae into both CIVs	Fistulae sutured; iliac graft	Died, 10 days
8	F	73	Dyspnoea, 4 years; swollen legs, 3 years	Pulsating RIF mass – machinery bruit; BP 130/60 mmHg; CVP+22 cmH$_2$O	Pelvic right kidney; right renal artery aneurysm; fistula into right renal vein	Right nephrectomy	Died, 25 days

Abbreviations: AAA, abdominal aortic aneurysm; IVC, inferior vena cava; CIA, common iliac artery; CIV, common iliac vein; LIF/RIF, left/right iliac fossa; BP, blood pressure; CVP, central venous pressure.
(Courtesy of Gilling-Smith GL, Mansfield AO: *Br J Surg* 78:421–426, 1991.)

the diagnosis may be confirmed and the fistula localized by angiography. However, this should not delay operation.

Treatment.—In stable patients, it may be advisable to clamp the aorta gradually; a sudden increase in cardiac afterload and an abrupt fall in ve-

TABLE 2.—Site of Spontaneous Abdominal Arteriovenous Fistula
in 148 Cases Reported Since 1955

Aneurysm	Vein	n	References
Aorta	IVC (right-sided)	113	
	IVC (left-sided)	2	21, 47
	Left renal vein (retroaortic)	7	30, 34, 37, 49, 56, 59, 82
	Left renal vein (preaortic)	1	74
	Lumbar vein	1	27
	Right CIV	2	1, 48
	Left CIV	2	18, 20
Right CIA	Right CIV	5	9, 41, 54, 65, 83
	Left CIV	2	9, 43
	Both CIVs	1	Case 7
	IVC	4	Case 5, refs. 9, 57, 80
Left CIA	Left CIV	7	Case 6, refs. 11, 20, 25,27, 39, 64
Renal renal artery	Right renal vein	1	Case 8

Abbreviations: IVC, inferior vena cava; CIA, common iliac artery; CIV, common iliac vein.

(Courtesy of Gilling-Smith GL, Mansfield AO: *Br J Surg* 78:421–426, 1991.)

nous return could result in cardiac arrest. "Paradoxical" pulmonary embolization should be avoided by careful evacuation of the aneurysm thrombus. Usually, digital compression of the vein at the fistula site allows suturing of the fistula from within the aneurysm sac. Routine aortoiliac grafting completes the operation. The patient may need ventilatory and inotropic support postoperatively.

Conclusion.—The 8 current cases (Table 1) and the 148 reported in the literature (Table 2) demonstrate the variety of clinical presentations and the difficulty of diagnosing this condition.

▶ This is an excellent review of a relatively rare lesion. As the authors stress, early diagnosis is the key to successful management. The review of the literature is certainly complete, and the authors' personal experience provides meaningful information. It is of historical interest that the femorofemoral anastomosis truly represents the first extra-anatomical vascular bypass. The theoretical adverse consequence, the steal phenomenon, is rarely defined. The most subsequent operations in patients undergoing femorofemoral anastomosis relate to the distal runoff. The authors' findings of similar patency rates for femorofemoral bypass grafts, compared to balloon angioplasty, emphasize the need for selection in applying 1 of the 2 procedures. Alexander and Imbembo reported on aorta-vena cava fistulas (1). They pointed out that spontaneous aorta-vena cava fistulas are now seen more frequently and comprise 80% to 90% of all cases, with traumatic injury accounting for the others. Surgical repair of spontaneous aortocaval fistulas had a mortality rate of 22% to 51%.—S.I. Schwartz, M.D.

Reference

1. Alexander JJ, Imbembo AL: *Surgery* 105:1, 1989.

Randomized Trial of Intra-Arterial Recombinant Tissue Plasminogen Activator, Intravenous Recombinant Tissue Plasminogen Activator, and Intra-Arterial Streptokinase in Peripheral Arterial Thrombolysis
Berridge DC, Gregson RHS, Hopkinson BR, Makin GS (Univ Hosp, Nottingham, England)
Br J Surg 78:988–995, 1991   18–5

Background.—When systemic thrombolysis is used to treat peripheral arterial thrombosis, a fibrin-specific agent must be given for several hours without producing a profound systemic lytic effect. Recombinant tissue plasminogen activator (rt-PA) has this potential. A randomized trial of intra-arterial rt-PA, intravenous rt-PA, and intra-arterial streptokinase in peripheral arterial thrombolysis was carried out.

Methods.—Sixty patients were assigned randomly in equal groups to the 3 treatments. The groups did not differ significantly in age, duration of history, length of occlusion, or presence of neurosensory deficit.

Results.—Initially, lysis was significantly more successful with intra-arterial rt-PA than with other 2 treatments. The treatment duration varied from a median of 35 hours with intra-arterial rt-PA to 40 hours with streptokinase. The median increase in ankle:brachial pressure index after intra-arterial rt-PA was significantly greater than for the other treatments. Limb salvage at 30 days was obtained in 80% of those in the group given intra-arterial rt-PA, 60% in those given streptokinase and 45% in the group given intravenous rt-PA. Bleeding complications occurred in 6 pa-

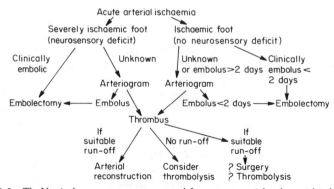

Fig 18–2.—The Nottingham management protocol for an acute peripheral arterial ischemia. (Courtesy of Berridge DC, Gregson RHS, Hopkinson BR, et al: *Br J Surg* 78:988–995, 1991.)

tients after streptokinase therapy and in 13 after intravenous rt-PA. Only 1 minor hemorrhage occurred, this after a catheter perforation in a patient who received intra-arterial rt-PA (Fig 18–2).

Conclusions.—Intra-arterial rt-PA is a safer, more effective fibrinolytic regimen than conventional streptokinase treatment. The less successful intravenous rt-PA treatment is associated with a significantly greater risk of bleeding complications.

▶ Towne and Bandyk (1) review the application of thrombolytic therapy in vascular occlusive disease. Clinically successful fibrinolysis was achieved in only 50% to 80% of patients, and the duration of drug infusion required to lyse an arterial thrombus could not be predicted. Sicard et al. (2) reported a series in whom treatment of the native artery occlusion led to complete lysis in 45%, but only 21% of graft occlusions were treated successfully. In comparing the effects of streptokinase and rt-PA, more recent literature suggests that there is no advantage to the latter, and that the rt-PA activator is associated with a higher incidence of complications, particularly hemorrhage (3).—S.I. Schwartz, M.D.

References

1. Towne JB, Bandyk DF: *Am J Surg* 154:548, 1987.
2. Sicard GA, et al: *J Vasc Surg* 2:65, 1985.
3. Marder VJ, Sherry S: *N Engl J Med* 318:1512, 1988.

Percutaneous Intraarterial Thrombolysis in the Treatment of Thrombosis of Lower Extremity Arterial Reconstructions
Seabrook GR, Mewissen MW, Schmitt DD, Reifsnyder T, Bandyk DF, Lipchik EO, Towne JB (Med College of Wisconsin; Clement J Zablocki VA Med Ctr, Milwaukee)
J Vasc Surg 13:646–651, 1991   18–6

Background.—Acute thrombosis of vascular bypass grafts in the lower extremities can lead to loss of the limb. One alternative to balloon catheter thrombectomy salvage is intra-arterial thrombolytic therapy under angiographic guidance. Fifteen patients with 30 acute occlusions of an autologous or prosthetic vascular graft were evaluated. All 15 were treated with intra-arterial urokinase.

Results.—The origins of the graft occlusion included morphological defects, pseudoaneurysm, disease progression distal to the graft, or coagulation disorders. In 13 occlusions a cause could not be determined. Patency was restored initially in all cases. However, in 6 patients adjunctive surgical thrombectomy was required to remove persistent thrombus. One graft could not be salvaged and amputation was performed. Five significant hemorrhagic complications occurred and 1 patient died.

Conclusion.—Percutaneous intra-arterial thrombolysis allows the salvage of some grafts that would not remain patent after balloon catheter thrombectomy. Thrombolytic therapy can be associated with serious complications and should be used only when the benefits of graft salvage outweigh the risk of hemorrhage.

▶ Sicard et al. (1) reported a series of 40 patients. In 45%, treatment of native artery occlusion lead to complete lysis of clot without the need for further surgical intervention. But only 21% of the treatments for graft occlusion were successful. Ricotta et al. (2), after polling vascular surgeons, reported that a successful outcome was achieved by thrombolytic therapy for vascular occlusive disease in only 50% of patients and there was significant morbidity, leading to a general lack of enthusiasm for the procedure.—S.I. Schwartz, M.D.

References

1. Sicard GA, et al: *J Vasc Surg* 2:65, 1985.
2. Ricotta JJ, et al: *J Vasc Surg* 6:45, 1987.

Limitations to the Widespread Usage of Low-Dose Intra-Arterial Thrombolysis
Browse DJ, Barr H, Torrie EPH, Galland RB (Royal Berkshire Hosp, Reading, England)
Eur J Vasc Surg 5:445–449, 1991   18–7

Introduction.—Although low-dose intra-arterial thrombolysis (IAT) has given encouraging results in patients with acute and chronic ischemia, British surgeons have been slow to use this technique. British vascular surgeons were surveyed as to their opinions about IAT.

Survey.—A questionnaire concerning the use or reasons for nonuse of IAT was sent to 232 vascular surgeons, of whom 134 (58%) responded. Of the respondents, 38% never used IAT and 45% used it only on occasion. Reasons for not using IAT included lack of backup in 47% of patients—either radiologic, intensive care unit, or staff; 45% had doubts concerning the efficacy of the technique. Surgeons in teaching hospitals were more likely to use IAT than those in district hospitals.

Clinical Experience.—Data were reviewed on IAT used to treat 82 occlusions in 73 patients during a 22-month period. The most common symptom was rest pain, and the most common site was the superficial femoral artery. Streptokinase was used in 74 patients and rt-PA in 8. When treatment was started within 1 week of symptom onset, lysis was successful in 82% of the patients. With symptoms of longer duration, the success rate was 62%. No further treatment was needed after IAT in 44% of the patients; reconstruction was needed in 26%, angioplasty in 23%, and major amputation in 1. Major complications included a fatal cerebrovascular accident and bleeding from the catheter insertion site in 5 cases. Emergency operation was needed in 2 of these patients, and 1 who had an angioplasty immediately after lysis died. In 16 patients, there were local hematomas, 6 had catheter problems, and 2 had allergic reactions. A median of 4 angiograms were obtained at intervals and the catheter repositioned as necessary until lysis was complete. Of these angiograms, 46% were performed outside of normal working hours.

Conclusion.—Low-dose IAT appears to be a safe and effective form of treatment in carefully selected and monitored patients. The need for substantial radiologic support appears to be a limiting factor in the use of this technique. Surgeons and vascular radiologists must be trained in the use of this procedure.

▶ As Towne and Bandyk have pointed out (1), acute arterial occlusions are more likely to respond to thrombolytic therapy. The duration of drug infusion required to lyse the thrombosis cannot be predicted, and hemorrhage remains a significant complication.—S.I. Schwartz, M.D.

Reference

1. Towne JB, Bandyk DR: *Am J Surg* 154:548, 1987.

Femorofemoral Bypass: A Profile of Graft Failure
Farber MA, Hollier LH, Eubanks R, Ochsner JL, Bowen JC (Ochsner Clinic and Alton Ochsner Med Found, New Orleans)
South Med J 83:1437–1443, 1990   18–8

Background.—Femorofemoral bypass grafting is popular for the surgical treatment of unilateral iliac artery occlusive disease. It is associated with low morbidity and mortality and acceptable long-term patency. The causes of graft failure in cases of femorofemoral bypass were reviewed.

Methods.—Seventy-one patients who had a femorofemoral bypass for unilateral iliac artery occlusion or stenosis were assessed for morbidity, mortality, initial symptom relief, early patency, and long-term primary and secondary patency. The causes of graft failure also were evaluated.

Results.—The overall postoperative hospital mortality was 4%. Survival at 1 year and 2 years was 84% and 81%, respectively. At 1 month, patency was 98.5%. Late patency at 1 year and 5 years was 91% and 82%, respectively. Inadequate run-off and outflow disease progression were the major causes of graft failure. There were no significant differences in graft failure between polytetrafluoroethylene grafts and other materials used.

Conclusions.—The morbidity and mortality in this series of patients were comparable to that in a cohort undergoing balloon angioplasty.

However, the patients having femorofemoral bypass were usually not candidates for balloon angioplasty.

▶ The hemodynamic results of femorofemoral bypass graft surgery were assessed in 54 patients by Lamerton et al. (1). The majority had bilateral superficial femoral occlusion in addition to iliac occlusion. Significant improvements in the recipient limb pressure index at rest were seen in patients with patent grafts 6 weeks after operation. The early graft failure rate was 13%, and the cumulative patency rate at 5 years was 60%. Femorofemoral bypass remains a valuable operation in the management of selected patients. The issue of significant diversion away from the donor limb after operation, either after rest or after exercise, has not been resolved.—S.I. Schwartz, M.D.

Reference

1. Lamerton AJ, et al: *Arch Surg* 120:1274, 1985.

Popliteal Artery Aneurysms: Long-Term Follow-Up of Aneurysmal Disease and Results of Surgical Treatment
Dawson I, van Bockel JH, Brand R, Terpstra JL (Univ Hosp Leiden, The Netherlands)
J Vasc Surg 13:398–407, 1991   18–9

Introduction.—Popliteal artery aneurysms have been associated with thromboembolic complications, a risk of new aneurysms developing, and possibly decreased life expectancy. To evaluate the long-term results of popliteal aneurysms, data were reviewed on a series of 50 consecutive patients.

Patients.—Between 1958 and 1985, 50 men were treated at the study institution for arteriosclerotic popliteal aneurysm. The patients' mean age at diagnosis was 65 years. Twenty-one patients had a contralateral popliteal aneurysm at the time of presentation.

Treatment.—Forty-six of the 71 aneurysms were initially treated by surgery. Of the remaining popliteal aneurysms not treated by surgery, 21 were asymptomatic and 4 were in patients not judged to be medically fit for surgery. Eleven patients treated conservatively subsequently underwent surgery because of complications or a risk of complications. In most cases the operative procedure consisted of bypass surgery with exclusion of the aneurysm.

Outcome.—Twelve of the 21 asymptomatic, conservatively treated patients had complications, most within 2 years. During a mean follow-up of 5 years, 23 new aneurysms developed in 16 patients. The probability of new aneurysm formation rose from 6% at 1 year to 49% at 10 years. In patients who underwent reconstruction of a popliteal aneurysm, rates of graft patency and foot salvage were 64% and 95% at 10 years, respectively. Overall survival, however, was poor. Within a mean follow-up of 5 years, 33 patients (66%) died.

Implications.—The presence of multiple isolated aneurysms at the initial examination had the most significant influence on patient survival, even though most of the deaths resulted from myocardial infarction and not from complications of these aneurysms. Surgical reconstruction is recommended for all asymptomatic, as well as symptomatic, popliteal aneurysms. Patients with multiple aneurysms should undergo regular, lifelong follow-up.

▶ The experience at Strong Memorial Hospital is similar to that reported by these authors. Studies confirm the need for prophylactic reconstruction and long follow-up of the patient. Schellack et al. (1) reported 46 asymptomatic popliteal artery aneurysms. Twenty-six were managed initially without operation; only 2 of the 26 had significant complications as a result of conservative management. The 5-year cumulative patency rate in these patients was 93%. The authors concluded that, when faced with a high-risk patient having a small asymptomatic popliteal aneurysm, the conservative approach is reasonably safe.—S.I. Schwartz, M.D.

Reference

1. Schellack J, et al: *Arch Surg* 122:372, 1987.

Femoral-Distal Bypass With In Situ Greater Saphenous Vein: Long-Term Results Using the Mills Valvulotome
Donaldson MC, Mannick JA, Whittemore AD (Brigham and Women's Hosp, Boston)
Ann Surg 213:457–465, 1991   18–10

Introduction.—The autologous greater saphenous vein is widely used as a conduit for revascularization below the inguinal ligament. This vein was originally used in reversed fashion, but refinement of the valvulotome and small-vessel surgical techniques has led to widespread use of the in situ greater saphenous vein for infrainguinal arterial reconstruction.

Methods.—During a 7-year period 371 patients underwent 440 in situ greater saphenous vein bypass operations in the treatment of atherosclerotic occulsive disease. Saphenous vein bypass was the primary reconstruction in 406 procedures (92%), whereas previous infrainguinal revascularization had been performed in the remaining 34 cases. A modified Mills valvulotome was used for all operations. In all procedures the proximal anastomosis was at the groin level. An infrapopliteal artery was the site of distal anastomosis in 200 procedures (45%). Indications for arterial bypass were critical ischemia in 299 extremities and disabling claudication in 141.

Results.—Surgical complications—cardiopulmonary, renal, or cerebro-vascular—occurred in 104 patients (24%); these were major in 33 patients. Technical problems attributable to the in situ method occurred in 5 of 27 early occlusions. Nine patients (2%) died within the first 30 days after operation. The mean postoperative follow-up was 20.4 months. Of the 440 grafts, 352 (80%) were followed to known end points. Graft surveillance identified 18 stenotic grafts (4%); these were revised while still patent, but these grafts required 30 revisions to maintain patency during follow-up. Sixty-eight grafts (15%) occluded during follow-up; 36 of these underwent initial disobliteration and required a total of 52 revisions during follow-up. Five-year life-table analysis showed an overall primary patency rate of 72%, a primary revised patency rate of 78%, secondary patency of 83%, extremity salvage of 88%, and patient survival of 66%.

Conclusion.—In contrast to reversed vein grafts, long infrapopliteal in situ grafts have long-term secondary patency similar to that of shorter femoropopliteal bypass grafts. In situ greater saphenous vein grafting is therefore the procedure of choice for long infrapopliteal bypass.

▶ These excellent results represent a gold standard. It is to be pointed out that equivalent results have been achieved by Taylor et al. (1) using a reverse vein bypass grafting. Although there will continue to be champions of both techniques, results associated with each can be approved by monitoring of functional patency postoperatively but identifying grafts with correctable lesions before thrombosis occurs (2). Bergmark et al. (3) reported significantly higher patency for in situ grafts anastomosed to infrapopliteal arteries.—S.I. Schwartz, M.D.

References

1. Taylor LM, et al: *J Vasc Surg* 11:193, 1990.
2. Bandyk DF, et al: *J Vasc Surg* 9:286, 1989.
3. Bergmark C, et al: *J Cardiovasc Surg* 32:117, 1991.

Infrapopliteal Prosthetic Graft Patency by Use of the Distal Adjunctive Arteriovenous Fistula
Dardik H, Berry SM, Dardik A, Wolodiger F, Pecoraro J, Ibrahim IM, Kahn M, Sussman B (Englewood Hosp, Englewood, NJ)
J Vasc Surg 13:685–691, 1991   18–11

Background.—The use of autologous saphenous vein for lower limb revascularization has produced excellent results and reduced the need for prosthetic arterial substitutes. However, in some cases, autologous tissue may not be available or suitable, necessitating the use of a prosthetic graft. The major surgical approaches to augmenting graft patency rates are construction of a sequential component to the bypass graft and creation of an arteriovenous fistula (dAVF) in relationship to the distal anastomosis of the prosthetic graft.

Patients.—Between 1979 and 1989, 210 dAVFs were constructed as adjuncts to tibial and peroneal vascular reconstructive procedures in 203 patients at risk of losing their limbs. Two-year cumulative patency rates were determined after grouping patients according to time of treatment. Group I consisted of 61 patients treated between 1979 and 1983; group 2, 80 patients treated from 1983 to 1986; and group 3, 69 treated from 1986 to 1989.

Outcomes.—Patency rates in these 3 groups were 18%, 33%, and 44%, respectively. Arteriography done after surgery demonstrated that flow was prograde in the distal vessels beyond the dAVF. Duplex ultrasonographic graft surveillance also showed that flow in the distal arteries was prograde and that "steal" did not occur. Peak systolic velocity and mean velocity flow rates were increased in grafts with patent dAVFs when compared with bypasses with closed dAVFs. No differences occurred in flow measures for arteries beyond the distal anastomoses and dAVFs, which confirmed the prograde nature of the distal flow. Analysis of graft and fistula patency by duplex sonography in 22 patients demonstrated that 25% of all grafts were patent without fistulas 1 year and 2 years after surgery. At 1 year, 68% of patent grafts had patent fistulas, as did 58% at 2 years (Fig 18–3).

Conclusions.—The dAVF increases graft flow and prevents distal arterial overload without resulting in "steal." This method should be considered when a prosthetic graft is needed for crural reconstruction and in selected cases of revascularization with autologous veins.

▶ The use of dAVF is usually a "last resort" approach in a patient who has

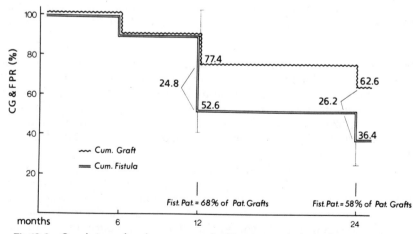

Fig 18–3.—Cumulative graft and patency rates for 22 patients with duplex follow-up studies. One fourth of all the grafts were patent without fistula patency at 1 and 2 years. Of those grafts patent at 1 year, 68% still had patent fistulas. At 2 years, fistula patency occurred in 58% of the grafts patent at that time. (Courtesy of Dardik H, Berry SM, Dardik A, et al: *J Vasc Surg* 13:685–691, 1991.)

undergone other, or conventional, procedures. In the discussion, Shah reported that his group in Albany created a remote dAVF in 22 patients in whom previous vein and synthetic graft bypasses had failed. The 1-year graft patency rate was 77%, and limb salvage was achieved in these patients. In the conclusion, Dardik et al. point out that complications in the venous circulation have not been noted.—S.I. Schwartz, M.D.

Chronic Visceral Ischemia: Three Decades of Progress
Cunningham CG, Reilly LM, Rapp JH, Schneider PA, Stoney RJ (Univ of California, San Francisco)
Ann Surg 214:276–288, 1991   18–12

Introduction.—Symptomatic visceral atherosclerosis is a life-threatening condition requiring complex surgical management. The safety and efficacy of visceral revascularization by transaortic endarterectomy (TA TEA) or antegrade bypass, and the adjunctive measures contributing to long-term survival and relief of symptoms, were reviewed.

Methods.—Patients had chronic symptoms of intestinal ischemia. The group included 69 women and 16 men (mean age, 61 years); 48 underwent TA TEA and 26 had an antegrade visceral bypass. Vascular reconstruction was performed in the remaining 11 patients using a variety of other techniques.

Technique.—Initially, TA TEA was performed through a thoracoretroperitoneal approach, but more recently a transabdominal route has been used with medial rotation of the viscera from the left. A trapdoor aortotomy circumscribes the visceral orifices before the endarterectomy. Medial visceral rotation has replaced a transabdominal, transcrural approach to the aorta in antegrade visceral bypass. The proximal anastomosis requires temporary total aortic occlusion, and a small ellipse of aorta is excised to facilitate the end-to-side anastomosis.

Results.—In the perioperative period, 9 patients (12.5%) died, 5 of complications of bleeding. Neither the mortality rate nor the overall complication rate differed significantly between the 2 operative groups. Of 63 patients who were followed for a mean of 71 months, 9 had recurrent symptoms of visceral ischemia. At 5 years, 88% of the patients having antegrade bypass and 86% who had TA TEA remained asymptomatic.

Conclusion.—Both TA TEA and antegrade bypass offer durable symptom relief with acceptable rates of operative morbidity and mortality. Success is attributed to intraoperative transesophageal echocardiography, intraoperative assessment of the visceral reconstruction with Duplex ultrasonography, and the increasing use of the transabdominal approach to provide aortic exposure.

▶ This represents one of the largest reported experiences with surgical management of chronic visceral ischemia. In the discussion, Dr. DeBakey reported the results from Houston, demonstrating that the Kaplan-Meier survival curve for 10 years was about 70% and for 20 years a little more than 50%. He also stressed that gratifying results should be anticipated in about 25% of the cases.—S.I. Schwartz, M.D.

Long-Term Results After Percutaneous Transluminal Angioplasty of Atherosclerotic Renal Artery Stenosis: The Importance of Intensive Follow-Up

Weibull H, Bergqvist D, Jonsson K, Hulthén L, Mannhem P, Bergentz S-E (Malmö Gen Hosp, Sweden)
Eur J Vasc Surg 5:291–301, 1991   18–13

Introduction.—The long-term results of percutaneous transluminal renal angioplasty (PTRA) on isthmus and juxta-aortic artherosclerotic renal artery stenoses in patients with renovascular hypertension, with or without renal insufficiency, were reviewed with regard to patency, the effect on blood pressure and renal function, and the necessity of reintervention.

Methods.—In 65 patients, 71 atherosclerotic renal artery stenoses were treated. All patients had renovascular hypertension and 37 also had impending renal insufficiency. Diagnostic studies included angiography and measurement of pressure gradient and renal venous renin. Patients were followed up at least 4 times a year. The indication for reevaluation and possible reintervention was deterioration in blood pressure or renal function. The median follow-up period was 56 months.

Results.—Treatment with PTRA was successful in 59 stenoses and 2 occlusions and failed in 10 (Fig 18–4). The primary patency rate at fol-

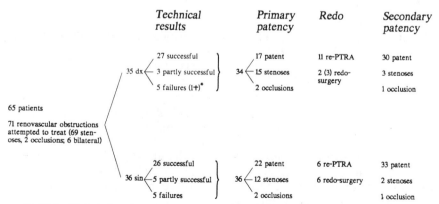

Fig 18–4.—Technical results, primary patency, redo-procedures performed and secondary patency on right and left side, separately. (Courtesy of Weilbull H, Bergqvist D, Jonsson K, et al: *Eur J Vasc Surg* 5:291–301, 1991.)

low-up was 55%. There were 27 restenoses and 4 occlusions, all but 2 of which occurred within 1 year. Further PTRA was performed in 17 patients and surgical reconstruction in 8. After all interventions, the secondary patency rate was 90%. By the end of follow-up, 21 patients (32%) had died, usually of cardiovascular disease. Survival was significantly reduced in patients with multilocular atherosclerosis, renal insufficiency, contralateral renal artery stenosis, and ischemic heart disease. Blood pressure problems were cured or improved in 90% of the patients. Improvement of renal function was achieved in 50% who had impending renal insufficiency but was unchanged in 39%. Only 1 PTRA was needed in 55% of the patients, a repeated procedure in 25%, and operation in 20%.

Conclusion.—Percutaneous transluminal angioplasty may be used as the initial treatment for atherosclerotic renal artery stenosis. Follow-up must be intensive, with angiography performed if there are symptoms or signs of recurrence. A repeated procedure or reconstructive surgery should be performed if the PTRA is a technical failure or if the condition recurs.

▶ The results reported are most encouraging. The authors' results with primary percutaneous transluminal angioplasty of the renal artery are certainly equivalent to the best surgical results. Geyskes (1) reported similarly good results with this technique, whereas others such as Brawn and Ramsay (2) found the technique of transluminal angioplasty unsuitable for renal atherosclerosis. This selected article certainly suggests that it is appropriate, in the algorithm of therapy to begin with this approach.—S.I. Schwartz, M.D.

References

1. Geyskes GG: *Am J Kidney Dis* 12:253, 1988.
2. Brawn LA, Ramsey LE: *Lancet* 2:1313, 1987.

The Role of Microvascular Free Flaps in Salvaging Below-Knee Amputation Stumps: A Review of 22 Cases
Kasabian AK, Colen SR, Shaw WW, Pachter HL (New York Univ)
J Trauma 31:495–501, 1991   18–14

Introduction.—Because of the greater physical capacities of below-knee amputees, the longest possible functional amputation level should be preserved when handling severe injuries to the leg and traumatic amputations. Evaluation was made of the results of using microvascular free flaps to attain adequate tissue coverage of the below-knee stump in patients who would have needed an above-knee amputation had coverage not been supplemented in this way.

Methods.—Below-knee salvage of functional knees with inadequate soft tissue for coverage may be immediate or delayed, depending on the

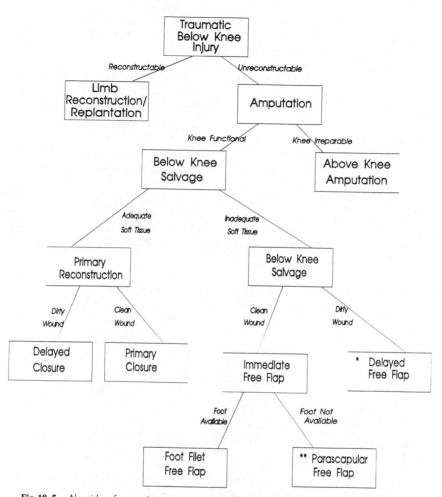

Fig 18–5.—Algorithm for treating severe traumatic below-knee injuries. If the knee is functional, a below-knee amputation can be preserved with microvascular free flaps, even if there is inadequate soft tissue. *Asterisk* indicates selected cases where, even if the wound is heavily contaminated, consideration should be given for a foot filet flap if the foot is available as a donor site. *Double asterisk,* the para-scapular free flap is the flap of choice, although other donor sites are available. (Courtesy of Kasabian AK, Colen SR, Shaw WW, et at: *J Trauma* 31:495–501, 1991.)

state of the wound (Fig 18–5); plastic surgery, trauma, and orthopedic teams collaborate on all decisions. During a 9-year period 24 flaps were used in 22 patients. In 29%, surgery was performed within the first week after injury; in 50% it was performed 1–3 months after injury, and the remainder were operated on 3 or more months after injury. The donor tissues of choice were filet of the amputated foot when available (25%), or parascapular free flaps (46%). Half of the patients had serious con-comitant injuries. Follow-up lasted for 12–116 months.

Results.—The 22 patients underwent 107 operations (average, 4.9 operations), 25% of which involved revisions or were necessitated because of complications. The most common complication was partial necrosis (25%), followed by neuroma (13%), hematoma (8%), and donor site morbidity (8%). These rates are similar to those for standard below-knee amputations and free flaps to lower limb trauma sites. The average hospital stay was 51 days, and the average time to walk with a prosthesis was 5.75 months. Knee function was excellent in all patients. Most patients who were employed before their injury were able to return to work.

Conclusions.—Although the prolonged term of recovery and delay before ambulation are of some concern, the significantly greater functional capacity achieved after below-knee amputation compared with above-knee amputation warrants the initially greater investment of time and surgical skill. If a functional knee can be salvaged, even in unsteady patients with multiple serious injuries, it is not necessary to perform a more proximal amputation just to provide adequate soft tissue coverage of the stump.

▶ This represents the largest North American series of free tissue transfers to salvage below-knee amputations. The results are outstanding. The modality of free tissue transfer was combined with distal revascularization to achieve limb salvage despite extensive tissue loss. Cronenwett et al. (1) reported 15 patients with extensive tissue loss exposing bone or tendon. The patients underwent distal arterial revascularization after free tissue transfer. Limb salvage was achieved in 93% of the cases.—S.I. Schwartz, M.D.

Reference

1. Cronenwett JL, et al: *Arch Surg* 124:609, 1989.

Thromboembolic Complications in Patients With Advanced Cancer: Anticoagulation Versus Greenfield Filter Placement
Calligaro KD, Bergen WS, Haut MJ, Savarese RP, DeLaurentis DA (Univ of Pennsylvania)
Ann Vasc Surg 5:186–189, 1991   18–15

Introduction.—Patients with cancer who have thromboembolic disease when treated with anticoagulation have a high incidence of bleeding, recurrent thromboembolism, and other complications.

Methods.—To determine whether treatment with anticoagulation or with a Greenfield filter is most effective in patients with advanced cancer and deep vein thrombosis (DVT) or pulmonary embolism (PE), studies were made in 15 men and 15 women aged 47–83 years with stage III or IV cancer and DVT or PE. In 12 patients, the DVT was proximal to the calf and was diagnosed by duplex scanning or contrast venography; in 15, PE was diagnosed by a high-probability pulmonary ventilation/perfusion scan or arteriography; 3 patients had both DVT and PE. Anticoagulation was the primary treatment in 20 patients, and 10 underwent Greenfield filter placement.

Results.—Of the 20 patients treated primarily with anticoagulation, 20 had bleeding or thrombosis-related complications, including major bleeding, recurrent DVT or PE, the inability to attain consistent therapeutic anticoagulation levels, heparin-induced thrombocytopenia, or progression of DVT. Of these patients, 10 eventually had a Greenfield filter placed without complications; in 3 of these 10 patients, DVT progressed and anticoagulation was necessary. One other patient died of guidewire-induced arrhythmia.

Conclusion.—Patients with advanced cancer and venous thromboembolic disease have a high complication rate after either anticoagulation or Greenfield filter placement. However, initial treatment with a Greenfield filter appears more definitive. Anticoagulation should be limited to use in patients with progressive symptomatic DVT after Greenfield filter placement.

▶ Greenfield and Michna reported their experience in a 12-year period with the Greenfield vena caval filter (1). Long-term filter patency was 98%, and the recurrent PE rate was 4%. Others (2) confirmed the safety and effectiveness of the filter and indicated that its use should be expanded to include prophylactic insertion in certain high-risk patients.—S.I. Schwartz, M.D.

References

1. Greenfield LJ, Michna BA: *Surgery* 104:706, 1988.
2. Golueke PJ, et al: *Surgery* 103:111, 1988.

Pulmonary Embolectomy: A 20-Year Experience at One Center
Meyer G, Tamisier D, Sors H, Stern M, Vouhé P, Makowski S, Neveux J-Y, Leca F, Even P (Laennec Hosp, Paris)
Ann Thorac Surg 51:232–236, 1991   18–16

Background.—Thrombolysis is widely accepted as front-line therapy for most patients with massive pulmonary embolism (PE). It is contraindicated in some cases, however, and it fails in 15% to 20% of patients. In the most severe cases it can result in death. Pulmonary embolectomy under cardiopulmonary bypass was studied to gain a better understanding of the factors predicting outcomes.

Patients.—Ninety-six consecutive patients underwent pulmonary embolectomy under cardiopulmonary bypass because of acute massive PE between 1968 and 1988. The surgical mortality was 37.5%. Twelve clinical and hemodynamic factors were evaluated using univariate and multivariate analyses.

Results.—According to multivariate analysis, cardiac arrest and associated cardiopulmonary disease independently predicted operative death. Of the 55 patients followed for 2–144 months, 6 died and 5 complained of persistent mild or severe exertional dyspnea.

Conclusions.—These findings should help physicians to assess the preoperative risks in patients undergoing pulmonary embolectomy. In the few patients who do not benefit from medical treatment, pulmonary embolectomy is still an acceptable procedure.

▶ This report from Paris describes experiences with 96 patients undergoing pulmonary embolectomy in a period of 20 years. Operative mortality was 37%. Excellent results, however, were obtained in the majority of long-term survivors.

The authors emphasize that embolectomy was undertaken only when medical therapy was either contraindicated or proved ineffective. Pulmonary angiography was performed preoperatively in 92 of the 96 patients. Caval interruption was almost routinely performed.

Among the causes of death, preoperative cardiac arrest was the most significant predictor of mortality. This occurred in 25% of the patients before operation, well indicating that embolectomy was undertaken as a last resort.

For unknown reasons, massive pulmonary hemorrhage caused 8 of the 36 deaths. Recurrent PE was extremely rare, reflecting the effectiveness of vena caval interruption as well as anticoagulant therapy.—F.C. Spencer, M.D.

Leiomyosarcoma of the Inferior Vena Cava: Experience With 7 Patients and Literature Review
Cacoub P, Piette JC, Wechsler B, Ziza JM, Blétry O, Bahnini A, Kieffer E, Godeau P (Groupe Hosp La-Pitié-Salpétrière, Paris)
Medicine 70:293–306, 1991   8–17

Introduction.—Leiomyosarcoma (LMS) of the inferior vena cava is a rare malignant tumor; only 106 patients have been reported since it was first described in 1871. Prognosis is poor, although earlier diagnosis is now possible with the use of ultrasonography and CT. Data on 7 additional patients with LMS of the inferior vena cava and the literature on the tumor were reviewed.

Methods.—The main features of LMS of the inferior vena cava, including its clinical manifestations, methods of diagnosis, treatment, and prognosis were evaluated. Although most of the patients did not have sufficient follow-up, some treatment recommendations can be made. Follow-up for the 7 new patients ranged from 3 months to 120 months (table).

Results.—Of the 113 patients, women outnumbered men by a ratio of 6:1. Patients were aged 15–83 years (mean age, 56 years). The middle segment was the most frequent site of tumor development. In 30 pa-

Clinical Features of 7 Patients With Leiomyosarcoma of the Inferior Vena Cava

Patient	Age (at diagnosis)	Sex	Clinical Manifestations	Location (IVC segment)	Metastasis	Treatment	Follow-up (mo)
1	42	F	Abdominal pain, right flank palpable mass, weight loss	Middle	Liver, lungs	Radiotherapy, chemotherapy, surgery	24, died
2	73	M	Lumbar and right upper quadrant abdominal pain, gastrointestinal hemorrhage, right flank palpable mass, altered general condition	Middle and lower	No	Surgery	3, died
3	63	F	Edema of the lower extremities, right flank mass	Entire	Liver	Chemotherapy, surgery	10, lost to follow-up
4	42	F	Right flank pain	Lower	No	Surgery, chemotherapy	36, died
5	63	F	Right flank pain, edema of the lower extremities	Middle	Lungs	Surgery, chemotherapy	72, died
6	28	F	Epigastric palpable mass, fever	Middle	Bone	Chemotherapy, surgery, radiotherapy	36, died
7	39	F	Right flank pain	Middle	Skin, liver, lungs, pancreas, shoulder	Surgery, chemotherapy, radiotherapy	120, alive

(Courtesy of Cacoub P, Piette JC, Wechsler B, et al: Medicine 70:293–306, 1991.)

tients, 2 segments of the inferior vena cava were involved, but only 9 patients had extension of the LMS to all 3 segments. Abdominal pain was the most common symptom when the middle segment was involved. Tumors involving segment I (the lower segment) were more likely to pres-

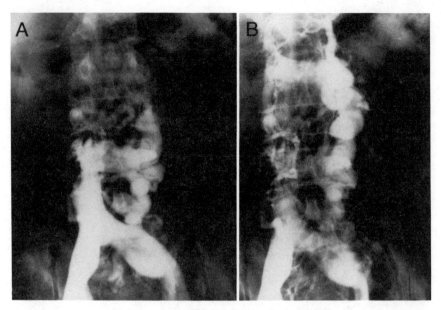

Fig 18–6.—Patient 2. Inferior cavography. **A,** frontal image showing in early phase a complete thrombosis of vena cava and the marked collateral circulation. On the right border of vena cava, several centimeters from its origin, a lacuna image caused by tumor is visible. **B,** frontal image in late phase showing opacification of suprahepatic segment of the IVC by marked collateral circulation. (Courtesy of Cacoub P, Piette JC, Wechsler B, et al: *Medicine* 70:293–306, 1991.)

ent as a palpable mass than tumors involving segments II and III. Edema of the lower limbs was common in patients with LMS of segment III. Invasion of hepatic veins led to Budd-Chiari syndrome in 27 patients. A specific treatment was used in 78 patients; 28 of 48 patients who underwent surgery alone died within a mean of 15 months.

Conclusion.—Diagnosis of LMS of the inferior vena cava remains difficult. The tumor has never been diagnosed by the presence of metastases. Ultrasonography may be helpful, but a CT scan clearly delineates the tumor (Fig 18–6). Both arteriography and contrast studies of the gastrointestinal, biliary, and urinary tract are nondiagnostic. Location is the main prognostic factor; patients with upper segment tumors have the poorest outcome. Complete surgical resection is the treatment of choice, but adjuvant radiotherapy, chemotherapy, or both, may be necessary. Large doses of preoperative chemotherapy are recommended to reduce tumor size.

▶ This is an excellent review of the literature related to a rare, malignant tumor. Leiomyoma and leiomyosarcoma have occurred in other veins, including the iliac, femoral, and even the saphenous (1). The data suggest that surgery should be followed by adjuvant chemotherapy and, perhaps, radiation therapy to improve the results.—S.I. Schwartz, M.D.

Reference

1. DeWeese JA, et al: *Ann Surg* 148:859, 1958.

19 The Esophagus

Laparoscopic Cardiomyotomy for Achalasia
Shimi S, Nathanson LK, Cuschieri A (Univ of Dundee, Scotland)
J R Coll Surg Edinb 36:152–154, 1991   19–1

Introduction.—Achalasia may be treated with medication or balloon dilatation of the lower esophageal sphincter, or surgically by a short 5- to 6-cm myotomy, which includes the entire extent of the lower esophageal high pressure zone and an adjacent 1 cm of stomach. A comparative study of balloon dilatation and myotomy reported that myotomy was successful in 95% of patients and balloon dilatation in 65%. However, precipitation of gastroesophageal reflux is an important disadvantage of surgical myotomy.

Technique.—After the pneumoperitoneum is established, the laparoscopic cannula is inserted above and to the left of the umbilicus. Of 3 other cannulas inserted under vision, 1 is used to lift up the left lobe of the liver and 2 are used as operating cannulas. Adequate retraction of the left lobe of the liver is essential. After division of the peritoneum over the hiatal margin, the right posterolateral wall of the gullet is dissected high up above the gastroesophageal junction until the mediastinum is reached. The anchoring bands of the phrenoesophageal membrane and the posterior vagus nerve are preserved. Myotomy is then initiated. The key to myotomy is high dissection to avoid branches of the left gastric artery and vein.

Case Report.—Woman, 30, with manometrically confirmed classic achalasia underwent laparoscopic cardiomyotomy. She experienced complete relief of episodic total dysphagia without any untoward symptoms, including gastroesophageal reflux. She had minimal postoperative discomfort and was discharged on the third postoperative day.

Conclusion.—Laparoscopic cardiomyotomy in the treatment of achalasia constitutes definitive therapy comparable to standard myotomy. The procedure is less disruptive of the lower esophageal fixation and is less likely to precipitate gastroesophageal reflux than standard myotomy is.

▶ This intriguing approach offers some advantage because it traumatizes the hiatus to a lesser extent. Personal communication with several surgeons indicates that they have used it successfully in the United States. It can include fundoplication, which, with new instrumentation, can be performed laparoscopically.—S.I. Schwartz, M.D.

Spontaneous Rupture of the Esophagus: Immediate and Late Results
Justicz AG, Symbas PN (Emory Univ)
Am Surg 57:4–7, 1991   19–2

Background.—Controversy exists over the management of spontaneous esophageal rupture. However, the mainstay of surgery is still primary repair with or without suture line plication. Results of 18 patients treated in a 16-year period were reviewed.

Methods.—The mean time from onset of symptoms to arrival in the emergency department was 29 hours. Six patients had primary repair within 12 hours and were termed "early"; 12 patients seen more than 18 hours after rupture were termed "late." Usually, primary repair with or without suture line plication was done. Follow-up esophagography was done in 8 of 11 survivors at a mean of 28 months.

Results.—Primary repair was carried out in 15 patients; 1 had cervical esophagostomy in continuity and exclusion of the repair, 1 was managed with chest tube drainage, and 1 was treated with T tube drainage. Survival in the early group was 83%, and that in the late group, 55%. In the early group, 1 patient died of gastric ulcer perforation, renal failure, and cardiac arrest, and 1 nonoperatively treated patient died of progressive sepsis and multiorgan failure. In the late group, the patient treated with T tube drainage died of sepsis. Gastric fundus plication was done in 8 primary repairs, with 6 recoveries. Pleural flap plication was done in 3 cases, with 1 recovery. No plication was done in 4 cases, with 3 recoveries. Esophagography was normal in 4 patients with fundoplication and 1 without plication. Stricture was present in the lower esophagus in 2 patients with fundoplication, in both of whom the fundoplicated segment was left above the diaphragm.

Conclusions.—Management of spontaneous rupture of the esophagus should be individualized. Excellent immediate and acceptable late results may be achieved by plication of the esophageal suture line with gastric fundus; this technique may be used when pleural or other tissue flaps are unavailable.

▶ Pate et al. (1) reviewed data concerning 34 patients with spontaneous rupture of the esophagus. Twenty-six underwent a primary surgical repair. Thoracotomies were performed in all but 4 patients. The 14 patients who died included all 4 who did not have thoracotomy. Delay in treatment (24 hours or more) did not significantly affect the mortality rate, but it did cause an increase in complications.—S.I. Schwartz, M.D.

Reference

1. Pate JW, et al: *Ann Thorac Surg* 47:689, 1989.

Barrett's Esophagus and Adenocarcinoma of the Esophagus and Gastroesophageal Junction

Duhaylongsod FG, Wolfe WG (Duke Univ)
J Thorac Cardiovasc Surg 102:36–42, 1991

19–3

Background.—"Barrett's esophagus" refers to the presence of columnar epithelial lining within the distal tubular esophagus. Barrett's esophagus and adenocarcinoma of the esophagus and gastroesophageal (GE) junction were studied in 1 series of patients.

Patients.—Fifty-seven patients with adenocarcinoma of the esophagus and GE junction underwent surgical resection during the past 7 years. Sixteen tumors arose in a Barrett's esophagus. In this subgroup, there was a predominance of white men older than 55 years (94%). The mean proximal extent of abnormal columnar involvement above the GE junction was 5.4 cm, with a range of 2.5–11 cm. The mean location of neoplasm centered in the distal esophagus 1.8 cm above the GE junction. During this same period, 30 patients with Barrett's esophagus were seen without adenocarcinoma.

Findings.—There were no significant differences between these 2 groups in the proximal extent of columnar involvement or the presence of reflux symptoms. Also, no significant differences were found in age, smoking history, and alcohol intake between patients with benign or ma-

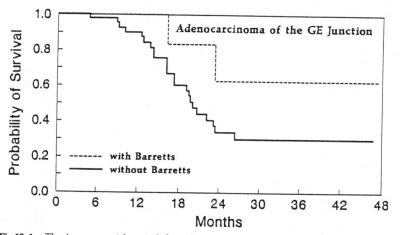

Fig 19–1.—The 4-year actuarial survival, from date of diagnosis, of patients with Barrett's adenocarcinoma and patients with adenocarcinoma of the esophagus and gastroesophageal (GE) junction, without recognized Barrett's carcinoma. (Courtesy of Duhaylongsod FG, Wolfe WG: *J Thorac Cardiovasc Surg* 102:36–42, 1991.)

lignant Barrett's esophagus; compared with patients with adenocarcinoma of the GE junction not associated with Barrett's mucosa. The predominance of white men observed in the group with malignant Barrett's esophagus was not observed in the benign group; however, it did occur in the adenocarcinoma group without recognized Barrett's esophagus. The patients with non-Barrett's adenocarcinoma had a 4-year survival rate of approximately 30%, compared with 60% in the group with Barrett's adenocarcinoma (Fig 19-1).

Conclusions.—The sensitivity of endoscopic surveillance may be increased if the biopsy specimens are concentrated in the distal 6 cm of the tubular esophagus. Although the reason for the current difference in survival between patients with Barrett's and non-Barrett's adenocarcinoma is not known, it may be related to endoscopic surveillance permitting earlier diagnosis and treatment.

▶ It's probably true that the difference in survival between the Barrett's and non-Barrett's adenocarcinoma is related to endoscopic surveillance, which permits earlier diagnosis and treatment. Altorki et al. (1) indicated that esophageal resection for a Barrett's esophagus is indicated in selected patients, including those with high-grade dysplasia and strong suspicion of cancer. The issue of progression of Barrett's epithelium after an antireflux operation remains a controversial topic. Williamson et al. (2) reported that cancer developed in 8 patients with Barrett's esophagus who had undergone an antireflux procedure. This stresses the need for continued surveillance of these patients.—S.I. Schwartz, M.D.

References

1. Altorki NK, et al: *Ann Thorac Surg* 49:724, 1990.
2. Williamson, WA et al: *Ann Thorac Surg* 49:537, 1990.

Postoperative Radiation Therapy Does Not Increase Survival After Curative Resection for Squamous Cell Carcinoma of the Middle and Lower Esophagus as Shown by a Multicenter Controlled Trial
Ténière P, Hay J-M, Fingerhut A, Fagniez P-L (French Univ Assoc for Surg Res, Bois-Colombes, France)
Surg Gynecol Obstet 173:123–130, 1991   19–4

Introduction.—Although immediate postoperative morbidity and mortality after surgical treatment of squamous cell carcinoma of the esophagus have improved, the long-term results remain poor. In 1978 it was reported that postoperative radiation therapy increased the 5-year survival rates in patients undergoing curative resection. The effect of adjuvant postoperative radiation therapy on long-term survival after surgical treatment for epidermoid carcinoma was assessed in a multicenter trial.

Methods.—Of 221 patients with squamous cell carcinoma in the lower two thirds of the thoracic esophagus, 119 underwent isolated surgical treatment and 102 had surgical treatment followed by radiation therapy. Randomization was done by institution and was stratified according to lymph node status. All resections were performed with curative intent. In 87 patients there was no lymph node invasion and in 131 patients there was invasion of paraesophageal lymph nodes or of distal lymph nodes.

Results.—The 5-year survival rate for patients without lymph node invasion was 38% compared with 7% for patients with lymph node invasion. Postoperative radiation treatment did not improve survival. The lack of improvement in survival was present irrespective of lymph node status. However, patients who underwent postoperative irradiation had significantly fewer recurrences than those who did not.

Conclusion.—Postoperative irradiation after curative resection of squamous cell carcinoma of the mid and lower esophagus does not improve postoperative survival, irrespective of lymph node status. Absence of lymph node involvement is the most influential single prognostic factor with respect to survival.

▶ Throughout the literature there has been uncertainty about the efficacy of radiotherapy on squamous cell esophageal carcinoma. Earlam and Johnson (1) treated 22 patients with radical radiotherapy for operable squamous cell carcinoma of the esophagus. Only 14% survived for 5 years. Bluett et al. (2) assessed the effect of radiation therapy and noted no improvement in survival, and also that preoperative radiation therapy did not significantly affect the postoperative complication rate.—S.I. Schwartz, M.D.

References

1. Earlam RJ, Johnson L: *Ann R Coll Surg Engl* 72:32, 1990.
2. Bluett MK, et al: *Am Surg* 53:126, 1987.

20 The Stomach and the Duodenum

Leukotriene Receptor Blockade Reduces Bile Acid-Induced Superficial Gastric Mucosal Injury
Mercer DW, Milner R, O'Neill S, Ritchie WP Jr, Dempsey DT (Temple Univ Hosp)
J Surg Res 50:602–608, 1991   20–1

Introduction.—Leukotrienes reduce gastric mucosal blood flow in experimental animals and may serve as mediators of necrosis from cytotoxic agents. Increased leukotriene production has been demonstrated with ethanol, taurocholic acid, and aspirin.

Methods.—Pretreatment with topical leukotrienes C_4 and D_4 was evaluated in the setting of superficial injury caused by low concentrations of bile acid in rats. Injury was induced with topically applied 5-mM acidified taurocholate (pH 1.2). Hydrogen ion flux and DNA efflux were measured to determine a marker of mucosal cell exfoliation. The effects of the leukotriene D_4 receptor antagonist SKF-104353 also were studied.

Results.—Both leukotrienes significantly increased luminal hydrogen ion loss and DNA efflux after exposure to bile acid. Leukotriene receptor blockade significantly reduced these effects and also the injury from bile acid alone.

Conclusion.—The effects of topically applied leukotrienes and of leukotriene receptor blockade suggest that leukotrienes may mediate the gastric mucosal injury induced by exposure to bile acid.

▶ We should approach the idea of gastric mucosal injuries caused by bile with some healthy skepticism, i.e., we must remember that the gastric mucosa varies greatly in its response to contact with bile. In years past, the palliative bypass route for bile in patients with obstructing carcinoma of the head of the pancreas was frequently created by an anastomosis between the gallbladder and the stomach. Patients seem to tolerate that anastomosis fairly well. Their other troubles may have been of such magnitude that the background noise obscured any problems caused by bile injury to the mucosa.

In vitro studies clearly show that bile salts damage the membranes of gastric epithelial cells. The mechanism for this injury was addressed in this study from Temple University. Dr. Ritchie is a renowned student of mucosal injury, and the suggestion that the mechanism may involve leukotrienes is attractive. What is demonstrated here is a possible route by which this injury might occur. We need additional studies to tell us whether it is clinically relevant. Could injury be prevented by blocking the actions of leukotrienes? Do known releasors of leukotrienes cause similar mucosal damage?—J.C. Thompson, M.D.

Proximal Gastric Vagotomy in the Emergency Treatment of Bleeding Duodenal Ulcer

Miedema BW, Torres PR, Farnell MB, van Heerden JA, Kelly KA (Mayo Clinic and Found, Rochester, Minn)
Am J Surg 161:64–68, 1991   20–2

Background.—Proximal gastric vagotomy without drainage has an extremely low operative mortality rate and seldom causes postgastrectomy side effects. It has been used primarily to treat intractable peptic ulcer.

Methods.—Proximal gastric vagotomy was performed in 52 low-risk patients requiring emergency surgery for bleeding duodenal ulcer in 1973–1986. Their median APACHE II score was 3, and the patients were generally in good health apart from the ulcer.

Results.—No postoperative deaths occurred, and no patient required reoperation in the postoperative period. Six patients had complications, but none required intensive care for longer than 3 days. Four patients died later of disorders unrelated to duodenal ulcer disease. None had long-term severe postgastrectomy symptoms. Six patients had recurrent ulcer disease after a median follow-up of 3 years. No patient experienced pyloric obstruction.

Conclusions.—Proximal gastric vagotomy is an effective, safe approach to bleeding duodenal ulcer. However, because it is not a short operation, it may be used only in patients who are stable. The low rate of postgastrectomy syndrome makes proximal gastric vagotomy an attractive alternative to more traditional operations.

▶ The title of this paper is "Proximal Gastric Vagotomy in the Emergency Treatment of Bleeding Duodenal Ulcer." This idea has been around for a long time. David Johnson suggested that selective proximal vagotomy was safely applicable to bleeding peptic ulcer in 1973 (1), and Paul Jordan in a discussion of the present paper reported his series of 27 patients, 1 of whom died. This series from the Mayo Clinic is certainly one of the largest, and their mortality rate of zero cannot be improved upon. Even more impressive, perhaps, is that there were no significant complications other than a 12% recurrence rate in a mean follow-up of less than 3 years. Because the mean APACHE II score was 3, and only 1 or 2 of the patients were in shock, an obvious question is how many of these procedures were actually conducted on an emergency basis? The authors' statement that there were no postoperative sequelae must also be tempered by the long postoperative stay that several patients required before return of gastric emptying was achieved.—J.C. Thompson, M.D.

Reference

1. Johnson D, et al: *Br J Surg* 60:790, 1973.

Recurrent Peptic Ulceration After Highly Selective Vagotomy: Long-Term Outcome

Maddern GJ, Vauthey J-N, Devitt P, Britten-Jones R, Hetzel DJ, Jamieson GG
(Royal Adelaide Hosp, Adelaide, South Australia)
Br J Surg 78:940–941, 1991   20–3

Objective.—The course of peptic ulcer disease following highly selective vagotomy (HSV) was examined in a group of 27 patients, 16 of whom reported a previous symptomatic recurrence of disease. The other 11 patients had an asymptomatic recurrence. Patients were followed for at least 7½ years after HSV.

Findings.—The 16 patients with symptomatic recurrences included 5 who had a gastric ulcer, all of whom had undergone further surgery. One of these patients had Zollinger-Ellison syndrome. One of 8 patients who agreed to endoscopy was found to have an active duodenal ulcer. Seven of 10 evaluable patients were still taking regular H_2 receptor blocker treatment. None of the 11 patients with asymptomatic ulcer had undergone further surgery. When 4 later became symptomatic, they received H_2 receptor blocker treatment. Two of 8 patients having endoscopy were found to have a duodenal ulcer.

Conclusions.—Asymptomatic recurrences are not infrequent after HSV, and a substantial number of patients may become symptomatic. Most patients with recurrent ulcer, however, do well with H_2 receptor blocker therapy.

▶ One of the great surprises resulting from endoscopic control in clinical trials of the early H_2-receptor blockade drugs was the high incidence of asymptomatic duodenal ulcer. A confounding finding was the lack of symptoms of recurrent ulceration after "adequate" drug therapy. How should these patients be handled? If they were not undergoing routine endoscopy, no one would have known of the recurrence. The current paper from Adelaide reminds us that these asymptomatic recurrences will plague us after operative treatment of peptic ulcer disease. More than a third of the asymptomatic patients later experienced pain. In agreement with nearly all previous studies of postoperative recurrences after highly selective vagotomy, most patients were well managed by H_2-receptor blocker treatment.

Because such treatment preoperatively had failed in nearly all of the patients, the operation appears to contribute to the efficacy of H_2-receptor treatment. Another explanation would be that patients were more conscientious in taking their drugs postoperatively than they were preoperatively. We find that the main current cause of failure of medical treatment is lack of patient compliance. Undergoing an operative procedure may bring about improvement.—J.C. Thompson, M.D.

A Multifactorial Analysis of Mortality and Morbidity in Perforated Peptic Ulcer Disease

Bodner B, Harrington ME, Kim U (City Hosp Ctr, Elmhurst, NY; City Univ of New York)
Surg Gynecol Obstet 171:315–320, 1990   20–4

Introduction.—The optimal surgical treatment of perforated peptic ulcer would provide the best short-term survival as well as long-term control of the ulcer diathesis. Data were reviewed on 113 patients who were treated by operation from 1981 through 1986. A number of factors that influenced morbidity or mortality were identified. Twenty patients had severe complications and 11 died.

Findings.—Patients without complications were younger than the others, had fewer medical disorders, and received fewer transfusions. On multiple regression analysis, age, number of other medical disorders, and lower mean blood pressure predicted a higher rate of complications. Patients with duodenal ulcer did better than those with gastric or pyloric ulcers. The long-term results improved with definitive surgery, but the type of operation did not influence either morbidity or mortality.

Conclusions.—Definitive surgery for perforated peptic ulcer provides a better long-term quality of life than simple closure. Patients who can withstand the operation should undergo either resection or vagotomy and drainage.

▶ The import of this paper is that immediate results (mortality and morbidity) after surgical treatment for perforated peptic ulcer disease seem to depend on other coexisting health problems; perforated gastric ulcers had a worse outlook than did duodenal perforations.

Over the long haul, however, patients undergoing definitive acid-reducing procedures at the time of closure of their perforated ulcers fared much better in terms of their clinical responses and need for reoperation. We believe that patients who are operated on for perforated duodenal or gastric ulcers should have a definitive acid-reducing procedure unless there is absolutely no history of ulcer disease, or unless a clinical condition exists at operation that is so precarious that any prolongation of the operation is contraindicated.—J.C. Thompson, M.D.

Completion Gastrectomy for Refractory Gastroparesis Following Surgery for Peptic Ulcer Disease: Long-Term Follow-Up With Subjective

and Objective Parameters
McCallum RW, Polepalle SC, Schirmer B (Univ of Virginia)
Dig Dis Sci 36:1556–1561, 1991   20–5

Introduction.—Effective management of chronic nonmechanical gastric stasis after ulcer surgery often is difficult. As many as half of the patients with gastric outlet obstruction preoperatively may have persistent gastric stasis postoperatively. The results of completion gastrectomy were assessed in 8 patients with documented nonmechanical gastric stasis.

Patients.—The patients (mean age, 45 years) were followed for a mean of 30 months after completion gastrectomy. All of the patients initially had presented with evident gastric outlet obstruction secondary to gastric ulcer. They had a mean of 2.3 operations for relief of stasis symptoms before completion gastrectomy. The mean duration of symptoms was 32 months. Treatment with various prokinetic agents had been ineffective.

Outcome.—Completion gastrectomy was carried out successfully in all patients, leaving less than 1 cm of proximal stomach to ensure a nonleaking anastomosis. Two patients required reoperation—1 for anastomotic leakage and 1 for a kinked Roux-en-Y limb. One patient continued to have nausea/vomiting intermittently, and another required analgesia for abdominal pain. Three patients had mild bloating, dumping, or diarrhea. Body weight remained stable. In 2 of the 3 patients studied, a fed-state motility pattern was clearly observed after they ingested a solid meal.

Conclusion.—Completion gastrectomy is a reasonable approach to patients with chronic gastroparesis following surgery for gastric outlet obstruction secondary to peptic ulcer disease if mechanical obstruction is ruled out and there is no response to prokinetic drugs.

▶ Perhaps the most surprising thing in this paper is the authors' finding that 50% of patients who are operated on for gastric outlet obstruction require further operations in attempts to relieve symptoms caused by chronic nonmechanical postoperative gastric stasis. Every surgeon with experience in this field knows that the rate of delayed gastric emptying after operations for gastric outlet obstruction is high, but I have never seen an experience in which half of the patients went on to further operation. The present authors suggest, in concert with the experience from the University of Michigan reviewed in this section 3 years ago (1), that total gastrectomy proved a good solution to the problems of their most recalcitrant patients.

Let there be no mistake. These are among the most trying problems that any surgeon who operates on the stomach faces. Most of these patients underwent operation because the stomach was not emptying and, here, days or weeks after operation, the stomach still is not emptying. Anxiety levels are high in the patient, the family, and the surgeon. Initially, it is important to establish patency of the gut, and this can easily be done by endoscopy (the gastric outlet is nearly always patent). Barium-coated meals often reveal a great deal of churning and slow emptying. The problem is that the gastric corpus (or remnant) is atonic. A common cause of delayed emptying after selective proximal vagotomy is that denervation of the stomach was carried too far distally, a complication that led the originator of the procedure, Fritz Holle in Munich, to add a submucosal anterior pylorectomy to his operation.

The careful accounting of all of the problems that their patients had after total gastrectomy makes for restrained enthusiasm, but we and others, by and large, have been highly satisfied with the ultimate nutrition possible after Roux-en-Y esophagojejunostomy.—J.C. Thompson, M.D.

Reference

1. Eckhauser FE, et al: *Ann Surg* 208:345, 1988.

Efficacy of Octreotide Acetate in Treatment of Severe Postgastrectomy Dumping Syndrome

Geer RJ, Richards WO, O'Dorisio TM, Woltering EO, Williams S, Rice D, Abumrad NN (Vanderbilt Univ; VA Med Ctr, Nashville; Ohio State Univ; Oregon Health Sciences Univ)

Ann Surg 212:678–686, 1990　　　　　　　　　　　　　　　　　　20–6

Introduction.—It has been hypothesized that inhibition by somatostatin of hormonal secretion associated with dumping syndrome might ablate the symptoms of postgastrectomy dumping syndrome. The somatostatin analogue octreotide acetate was evaluated for this purpose on an acute and chronic basis in a double-blind, prospective, randomized study.

Study Design.—Subjects were 10 patients with severe dumping syndrome, the definition of which includes failure of dietary manipulation, loss of more than 10% of body weight, and significant alteration in lifestyle. Six postgastrectomy patients without dumping syndrome served as controls. Patients were studied on 2 consecutive days before and after eating a "dumping breakfast." Patients were given 100 µg of octreotide subcutaneously on 1 study day or the other. Neither the investigator nor the patient was aware of which day the patient was receiving octreotide.

Findings.—In test subjects who received placebo, the test meal caused immediate increases in pulse rate (Fig 20–1) and in plasma levels of glucose, glucagon, pancreatic polypeptide, neurotensin, and insulin. The controls who received placebo had a lesser increase in glucagon and neurotensin. Patients who received octreotide did not have vasomotor or gastrointestinal symptoms, nor did they have plasma peptide responses (Fig 20–2). Diarrhea was completely ablated. Treatment with octreotide suppressed the rise in insulin and thus ablated the late hypoglycemia. Octreotide also dealyed gastric emptying and transit time. Pa-

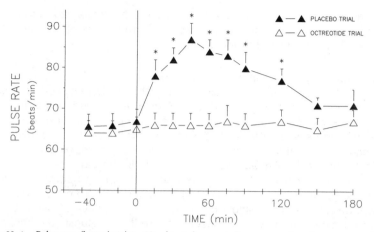

Fig 20–1.—Pulse rate (beats/min) in 10 subjects known to have severe dumping symptoms before and after high carbohydrate breakfast given at 0 minutes and consumed within 15 minutes. Thirty minutes before meal patients received a subcutaneous injection of 100 µg of octreotide acetate (*open triangles*) or vehicle (*filled triangles*). *Denotes differences between group at $P < .01$. (Courtesy of Geer RJ, Richards WO, O'Dorisio TM, et al: *Ann Surg* 212:7-678–687, 1990.)

tients who took octreotide daily over the long term had minimal side effects. They had stable fasting plasma levels of glucose, normal findings on liver function tests, and an average weight gain of 11% in 1 year; in addition, 7 patients were able to return to work.

Conclusions.—Octreotide acetate prevents the vasomotor and gastrointestinal symptoms of severe postgastrectomy dumping syndrome.

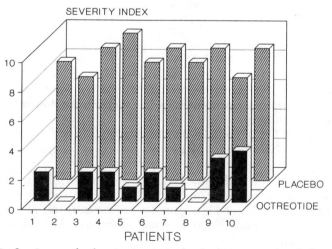

Fig 20–2.—Severity score for dumping symptoms of each of 10 patients described in Figure 20–1 who were treated with octreotide (*filled bars*) or placebo (*striped bars*). Score of zero denotes no symptoms and score of 10 denotes severe symptoms. (Courtesy of Geer RJ, Richards WO, O'Dorisio TM, et al: *Ann Surg* 212:678–687, 1990.)

Long-term treatment is successful and causes no major side effects. Octreotide appears to reduce gastrointestinal motility, probably by inhibiting the release of several humoral agents.

▶ This study follows the initial report by Hopman et al. (1) that was reviewed in this section in 1989. In agreement with the study reviewed in Abstract 20–7, patients with dumping syndrome in the present study were greatly improved by administration of the long-acting somatostatin analog. The present study was addressed, in part to study the possible mechanisms involved. In this regard, the authors noted that elevations in glucose, glucagon, pancreatic polypeptide, insulin, and neurotensin seen in the patients with dumping syndrome who received placebo were blocked entirely by somatostatin. The authors suggest that amelioration of symptoms results from this suppression of peptide release. They single out prevention of release of neurotensin as important. Some of the very earliest studies with neurotensin did implicate a role in the dumping syndrome, but as far as I know that has not been substantiated. The authors certainly demonstrate remarkable suppression of postprandial glucose, insulin, glucagon, pancreatic polypeptide, and neurotensin, and they are able to show significant elevations of the somatostatin analog after injection. To fulfill Koch's postulates, however, the authors must show that dumping symptoms are ameliorated by blocking the release or actions of 1 or more of these peptide agents. These studies, involving receptor antagonist or antibody neutralization, are difficult to perform in humans. Animal models have not been particularly successful.

Treatment of the dumping syndrome goes back to the original problem: why is it, in fact, that symptoms of the dumping syndrome develop in only a fraction of those patients who meet the anatomical requirements for jejunal hyperosmolarity?—J.C. Thompson, M.D.

Reference

1. Hopman WPM, et al: *Ann Surg* 207:155, 1988.

Control of Dumping Symptoms by Somatostatin Analogue in Patients After Gastric Surgery
Gray JL, Debas HT, Mulvihill SJ (Univ of California, San Francisco)
Arch Surg 126:1231–1236, 1991   20–7

Background.—The pathophysiology of postgastrectomy dumping syndrome remains incompletely understood. The factors implicated include rapid gastric emptying of hyperosmolar chyme into the proximal small bowel, release of peptide hormones, and postprandial hypoglycemia secondary to a high serum insulin level.

Objective.—The somatostain octreotide acetate has most of the gastrointestinal actions of somatostatin and a longer serum half-life. A double-blind, crossover trial of octreotide was carried out in 9 patients who

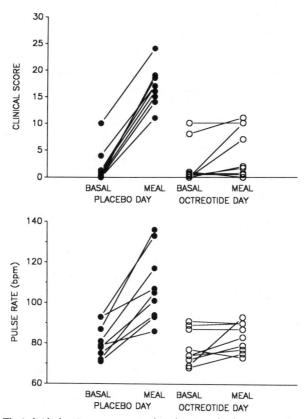

Fig 20–3.—The individual patient responses in clinical score and pulse rate to a provocative meal on the placebo (*closed circles*) and octreotide (*open circles*) treatment days are pictured. Octreotide treatment significantly reduced the number of patients experiencing symptoms or an increase in pulse rate greater than 10 beats per minute (BPM). (Courtesy of Gray JL, Debas HT, Mulvihill SJ: *Arch Surg* 126:1231-1236, 1991.)

had severe dumping symptoms after gastric surgery and had failed to respond to dietary or pharmacologic measures. Subcutaneous injections of 100 μg of octreotide acetate or a saline placebo were given in random order.

Findings.—Ingestion of a test meal was not followed by significantly increased dumping scores when octreotide was injected. Only 2 of the 9 patients had any substantial increase in symptoms (Fig 20–3). Pulse rates differed significantly on treatment and control days. The rise in osmolality was similar on the 2 days. Patients received octreotide for an average of nearly 6 months after the trial. Two patients required pancreatic enzyme replacement for steatorrhea.

Conclusion.—Octreotide acetate is a useful treatment for severe, refractory dumping syndrome in patients who have had gastric surgery. Injection site pain, however, may be a significant problem.

▶ This and the preceding paper (Abstract 20–6) demonstrate the efficacy of somatostatin in treatment of the dumping syndrome. Although the mechanism responsible appears to be rapid emptying of hyperosmolar chyme into the jejunum, the major conundrum is why the dumping syndrome does not develop in everyone who has their pylorus destroyed, removed, or bypassed. Certainly, the criteria are met in any patient who has gastric surgery for ulcer disease, with the exception of selective proximal vagotomy. For that matter, why is it that patients who undergo total gastrectomy and esophagojejunostomy have a rate of dumping of only about 30%, and fewer than 10% have severe symptoms? The mechanism by which somatostatin ameliorates symptoms of the dumping syndrome is unclear; patients with high levels of somatostatin (those with somatostatinomas or those receiving long-term treatment for acromegaly) do not exhibit gut stasis. We and others have great experience in the use of somatostatin in management of pancreatic and gut fistulas, and these patients rarely have ileus.

Of the 9 patients, only 3 have chosen to continue receiving somatostatin. Two have elected to undergo reversal of their pyloroplasty and 2 stopped because pain at the injection site proved more troublesome than the dumping symptoms. What was the incidence of "cure" in those who stopped taking the drug?

If anastomoses are patent, it is wise to avoid reoperating on patients with the dumping syndrome. Somatostatin is helpful in achieving that avoidance.—J.C. Thompson, M.D.

Helicobacter pylori Infection and Gastric Carcinoma Among Japanese Americans in Hawaii

Nomura A, Stemmermann GN, Chyou P-H, Kato I, Perez-Perez GI, Blaser MJ (Kuakini Med Ctr, Honolulu; Vanderbilt Univ)
N Engl J Med 325:1132–1136, 1991   20–8

Background.—It is not clear why deaths from gastric cancer have declined since 1930 in the United States, but epidemiologic findings suggest that environmental factors are important pathogenetically. The presence of *Helicobacter pylori* is thought to have a causative role in gastritis, which may progress to chronic atrophic gastritis, a precursor of gastric carcinoma. Because gastric cancer and *H. pylori* infection share similar epidemiologic features, the infection may be a risk factor for the malignancy.

Study Plan.—An attempt was made to relate *H. pylori* infection to the development of gastric cancer in a cohort of 5,908 Japanese-American men living in Hawaii between 1967 and 1970. By 1989, a total of 109 cases of confirmed gastric carcinoma had been collected. Sera from patients and age-matched controls were analyzed for serum IgG antibody to *H. pylori*.

Findings.—Antibody to *H. pylori* was found in 94% of the men with gastric cancer and in 76% of the matched controls, for an odds ratio of

6.0. The estimated population-attributable risk of gastric cancer attributable to *H. pylori* infection was 63%. The risk increased with the antibody titer. A strong association was evident even in patients in whom the disease was diagnosed 10 years or longer after serum sampling. Relatively few patients who had cancer of the gastric cardia were antibody positive.

Implications.—Although *H. pylori* infection is strongly associated with an increased risk of gastric cancer, most of those infected do not progress to malignancy. It seems likely that other factors are important in the development of gastric carcinoma.

▶ Similar to its epidemiologic association with peptic ulcer disease, *H. pylori* infection shows a strong association with gastric cancer. But because thousands of individuals harbor the infection without ulcer or cancer, the etiology of both diseases is clearly based on multiple factors, only 1 of which is *H. pylori.*—J.C. Thompson, M.D.

Association Between Infection With *Helicobacter pylori* and Risk of Gastric Cancer: Evidence From a Prospective Investigation
Forman D, Newell DG, Fullerton F, Yarnell JWG, Stacey AR, Wald N, Sitas F (Radcliffe Infirmary, Oxford; PHLS Ctr for Applied Microbiology Research, Salisbury; St Bartholomew's Hosp Med College, London; Llandough Hosp, Penarth, Wales)
BMJ 302:1302–1305, 1991   20–9

Introduction.—*Helicobacter pylori* is a cause of chronic antral gastritis. Because this disorder disposes to precancerous changes in the stomach, *H. pylori* may be involved in the development of gastric cancer.

Methods.—A case-control study was conducted of 29 men in whom gastric cancer was diagnosed and 116 age-matched male controls. The presence of *H. pylori* antibody was determined by an enzyme-linked immunosorbent assay.

Results.—Specific *H. pylori* antibody was identified in 69% of men in whom gastric cancer developed and in 47% of controls. The respective median specific IgG concentration was significantly greater in the patients. The odds ratio for gastric cancer developing in patients with a history of *H. pylori* infection was 2.8.

Conclusion.—A significant association was found between *H. pylori* infection and the risk of gastric cancer. It remains unclear how *H. pylori* infection develops, but it is possible that controlling this infection can prevent gastric cancer.

▶ Clearly, *H. pylori* is up to no good. After 3 or 4 years of publication of sufficient numbers of studies on the role of *H. pylori* in peptic ulcer disease, so as to be regarded almost as a cottage industry, this year the great interest is in control in gastritis-type intestinalization of gastric mucosa and the development of gastric neoplasms [see Abstract 20–9 and some of the relevant articles (1–3)]. All papers report a highly suggestive relationship between *H. pylori* and either gastric cancer or primary β cell gastric lymphoma. The present article suggests that treatment of *H. pylori* might diminish the incidence of gastric cancer, but neither the factors that govern the risk of an individual acquiring *H. pylori* infection, nor the risk of cancer once the infection is present, nor the efficacy of prophylaxis, have yet been identified.—J.C. Thompson, M.D.

References

1. Loffeld RJLF, et al: *Histopathology* 17:537, 1990.
2. Wotherspoon AC, et al: *Lancet* 338:1175, 1991.
3. Friedman GD, et al: N *Engl J Med* 325:1127, 1991.

Lack of Relationship Between Perioperative Blood Transfusion and Survival Time After Curative Resection for Gastric Cancer
Moriguchi S, Maehara Y, Akazawa K, Sugimachi K, Nose Y (Kyushu Univ, Fukuoka, Japan)
Cancer 66:2331–2335, 1990   20–10

Background.—Several reports have suggested an adverse relationship between perioperative blood transfusion and survival after various types of major surgery. Other studies have failed to support such a relationship.

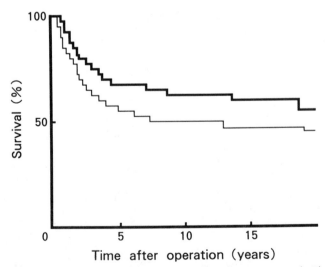

Fig 20–4.—Survival times of all 373 patients given blood transfusions, compared with those of 195 patients who did not receive transfusions. Light line indicates patients who received transfusions; heavy line indicates patients who did not receive transfusions. (Courtesy of Moriguchi S, Maehara Y, Akazawa K, et al: *Cancer* 66:2331-2335, 1990.)

Study.—A review was made of data on 568 patients who had curative gastrectomy for primary advanced gastric cancer from 1965 through 1983. About one third of the patients required no blood transfusion in the perioperative period.

Observations.—Nearly two thirds of the patients died during a median follow-up of 12 years, most of gastric cancer. When deaths from other causes were considered, transfusion recipients lived a significantly shorter time than those who did not receive transfusions (Fig 20–4). The patients with transfusions tended to be older and were more likely to have large and invasive tumors. Surgery lasted longer in this group and operative blood loss was greater. Multivariate analysis failed to support a relationship between survival time and perioperative blood transfusion. The most prominent factors were tumor size, extent of gastric wall invasion, and node status.

Conclusion.—Blood transfusion itself does not influence survival after gastrectomy for gastric cancer.

▶ This all started with the observation that kidney allografts had a higher rate of survival in patients who had received blood transfusion, which suggested an immunosuppressive effect of blood transfusion, followed next by the initial observation of a shortened postoperative survival of patients with bowel cancer who had received perioperative blood transfusions (1). There were multiple reports of adverse postoperative survival in patients who received transfusions during operations for a variety of cancers; other reports denied a harmful effect (the present abstract reviews this literature). This careful study from Fukuoka, Japan, found no difference in the postoperative survival of patients operated on for gastric cancer between a group of 195 patients who required no transfusion as compared with 373 patients who did require it.

This study points out 2 important aspects of gathering information. One of them, of course, is that a negative study can be valuable. The other one, however, is that when the number of papers in favor of a proposition outnumber those against the proposition (by 11 to 5 in the literature review provided by the authors), the addition of one more negative paper changes the ratio only to 11 to 6. Probably, the best thing is for everyone involved to get together and do a multicenter study, because sporadic reports from individual institutions (even with a large number of patients as reported here) will not necessarily solve the problem.—J.C. Thompson, M.D.

Reference

1. Burrows L, Tartter P: *Lancet* 2:662, 1982.

Meta-Analysis of the Risk of Gastric Stump Cancer: Detection of High Risk Patient Subsets for Stomach Cancer After Remote Partial Gastrectomy for Benign Conditions

Tersmette AC, Offerhaus GJA, Tersmette KWF, Giardiello FM, Moore GW, Tytgat GNJ, Vandenbroucke JP (University Hosp, Leiden, The Netherlands; Johns Hopkins Univ; Academic Med Ctr, Amsterdam)
Cancer Res 50:6486–6489, 1990
20–11

Background.—The risk of gastric cancer after partial gastrectomy is controversial, especially in the United States. A meta-analysis was done to determine the overall relative risk and weighted mean relative risk for subgroups of postgastrectomy patients.

Methods.—Studies published from 1982 to 1988 were surveyed, and 22 were chosen for analysis. Gastric stump cancer was defined as an adenocarcinoma of the stomach that occurred at least 55 years after gastric surgery for benign disorders.

Results.—When 2 studies were excluded because of heterogeneity, the overall relative risk for gastric stump cancer was 1.66. When these 2 studies were included, the relative risk summarized with a random effects model to account for heterogeneity was 1.46. There was no clear evidence of publication bias. Fifteen or more years after surgery patients had a weighted mean relative risk of 1.48. Five to 14 years after surgery the relative risk was .91. Patients who had surgery for gastric ulcer had a weighted mean relative risk of 2.12, and those with duodenal ulcers had a relative risk of .84. Women had a weighted mean relative risk of 1.79, and men had a risk of 1.43. The weighted mean relative risk for Billroth II and Billroth I gastrectomy was 1.6 and 1.2, respectively.

Conclusions.—There are differences in relative risk between subgroups of postgastrectomy patients. The postoperative interval is apparently a significant risk factor. The type of ulcer for which surgery was done may also be important.

▶ This problem was discussed in this section 5 years ago, at which time I asked that, if this problem is real, why is it so difficult to demonstrate? As paper after paper after paper has appeared in the past 5 years, the reason for the difficulty has become clear—differences in the rate of development of gastric cancer in the control population vs. postgastrectomy patients begin to appear only 15 to 20 years after gastrectomy, at which time we might expect as high as a 4.5-fold increase in gastric cancer (1). The present study is a compilation of 28 publications, some of which did and some of which did not support the concept of an increased risk. Those studies that follow patients for more than 20 years, however, report almost uniformly an increased incidence of gastric cancer. The cutoff does seem to be about 15 years, i.e., the increased risk does not really appear before that interval. The authors report that there seems to be a higher (but not statistically significant) risk of stump cancer in women than in men, and after Billroth II than after Billroth I. There is a report in rats that the frequency of gastric cancer increased with bile reflux (2).—J.C. Thompson, M.D.

References

1. Caygill CPJ, et al: *Lancet* 1:929, 1986.
2. Kobori O, et al: *J Natl Cancer Inst* 73:853, 1984.

Problems in the Definition and Treatment of Early Gastric Cancer

Inoue K, Tobe T, Kan N, Nio Y, Sakai M, Takeuchi E, Sugiyama T (Kyoto Univ, Japan)

Br J Surg 78:818–821, 1991   20–12

Introduction.—Early detection of gastric cancer through mass screening programs and developments in diagnosis have improved the 5-year survival rate from 60% to more than 90%. Although survival rates have increased, the problem of cancer recurrence remains. Radical surgery with extensive dissection of lymph nodes was performed in 245 of 257 patients with early gastric cancer.

Findings.—Lymph node metastases and the depth of cancer invasion can affect the prognosis of patients with early gastric cancer. The 5-year survival rate was 73.2% when lymph node metastases were present and 99.4% when they were not. The 5-year survival rate was also significantly lower in the 34 patients with lymph node metastases (Fig 20–5).

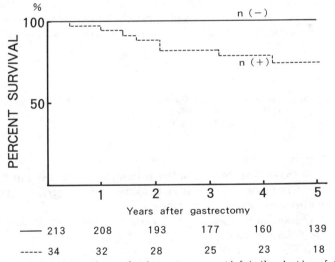

Fig 20–5.—Cumulative survival rate of early gastric cancer with [n(+)] and without [n(−)] lymph node metastases (total number of patients 247). *Solid Line* n(−) (213); *dashed line* n(+) (34): $P < .01$. The number of patients eligible for analysis at each of the time points is shown below the x-axis. (Courtesy of Inoue K, Tobe T, Kan N, et al: *Br J Surg* 78:818–821, 1991.)

Discussion.—In this study, when lymph node metastases were present, the survival rate of patients with early gastric cancer was almost as low as that of patients with the same stage of more advanced cancer. This finding may indicate a need for revision of the definition of early gastric cancer, which had predicted survival based on invasion of the cancer regardless of lymph node metastases. The definition should be modified to "carcinoma with invasion confined to the mucosa or submucosa and without evidence of lymph node metastases." Recommended treatment for mucosal cancer is R_1 operation with complete dissection of only the first group of lymph nodes. For submucosal cancer, R_2 operation with complete dissection of the first and second group of lymph nodes is the appropriate surgical treatment because of the relatively high frequency of lymph node metastases.

▶ Early gastric cancer seemed for years to be a disease limited almost entirely to Japan. Not so. Recent studies in western Europe and in the United States have nearly duplicated the extraordinary survival rate of more than 99% in patients without lymph node metastases. Because of the vastly inferior survival rate in patients with lymph node metastases, the authors pose in this scholarly presentation that early gastric cancer be defined as carcinoma in which the invasion is confined to the mucosa or submucosa without evidence of lymph node metastases. Few surgeons in America have adopted the rigorous techniques of R_0, R_1, R_2, and R_3 lymphadenectomies based on the extent of involvement of respective groups of lymph nodes. The general rules for this are summarized in an article from the Japanese Research Society for Gastric Cancer (1) that all of us should read, and are brought up to date in 2 articles in the *World Journal of Surgery* (2, 3). If we adopted this system in this country, we might well approach the excellent survival statistics achieved by Japanese surgeons in gastric cancer patients.—J.C. Thompson, M.D.

References

1. Japanese Research Society for Gastric Cancer: *Jpn J Surg* 11:127, 1981.
2. Soga J, et al: *World J Surg* 3:701, 1979.
3. Kodama Y, et al: *World J Surg* 5:241, 1981.

Splenectomy Does Not Correlate With Length of Survival in Patients Undergoing Curative Total Gastrectomy for Gastric Carcinoma: Univariate and Multivariate Analyses

Maehara Y, Moriguchi S, Yoshida M, Takahashi I, Korenaga D, Sugimachi K (Kyushu Univ, Fukuoka, Japan)

Cancer 67:3006–3009, 1991

20–13

Introduction.—Splenectomy often is performed at the time of total gastrectomy in patients with gastric cancer to dissect the hilar nodes.

Some claim longer survival for patients who undergo splenectomy, but others report that the prognosis is better if the spleen remains intact.

Methods.—The spleen was removed from 105 of 252 patients who underwent total gastrectomy with curative intent between 1965 and 1985. Patients who had splenectomy had larger tumors and more often had grossly infiltrative lesions. Node metastasis was documented in 8% of splenic hilar nodes and in 10% of splenic artery nodes.

Outcome.—The median follow-up period for the 75 survivors was 9.5 years. Patients who had splenectomy had a significantly shorter survival time than the others. The 10-year survival rates were 52% for patients who had an intact spleen and 37% for those who had splenectomy. Survival times did not differ significantly when patients were grouped by stage of disease.

Conclusion.—Splenectomy is not an independent prognostic factor in patients who undergo curative gastrectomy for gastric cancer.

▶ This paper, another negative study on factors affecting survival after operation for gastric cancer (in this instance, a total gastrectomy), found no difference in the survival of 103 patients who did not lose their spleens as compared with that of 149 patients who did. Again, this began with a series of observations (1) reporting prolonged survival in patients undergoing gastrectomy plus splenectomy for gastric cancer.

Wangensteen and others advocated splenectomy in the treatment of gastric cancer nearly 30 years ago, but were unable ultimately to demonstrate favorable results.—J.C. Thompson, M.D.

Reference

1. Noguchi Y, et al: *Cancer* 64:2053, 1989.

Multivariate Analysis of the Risk of Stomach Cancer After Ulcer Surgery in an Amsterdam Cohort of Postgastrectomy Patients

Tersmette AC, Goodman SN, Offerhaus GJA, Tersmette KWF, Giardiello FM, Vandenbroucke JP, Tytgat GNJ (Univ Hosp, Leiden, The Netherlands; Johns Hopkins Hosp; Academic Med Ctr, Amsterdam)
Am J Epidemiol 134:14–21, 1991
20–14

Introduction.—Deaths from gastric cancer in the Western world are steadily decreasing, presumably because of dietary changes. Early detection through screening programs can increase survival. However, persons who have undergone gastrectomy for benign ulcers appear to be at increased risk for stomach cancer. A group of patients who had undergone gastrectomy were followed, and the risks for stomach cancer among subgroups of this population were compared to those of the general population.

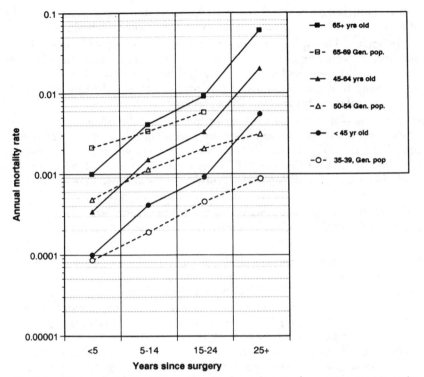

Fig 20–6.—*Filled symbols* and *solid lines* show fitted mortality rates from gastric cancer in an Amsterdam cohort of 2,633 postgastrectomy patients by postoperative interval and age at surgery for patients operated on between 1940–1960 for gastric ulcer disease. Fitted rates for patients with duodenal ulcer would be shifted downward by a factor of 2.6. *Dashed lines* and *open symbols* represent general population rates for males who were in the middle of each age range in 1952. (Courtesy of Tersmette AC, Goodman SN, Offerhaus GJA, et al: *Am J Epidemiol* 134:14-21, 1991.)

Methods.—The study population comprised 2,633 patients who had undergone surgery for benign conditions. The 15- to 40-year follow-up was 99.7% using the Dutch population register system.

Findings.—Compared with the general population, there was increased stomach cancer mortality among men 25 years or more after surgery and among women 15–24 years postoperatively. The most important risk factors for stomach cancer were postoperative interval and gastric vs. duodenal ulcer location (Fig 20-6).

Conclusions.—The risk of stomach cancer increased faster with time since surgery in the study population of patients who had undergone gastrectomy compared to the general population. Risk rates exceeded the general population rates 25 years after surgery for all patients and approximately 15–24 years after surgery for patients operated on for gastric ulcer disease. The subset of patients who have gastrectomy and are at high risk for stomach cancer may benefit from endoscopic surveillance.

▶ This article, with the same authors and a title remarkably similar to that of the article reviewed in Abstract 20–11, is included because of the great homogeneity of more than 2,500 patients studied (all Dutch, followed for 15–40 years, with a follow-up rate of 99.7%). In this group, the increased rate of cancer was not noted in men until 25 years postoperatively, although the differences appeared in women at 15 years.

The import of these 2 studies is, it appears, to nail down once and for all that there is in fact an increased risk of cancer after gastric operations, but that does not appear for 15–25 years. If the mechanism is prolonged achlorhydria, will we be seeing the same phenomenon in patients who take omeprazole?—J.C. Thompson, M.D.

Stapled or Manual Suturing in Esophagojejunostomy After Total Gastrectomy: A Comparison of Outcome in 379 Patients
Fujimoto S, Takahashi M, Endoh F, Takai M, Kobayashi K, Kiuchi S, Konno C, Obata G, Okui K (Chiba Univ, Japan)
Am J Surg 162:256–259, 1991   20–15

Objective.—The mechanical stapler has proved effective in limiting leakage from an esophagojejunostomy. The outcome was compared in 199 patients having esophagojejunostomy with stapling with that in 180 patients in whom manual suturing was carried out.

Technique.—A USSC EEA device was used for mechanical suturing of an end-to-side esophagojejunostomy. The other patients had a conventional 2-layer hand-sutured anastomosis constructed.

Results.—The stapling procedure required only about 10 minutes, compared with at least 30–45 minutes for manual suturing. More patients in the stapling group had a supradiaphragmatic anastomosis. Surgically related deaths were comparably frequent in the 2 groups. Seven patients who had stapling and 4 who had manual suturing had anastomotic leakage. In 6 stapled patients and 1 in the manually sutured group, anastomotic stenosis developed.

Conclusion.—Transabdominal stapled suturing of an esophagojejunostomy is an expeditious and reliable procedure, although stapler-related complications can occur.

▶ According to this study, the main advantage of the stapled esophagojejunostomy is that it can be done in 10 minutes compared to the 30–45 minutes required for a handsewn anastomosis. The overall duration of the entire operation was not significantly different, however. Also the rate of leakage was similar in the 2 groups with about a 1% death rate associated with leakage in both groups. The rate of stenosis was 6 to 1 (stapled to handsewn). We have found the stenosis to be easily managed with Maloney dilators. About one third of the patients in our experience required dilatation and, so far, only 1 patient has required more than 1—and that patient required 2.—J.C. Thompson, M.D.

21 The Small Intestine

The Effect of Intestinal Resection and Urogastrone on Intestinal Regeneration
Thompson JS, Bragg LE, Saxena SK (Omaha VA Med Ctr; Univ of Nebraska)
Arch Surg 125:1617–1621, 1990   21–1

Background.—Intestinal regeneration is observed when full-thickness bowel wall defects are patched with adjacent colonic serosa. The neomucosa forms through the proliferation of epithelial cells in mucosal crypts and the migration of cells across the patched defect. The roles of intestinal resection and urogastrone in intestinal regeneration were examined in the rabbit.

Methods.—The rabbits had 2 × 5 cm ileal defects patched with the adjacent colonic serosal surface. Treated animals had half of the small bowel resected or had mini-osmotic pumps implanted subcutaneously for infusion of recombinant urogastrone at a rate of 1.5 μg/kg/hr. Some animals had both resection and urogastrone infusion.

Results.—Intestinal resection, alone and combined with urogastrone, promoted epithelialization of the defects (Fig 21–1). Urogastrone inhibited contraction of the patched defect. Resection with or without urogastrone led to greater contraction than seen in controls or animals treated with urogastrone alone. Both interventions increased proliferative activity. Maltase and sucrase activities at 2 weeks were highest in urogastrone-treated animals.

Conclusions.—Both intestinal resection and urogastrone appear to stimulate epithelialization in full-thickness bowel wall defects patched with adjacent serosal surface. Intestinal resection may have a mechanical effect on contraction after patching. Its inhibitory effect on urogastrone-stimulated proliferation also may play a role.

▶ The purpose of the study was to determine whether small bowel resection and urogastrone (both shown to enhance regeneration of the intestine) have synergistic effects. The answer is no, and the authors conclude that urogastrone will probably not be of any help in enhancing adaptation in patients with massive small bowel resection. This is an important negative finding, and it is especially noteworthy because the authors have previously devoted great attention to stimulation of mucosal growth by the exogenous administration of urogastrone (1–3). Other candidates that we and others have been studying are enteroglucagon, neurotensin, and epidermal growth factor. We

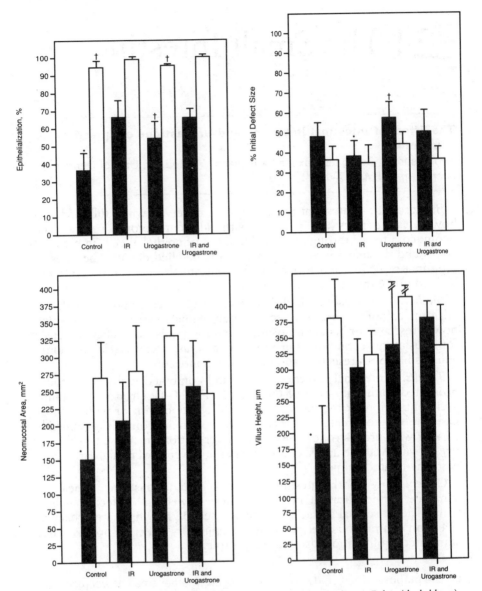

Fig 21–1.—Comparison of intestinal regeneration, with comparative values at 7 days (*shaded bars*) and 14 days (*open bars*). **Top left,** epithelialization. *Asterisk, P* <.05 vs. patients with intestinal resection (IR), urogastrone, and IR and urogastrone; *dagger, P* <.05 vs. patients with IR and those with IR and urogastrone. **Top right,** contraction. *Asterisk, P* <.05 vs. controls, those with urogastrone, and IR and urogastrone; *dagger, P* <.05 vs. controls. **Bottom left,** neomucosal area. *Asterisk, P* <.05 vs. patients with IR, urogastrone, and IR and urogastrone. **Bottom right,** villus height. *Asterisk, P* <.05 vs. IR, urogastrone, and IR and urogastrone. (Courtesy of Thompson JS, Bragg LE, Saxena SK: *Arch Surg* 125:1617–1621, 1990.)

believe that neurotensin is the strongest current candidate.—J.C. Thompson, M.D.

References

1. Thompson JS, et al: *J Surg Res* 42:402, 1987.
2. Thompson JS, et al: *Surg Forum* 34:180, 1988.
3. Thompson JS, et al: *Cell Tissue Kinet* 21:183, 1988.

Role of Intraoperative Enteroscopy in Obscure Gastrointestinal Bleeding of Small Bowel Origin

Desa LA, Ohri SK, Hutton KAR, Lee H, Spencer J (Royal Postgrad Med School, Hammersmith Hosp, London)
Br J Surg 78:192–195, 1991   21–2

Background.—Gastrointestinal bleeding of obscure origin continues to pose a major diagnostic problem. Bleeding from the small bowel usually is caused by a vascular malformation, tumor, ulcer, or Meckel's diverticulum. Intraoperative enteroscopy now makes it possible to visualize the entire gastrointestinal tract.

Methods.—Of 60 patients seen in a 5-year period with obscure gastrointestinal bleeding, 22 proved to have bleeding localized to the small bowel. Eighteen were operated on, and 12 had intraoperative enteroscopy.

Results.—It proved possible to reach the mid-ileum only because of adhesions from previous laparotomies. Fresh blood was observed in 7 patients, and discrete vascular lesions were observed in 3. Most of the patients underwent resection of the proximal 25 cm of jejunum as a primary procedure. One operative death resulted from chest infection and septicemia, and 1 late death resulted from chronic renal failure. Two patients later had laparotomy for recurrent bleeding, and 3 others had rebleeding during a median follow-up of 6 months.

Conclusions.—Intraoperative enteroscopy is a necessary adjunct to laparotomy for gastrointestinal bleeding localized preoperatively to the small bowel. Blind proximal jejunal resection is indicated only if bleeding is definitely localized to this site preoperatively and enteroscopy is negative in an elderly, poor-risk patient.

▶ Soon it will be possible preoperatively to endoscope the entire bowel (allowing, perhaps, for each endoscopist to examine the retina of his/her colleague). Until then (and even probably after then if the study were negative), intraoperative endoscopy will be helpful. We have been particularly impressed by our ability to visualize angiodysplastic lesions by transmural illumination in a darkened room (see illustration in the *Atlas of Surgery of the Stomach, Duodenum, and Small Bowel.* Mosby–Year Book, 1992, p 301). Any kind of "blind" resection is risky and the results are unpredictable, therefore often bad. Pre- and intraoperative endoscopy has greatly reduced the frequency of blind resection, *Gott sei dank.*—J.C. Thompson, M.D.

Recurrence of Crohn's Disease After Resection
Williams JG, Wong WD, Rothenberger DA, Goldberg SM (Univ of Minnesota)
Br J Surg 78:10–19, 1991   21–3

Background.—Recurrence of Crohn's disease after surgical resection is not infrequent, particularly on long-term follow-up. After colectomy with ileocolic or colocolic anastomosis, recurrent disease tends to develop in the ileum proximal to the anastomosis as well as in the remaining colon and rectum. Recurrences after proctocolectomy invariably are in the ileum proximal to the stoma but usually spare the actual stomal segment of ileum.

Factors in Recurrence.—Age at onset of illness does not seem to influence the risk of recurrence; and gender is not a factor. Patients with Crohn's colitis with ileal involvement are far more likely than those without ileal disease to have recurrences. Reports attempting to relate recurrences to the extent of resection have given conflicting results. Microscopic disease at the resection margin appears to be a factor in recurrence. Immunologic variables probably are markers for more severe disease and, therefore, a greater risk of early recurrence.

Conclusions.—In most patients, if observed long enough, overt recurrent disease develops after resection of Crohn's disease. Radical resection does not protect against recurrence, so that conservative removal is indicated to preserve the bowel.

▶ One basic thing to remember is that we have no cure, either medical or surgical, for Crohn's disease. We do not really know how it begins, we do not have a way to cure it, and we do not know why it usually gets better after the age of 50. Because the worst cases, usually, are those submitted to operation, we should not be too surprised at a high postoperative recurrence rate. Operations, in general, are limited to going in and fixing whatever is causing the current most prominent symptom. We often visualize other areas of diseased bowel but leave them in so that there is enough bowel to function. Those other areas of involvement may, unpredictably, proceed to mucosal ulceration, fistula formation, and cicatrization with gut obstruction. Because we do not attempt to eradicate the disease, it does not seem justified to ask for an intraoperative frozen-section determination of whether or not the bowel is involved at the site of resection. We are likely to be reoperating, thus it is important to leave as much bowel as possible, as the vanishing bowel syndrome is a true risk.—J.C. Thompson, M.D.

Risks of Intestinal Anastomoses in Crohn's Disease
Post S, Betzler M, von Ditfurth B, Schürmann G, Küppers P, Herfarth C (Univ

of Heidelberg, Germany)

Ann Surg 213:37–42, 1991   21–4

Background.—Intestinal resection of Crohn's disease frequently is associated with factors that increase the risk of complications. These may include obstruction, septic complications, poor nutrition, and the need for multiple anastomoses. Reported rates of complications tend to exceed those resulting from resection of noninflammatory disease.

Methods.—Complications were analyzed in a prospective series of 368 patients (mean age, 33 years) having 429 primary operations for Crohn's disease at a single center. In all, 658 intestinal anastomoses were done. Of these, 491 were fully circumferential. The patients had experienced symptoms for a mean of 8 years.

Findings.—Complications occurred in 9.7% of the patients, and 4% required reoperation. The overall rate of mortality was .5%. On multivariate analysis, the only factor significantly associated with overall complications was long-term steroid therapy. Serious complications occurred more often in patients with intra-abdominal abscess. The combination of abscess and preoperative steroid therapy increased the complication rate to 16%. Complications did not correlate with the site of anastomosis, the presence of inflamed anastomotic margins, or the performance of a diverting ileostomy or colostomy.

Conclusions.—These findings support a policy of limited surgery for Crohn's disease. It appears safe to suture bowel that is microscopically inflamed.

▶ The postoperative complication rate of 9.7% (4% required reoperation) is low. Because the authors made no attempt to go beyond areas of microscopic involvement, they frequently ended up anastomosing inflamed bowel, and these anastomoses usually were successful. This is certainly in concert with our own experience. The message is: Take out what is bad and make no attempt to eradicate the disease, and take out only the grossly diseased bowel and make no attempt at eradicating all areas of involvement. Anastomoses in bowel with microscopic involvement almost always heal.—J.C. Thompson, M.D.

Prevalence of Inflammatory Bowel Disease Among Relatives of Patients With Crohn's Disease

Monsén U, Bernell O, Johansson C, Hellers G (Huddinge Univ Hosp, Stockholm)

Scand J Gastroenterol 26:302–306, 1991   21–5

Introduction.—Although the cause of Crohn's disease remains unknown, a genetic factor appears to be involved in susceptibility to the disease. The prevalence of inflammatory bowel disease was investigated in the relatives of 1,048 patients with Crohn's disease.

Results.—There was a positive family history of Crohn's disease only in 88 patients, a history of both Crohn's disease and ulcerative colitis in 10, and a family history of ulcerative colitis only in 42. The overall prevalence of inflammatory bowel disease was 13.4%. The mean age at diagnosis was 25 years for index patients with a positive family history and 33 years for the others. Crohn's disease was more than 20 times more frequent in first-degree relatives than in nonrelatives. The prevalence of ulcerative colitis in first-degree relatives of patients with Crohn's disease was 6 times greater than in nonrelatives.

▶ This degree of association speaks for a causative or facilitative gene. Perhaps the most interesting finding is that those patients with a family history of Crohn's disease became symptomatic 8 years earlier than those with sporadic disease. Why does it usually get better with age? Many studies have suggested that poor people are less apt to get Crohn's disease than rich people. Is this true, and if so why? Is there a gene for wealth?—J.C. Thompson, M.D.

Short-Bowel Syndrome in Children: Quality of Life in an Era of Improved Survival

Weber TW, Tracy T Jr, Connors RH (St Louis Univ; Cardinal Glennon Children's Hosp, St Louis)
Arch Surg 126:841–846, 1991   21–6

Introduction.—A number of childhood disorders can lead to short bowel syndrome, with a short bowel length of less than 100 cm. Survival has improved with the advent of total parenteral nutrition (TPN) and balanced enteral feedings.

Methods.—Data were reviewed on 16 consecutive pediatric patients with 22–98 cm of small bowel who were followed for 2–10 years. The most common original diagnoses were necrotizing enterocolitis and multiple intestinal atresias. The mean amount of small bowel present was 49 cm. In 9 infants, an ileocecal valve was retained. All of the patients required multiple operations, which included combinations of adhesiolysis, tapering enteroplasty, reversed intestinal segments, and pull-through procedures. Total parenteral nutrition was administered to 9 patients at home and 12 required a home elemental diet, usually administered by pump.

Results.—All but 1 of the 16 patients survived; 2 survivors were deaf and 1 had mildly delayed development. At last follow-up, 10 patients no longer required nutritional support and 4 others were weaning. The presence or absence of an ileocecal valve did not influence the outcome. In general, growth and development were excellent.

Conclusion.—Modern nutritional support provides for excellent survival and a good quality of life in children with short bowel syndrome. However, patients must cope with many setbacks, reoperations, prolonged hospitalizations, and training in the use of technical equipment.

▶ Many of our greatest problems are compounded by our ignorance of eventual outcomes. What does happen to 900-g infants 10, 20, and 30 years after they survive the Neonatal Intensive Care Unit? What exactly is the limit of gut length that is compatible with life? How do children with 90% + burns fare in adulthood? The answers, usually, are that they survive, and that ultimate outcome depends on what criteria one chooses to define success. They certainly have to weather hundreds of vicissitudes, including enduring frequent trips back to the hospital, educating whole new generations of house staff in their problems, and coping with the response they elicit from society.

Many times, pediatric surgeons operating on children with midgut volvulus find nearly the entire gut infarcted and close the abdomen without resection, firm in the belief that the child has no chance. One of the toughest problems we face recurrently in our own Morbidity and Mortality Conferences is deciding what procedures are justified. When is it acceptable to cease further efforts at resuscitation? Studies like this one will help us make up our minds.

Wilmore (1) concluded that survival after massive small bowel resection in infancy was unlikely with less than 15 cm of bowel, and that less than 40 cm required the presence of an ileocecal valve for survival. The present series questions whether or not the ileocecal valve is any longer an important determinant. Anyone interested in this question would do well to read the entire article.—J.C. Thompson, M.D.

Reference

1. Wilmore DW: *J Pediatr* 80:88, 1972.

The Role of Tagged Red Blood Cell Imaging in the Localization of Gastrointestinal Bleeding

Bentley DE, Richardson JD (Univ of Louisville)
Arch Surg 126:821–824, 1991

21–7

Introduction.—Imaging of gastrointestinal tract bleeding with 99mTc-labeled red blood cells reportedly has excellent accuracy in many centers. Some radiologists refuse to perform visceral arteriography for bleeding unless a tagged red blood cell study is performed first.

Methods.—Data were reviewed on 162 patients who had 99mTc-red blood cell scans to localize gastrointestinal tract bleeding; 182 separate studies were performed. In 83 patients the ultimate diagnosis was made by endoscopy, angiography, or at operation.

Results.—Of 98 patients with positive scans, 48 had definitive identification of an anatomical site of bleeding. Nearly half of these scans identified an incorrect site as the source of bleeding. Scanning was most accurate in demonstrating colonic bleeding sites and least helpful where there was an upper gastrointestinal tract site. Of 15 patients operated on after red blood cell scanning, 6 had a site of bleeding identified only at operation.

Conclusion.—Scanning with tagged red blood cells is not an accurate means of localizing gastrointestinal tract bleeding. These findings call into question the value of red blood cell scanning as a screening tool before angiography.

▶ If bleeding is massive, it can usually be localized quickly. If it is a steady trickle, diagnosis is difficult; if it is an intermittent trickle, the diagnosis may not be made at all. Statistics for success can be manipulated by establishing entry criteria for any study that depends on loss of a lot of blood. When you start looking for small intermittent but persistent losses, everything is murky. A 52% rate does not look very good unless the diagnosis would not have been made any other way. The gold standard, of course, is to demonstrate bleeding by mesenteric angiography but, once again, success depends on the fortuitous coincidence of blood loss at exactly the time of injection of the dye.

The tagged red blood cell technique provides less precise localization, but gives a longer window of time. Like everything else, the results are better when the study is performed by someone who is enthusiastic and dedicated to the technique. That is why it is often difficult to replicate good results. In general, investigators publish results when they are good. When they are inferior to previously published results, most clinical investigators will decide they ought to study a few more patients or change their technique. This leads to a darwinian process of selection, i.e., better results get published, and less good results get restudied.—J.C. Thompson, M.D.

Expression of Neurotensin Messenger RNA in a Human Carcinoid Tumor

Evers BM, Ishizuka J, Townsend CM Jr, Rajaraman S, Thompson JC (Univ of Texas, Galveston)
Ann Surg 214:448–454, 1991   21–8

Objective.—Neurotensin is a distal gut peptide having important regulatory and trophic effects throughout the bowel. A human foregut carcinoid tumor line, BON, was used in athymic nude mice to examine the intracellular mechanisms regulating the expression and release of human neurotensin.

Methods.—The cells were maintained in tissue culture and examined by phase-contrast and electron microscopy. The effect of the cyclic

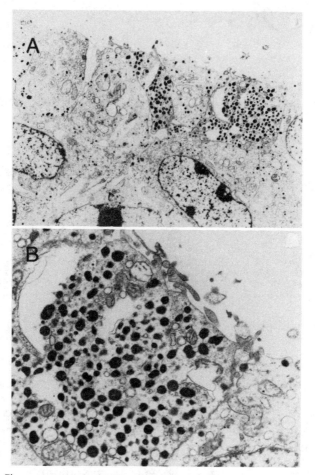

Fig 21–2.—Electron micrograph of BON cells showing abundant dense secretory granules. (**A,** original magnification, ×7,000) (**B,** original magnification, ×25,000). (Courtesy of Evers MB, Ishizuka J, Townsend CM Jr, et al: *Ann Surg* 214:448–454, 1991.)

adenosine monophosphate (cAMP) signal transduction pathway on neurotensin expression was studied, measuring neurotensin by radioimmunoassay; RNA was analyzed for neurotensin mRNA expression by Northern hybridization using a cDNA probe.

Findings.—Secretory granules were abundant in BON cells (Fig 21–2). Neurotensin mRNA transcripts were recognized in both BON cells and normal ileal mucosa (Fig 21–3). Forskolin induced release of neurotensin from BON cells in a dose-dependent manner. The addition of 5-hydroxytryptamine, which reduces intracellular cAMP in BON cells, lowered levels of neurotensin mRNA.

Implications.—The expression and release of human neurotensin is mediated in part by the cAMP signal transduction pathway. The BON

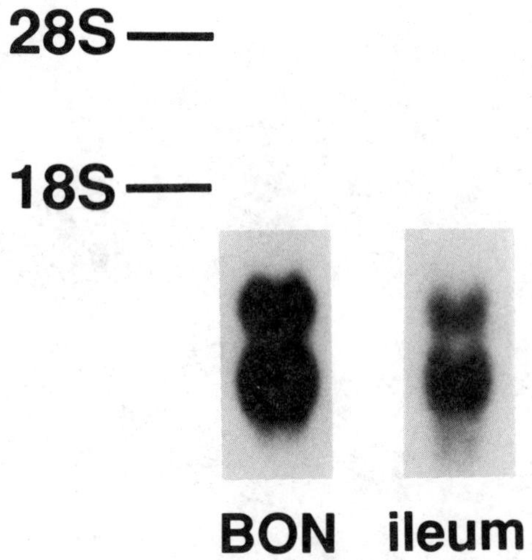

28S ——

18S ——

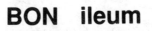

BON ileum

Fig 21–3.—Expression of neurotensin (NT) messenger RNA in BON and *human ileum*. Five micrograms of poly (A) + RNA from BON cells and ilial mucosa was analyzed by the Northern blot method. The blots were probed with a canine NT chromosomal RNA and were washed at high stringency. (Courtesy of Evers MB, Ishizuka J, Townsend CM Jr, et al: *Ann Surg* 214:448–454, 1991.)

cell line should prove helpful in defining the intracellular mechanisms involved in the transcriptional regulation and release of human neurotensin.

▶ This paper details the signal transduction pathway and the demonstration of mRNA for neurotensin in a transformed cell line of a human carcinoid tumor. Both demonstrations are important, but as Niederhuber observed in the question session after the paper, the real importance may be appreciated only after a similarity of actions is demonstrated between this cell line and appropriate normal cells. The ability of pluripotential neoplastic cells to elaborate vasoactive amines, regulatory peptides, and growth factors provides clues to their function and for studies on growth of the parent tumor. Small lung cancer cells have been shown to elaborate more than 40 agents, several of which appear to function as autocrine growth factors for the tumor. Knowledge of the mechanisms of control of tumor growth allows preparation of strategies to interfere, i.e., if a tumor is found to be dependent on, for example, bombesin for its growth, a likely strategy would be treatment with a bombesin receptor-blocking agent or bombesin antibodies. Or by interfering in the metabolic pathway that yields bombesin.—J.C. Thompson, M.D.

22 The Colon and the Rectum

Cecal Volvulus
Rabinovici R, Simansky DA, Kaplan O, Mavor E, Manny J (Hadassah Med Ctr, Jerusalem; Sheba Med Ctr, Tel Aviv; Rokach Med Ctr, Tel Aviv; Kaplan Med Ctr, Rehovot, Israel)
Dis Colon Rectum 33:765–769, 1990   22–1

Introduction.—Cecal volvulus is a surgical emergency caused by axial twisting of the cecum, distal ileum, and proximal colon in the absence of normal cecal fixation. The clinical features result from the subsequent closed-loop obstruction. Colonic ischemia, perforation, sepsis, and death may ensue unless an early diagnosis is made.

Methods.—Data were reviewed on 561 patients (mean age, 53 years) who were treated for cecal volvulus between 1959 and 1989. The clinical features were characteristic of distal closed loop obstruction. In more than half of the patients, the diagnosis was preoperative, but in only 17% was a definitive diagnosis made from plain abdominal radiographs. Necrosis was observed at exploration in 20% of the patients. Complications and recurrences were more frequent after resectional surgery than after detorsion or cecopexy. Resection gave comparable results in patients with necrotic and viable colon.

Current Series.—From 1973 to 1989, 7 patients (mean age, 43 years) were operated on for cecal volvulus. Abdominal pain and vomiting were the most common clinical features. In 5 patients, the diagnosis was preoperative. In 5 patients there was true volvulus, and 2 had anterior cephalad displacement of the cecum. There was 1 hospital death, but there were no recurrences during a mean follow-up of 44 months.

Conclusion.—Resection should be reserved for patients whose cecum is necrotic or perforated. Detorsion is adequate treatment when viable cecum is present.

▶ The frequency of colonic volvulus is greater in societies with high-fiber diets, diets that appear to cause lengthening of the colon. This effect is much more pronounced in sigmoid than in cecal volvulus. Sigmoid volvulus is said to be 3–4 times more common than cecal volvulus and occurs usually in patients older than age 60, whereas cecal volvulus has its highest incidence in the 25- to 30-year age group, with a mean age of 40 years (1). I was surprised, in this study, that there was no recurrence in this small series. The authors conclude that the treatment of choice in patients without gangrene is simple detorsion. I suspect the series is too small to make that conclusion.—J.C. Thompson, M.D.

Reference

1. Donhauser JL, Atwell S: *Arch Surg* 58:129, 1949.

Quality of Life of Patients With Ulcerative Colitis Preoperatively and Postoperatively
McLeod RS, Churchill DN, Lock AM, Vanderburgh S, Cohen Z (Toronto Gen Hosp; McMaster Univ)
Gastroenterology 101:1307–1313, 1991   22–2

Objective.—Changes in the quality of life after surgery for ulcerative colitis were examined in a prospective group of 20 patients who had no previous surgery for colitis and were assessed just before and a year after surgery. Another 93 patients who had surgery at least a year earlier participated in a cross-sectional study.

Methods.—The time trade-off technique is a measure of the perceived worth, or utility of a given health state. The patient is given a choice between 2 hypothetical options—one to continue in his present state of health, and the other to be in full health for a shorter time. In addition, the Direct Questioning of Objectives instrument was used to assess the quality of life.

Findings.—Both instruments suggested improvement postoperatively in the prospective series. In the cross-sectional study, no significant differences were found among patients given a conventional ileostomy, a Kock pouch, or an ileal reservoir.

Implication.—Surgery usually improves the quality of life in patients with ulcerative colitis, regardless of the operative procedure used.

▶ What the authors did was to study 20 patients who underwent colectomy for chronic idiopathic ulcerative colitis, before and at least 1 year after operation. These patients were studied by means of questionnaires developed to attempt to quantitate the patients' qualitiative assessment of life before and after operation. Another group of patients who had been operated on for at least a year also were interrogated. All assessments suggested postoperative improvement over the preoperative quality of life. All of us in this field have listened to surgeons tell us of the great joy their patients had when a conventional ileostomy was converted either to a Kock pouch or an ileal reservoir.

It should be mentioned that ileoanal anastomosis with mucosal proctectomy was not a part of this study. The surprising information here is that the quality of life did not seem to differ with the operation. One gathers the im-pression that once the sick colon is removed, the patient gets well, and that assessment of the quality of life is a direct reflection of the patient's improved state of health. The authors plan to "fine tune" the psychological testing procedures so as to attempt to differentiate between patient acceptance of different operations. When they do that, they certainly should include ileoanal anastomosis, but it may take years for people to be able to discern a perceived difference among the various operative procedures.—J.C. Thompson, M.D.

The Effects of Intracolonic EGF on Mucosal Growth and Experimental Carcinogenesis
Reeves JR, Richards RC, Cooke T (Univ of Liverpool; Univ of Glasgow)
Br J Cancer 63:223–226, 1991   22–3

Introduction.—The role of epidermal growth factor (EGF) in the adult intestine remains uncertain, but the finding of EGF receptors on gut epithelial cells suggests that the peptide may be involved in intestinal homeostasis.

Methods.—The effects of daily intracolonic EGF administration on the rat large bowel during colorectal carcinogenesis were investigated. Colon cancer was induced by injecting azoxymethane subcutaneously.

Results.—Treatment with EGF, 12 nM, stimulated growth of the intestinal mucosa as determined from crypt cell production rates in animals not given the carcinogen. Treatment with azoxymethane, .8 nM, was ineffective. Azoxymethane increased mucosal growth, but this effect was countered by the higher dose of EGF.

Conclusion.—Intraluminal EGF and azoxymethane each increase the proliferation of intestinal epithelial cells, but their combined effect is antagonistic. Although EGF may have a role in normal intestinal epithelial growth, it did not potentiate colonic carcinogenesis in this animal model.

▶ We are going to see a lot of these studies in which investigators attempt to demonstrate an etiologic or permissive role for various growth factors in the pathogenesis of gut cancer. At least 10 groups in the United States are working on the problem and have succeeded in uncovering small shards of information linking the 2. The basic concept is simple and has great biological precedent. You cannot help wondering whether cancers arising from the gut are not stimulated to grow by factors that promote growth of normal gut epithelium in a manner analogous to the way in which estrogen, which is a growth hormone for normal breast tissue, may stimulate breast cancers. The operative word is "may," because only a fraction of patients with breast cancer have true hormone dependency.

Dr. Townsend and his colleagues in our department have repeatedly shown that some gut cancer cells have receptors for certain growth factors and others do not. In the case of experimental pancreatic cancer, cells with receptors for cholecystokinin (CCK) are stimulated to grow by exogenous CCK; those without receptors do not grow. You cannot always predict how receptor activation will work. For example, CCK has been shown to suppress growth of certain human cholangiocarcinomas (that possess CCK receptors).—J.C. Thompson, M.D.

Carcinoid Tumor of the Appendix in the First Two Decades of Life
Moertel CL, Weiland LH, Telander RL (Mayo Clinic and Found, Rochester, Minn; Mayo Clinic Scottsdale, Ariz; Fargo Clinic, ND)
J Pediatr Surg 25:1073–1075, 1990   22–4

Background.—Carcinoid tumor is the most common gastrointestinal neoplasm in children and adolescents. Its discovery usually is an incidental encounter. The natural course of this tumor was examined in 23 patients seen from 1936 to 1988 aged 20 years or younger who had a histologically confirmed carcinoid tumor involving the appendix.

Findings.—The median age was 13.5 years; females predominated. Most patients had an acute abdomen at entry, but 3 initially had abdominal pain for about 6 months. None of the patients had symptoms of carcinoid syndrome. A majority of tumors were 1 cm or less in size; only 3 patients had lesions ≥ 2 cm in diameter. Seven tumors remained limited to the appendiceal mucosa, whereas 6 invaded to the mesoappendix or periappendiceal fat. Lymphatic invasion was observed in all patients, but vascular invasion was not seen in any. During follow-up (median, 26 years) 2 of 18 patients died, 1 of colonic adenocarcinoma and 1 of trauma. No recurrences of carcinoid tumor were observed.

Conclusions.—Appendiceal carcinoid tumor in children who lack metastasis at the time of diagnosis appears to be clinically benign. Conservative surgery is appropriate in these patients; "second-look" surgery is not called for.

► A good stand to take regarding carcinoid tumors is to consider those greater than 2 cm in size as bad actors. This large series of patients with appendiceal carcinoids from the Mayo Clinic, however, does not entirely support that concept and suggests a peculiarly benign outlook for carcinoids arising from the appendix. This has been appreciated for a long time, but the case study of a patient with a 2.5-cm carcinoid tumor of the appendix invading the serosa and mesoappendix who was treated by simple appendectomy and is free of disease at 31 years postoperatively is strong evidence in support of the concept of the benignity of appendiceal carcinoids. The authors conclude that carcinoid tumors of the appendix in children without gross metastases appear to be clinically benign and permit conservative management.—J.C. Thompson, M.D.

Long-Term Effects of Dietary Calcium on Risk Markers for Colon Cancer in Patients With Familial Polyposis

Stern HS, Gregoire RC, Kashtan H, Stadler J, Bruce RW (Mount Sinai Hosp, Toronto)

Surgery 108:528–533, 1990

22–5

Background.—There are epidemiologic indications that a high dietary calcium intake is associated with a low risk of colon cancer. Recent findings indicate that calcium may lower the rate of colonic mucosal proliferation in those belonging to kindreds with familial colon cancer. Patients undergoing ileorectal surgery for familial polyposis comprise a useful group in which to examine hypotheses for preventing colon cancer.

Methods.—A total of 31 patients with familial polyposis underwent subtotal colectomy and then were randomly assigned to a group receiving either 1,200 mg of calcium daily or a group receiving placebo daily for 9 months. The groups were similar in age, body size, macronutrient intake, and dietary fiber intake. There were more women in the placebo-treated group.

Results.—Fecal pH, weight, and bile acid levels were unchanged after intervention. Fecal calcium increased in the calcium-supplemented group. Thymidine labeling indices, estimated by rectal biopsies, were reduced in calcium-supplemented patients after 6 months but were at baseline levels after 9 months.

Conclusions.—No beneficial effect of calcium on rectal mucosal proliferation was evident in these patients with familial polyposis. The defective gene is now known to be on chromosome 5. Effective chemoprevention probably will depend on discovering what the gene normally codes for, or what triggers its expression.

▶ Learned cocktail party conversation in the past decade is unequivocal regarding the salutary effects of bran, low-fat diet, and high-calcium intake in the prevention of colon cancer. I am not sure that any of these could pass a rigorous submission to fulfillment of criteria for cause, and of the 3, calcium seems to be the weakest (that means that I lean toward bran and a low-fat diet). The question is whether a group of patients with familial polyposis forms a valid model for study of the induction of colon cancer in general. Nobody knows that, of course, but other questions are whether 9 months provides an adequate test for exclusion of calcium. What we can say is that in this group of patients with familial polyposis, a large daily intake of calcium for 9 months failed to affect the degree of proliferation of rectal mucosa.—J.C. Thompson, M.D.

Cancer and Polyps of the Colorectum and Lifetime Consumption of Beer and Other Alcoholic Beverages

Riboli E, Cornée J, Macquart-Moulin G, Kaaks R, Casagrande C, Guyader M (Internat Agency for Research on Cancer, Lyon; Nat Inst of Health and Med Research, Marseilles, France)
Am J Epidemiol 133:157–166, 1991   22–6

Introduction.—Case-control studies on drinking in relation to colorectal cancer have tended to be negative, although some studies suggest an increased risk of rectal cancer. Several case-control studies indicate a specific association between beer consumption and an increased risk of rectal cancer.

Methods.—In 1979–1985, 2 parallel case-control studies were conducted in the region of Marseilles, France. Incident cases included 389 patients with colorectal cancer and 252 with polyps. An equal number of controls were matched with the patients for age and gender.

Results.—The relative risk of rectal cancer for men who drank beer was 1.73, whereas men and women combined had a relative risk of 1.71. No association was evident between beer consumption and colon cancer. At neither site was cancer associated with total ethanol intake or the consumption of wine and spirits. Comparable results were obtained after adjusting for energy intake and fiber from fruits and vegetables.

Conclusion.—Epidemiologic findings of an association between beer drinking and rectal cancer relate to animal studies of nitrosamine carcinogenicity. Efforts are warranted to reduce the nitrosamine content of beer.

▶ This study from Marseilles concludes that the consumption of beer is associated with a higher risk of development of rectal, but not colon, cancer. This is in contrast to a study of brewery workers in Denmark who had no increase in mortality from colorectal cancer, as compared with that in the general population and in a group who abstained from alcohol (1, 2).

It is of interest that wine got off scot-free.—J.C. Thompson, M.D.

References

1. Jensen OM: *Int J Cancer* 23:454, 1979.
2. Jensen OM: *J Natl Cancer Inst* 70:1011, 1983.

Cholecystectomy as a Risk Factor for Colorectal Adenomatous Polyps and Carcinoma

Neugut AI, Murray TI, Garbowski GC, Forde KA, Treat MR, Waye JD, Fenoglio-Preiser C (Columbia Univ; Mt Sinai School of Medicine, New York; Univ of Cincinnati)
Cancer 68:1644–1647, 1991   22–7

Introduction.—The factors associated with colorectal cancer are largely unknown, but a possible relationship with previous cholecystectomy has been suggested, particularly in women and especially for right-sided colonic cancers.

Study Design.—A case-control study was carried out involving patients having colonoscopy in 3 private practices in New York City during a 2-year period. In all, 106 patients with colon cancer and 302 with adenomatous polyps were matched with 507 controls.

Findings.—No significant differences were found between cases and controls with respect to a history of cholecystectomy. This held true for females when analyzed separately.

Conclusion.—Cholecystectomy is not likely to be a significant risk factor for colorectal neoplasia.

▶ This abstract was included because it so satisfied my preconceptions. The authors reviewed 34 papers that examined the relationship between cholecystectomy and cancer of the large bowel; exactly half of these found an elevated risk associated with previous cholecystectomy. The other half of the studies, however, failed to find a relationship. The score was 17 to 17; now it is 17 to 18, with the current paper also failing to show a relationship.

One of the most difficult achievements is to demonstrate a true relationship between clinical variables. The question always centers about what is the proper control. For example, a putative increase in the incidence of peptic ulcer has been reported in patients with cirrhosis, portacaval shunt, obstructive pulmonary disease, hyperparathyroidism, and probably falling hair. The question is, who are the proper controls for these chronically ill patients? The answer is, another group of chronically ill patients who do not happen to include this group. When appropriate studies are carried out, we find that peptic ulcer disease is associated with chronic illness, not, apparently, with any specific chronic illness.

Anyway, no matter how I sliced the teleologic question, I could not arrive at a logical answer of why cholecystectomy should lead to colon cancer.—J.C. Thompson, M.D.

Adenocarcinoma of the Colon and Rectum in Patients Less Than 40 Years of Age

MacGillivray DC, Swartz SE, Robinson AM, Cruess DF, Smith LE (Uniformed Univ of the Health Sciences; George Washington Univ)
Surg Gynecol Obstet 172:1–7, 1991   22–8

Introduction.—Because colorectal adenocarcinoma is infrequent in patients younger than 40 years, data were reviewed on 50 such patients among a total of 801 treated from 1962 to 1988. The patients younger than 40 years included 33 men and 17 women (median age, 30.5 years).

Follow-up data were complete for 45 patients, the mean duration of follow-up being 62 months.

Characteristics.—The mean duration of symptoms before diagnosis was 5 months. Risk factors for colorectal cancer were present in 14 patients. Significantly more of the younger patients than older patients had stage C disease, whereas stage B disease was more frequent in the older group. Of the 50 younger patients, 42 underwent regional removal of involved bowel and lymphatic drainage. There were no operative deaths.

Results.—Cumulative survival rates were 43% at 5 years and 34% at 10 years. All patients with stage D disease were dead at 28 months, but 76% of those with stage B disease lived for 5 years. Of 46 patients without polyposis coli, 6 had synchronous or metchronous colonic lesions.

Conclusion.—Most younger patients with colorectal cancer are symptomatic at the time of diagnosis. Survival times have been similar to those in the overall patient population.

▶ Anecdotes abound as to the increasing frequency in the past 2 decades of young patients with colon cancer and the relatively bad prognosis of the disease in these young people. This careful study of 801 patients from the National Naval Medical Center shows that 6.25% were younger than age 40, and that the survival time for each stage of the disease in this younger group is similar to that in the overall population of patients with colorectal cancer. This survival was in spite of the fact that a significantly greater proportion of younger patients had stage C disease (42% vs 22% in the older group). Griffin and colleagues (1) also studied colorectal cancer in patients younger than 40 years of age and found a higher incidence in blacks than in whites and a later detection of cancer in black males. The younger patients also had a higher proportion of mucinous and signet ring tumors. Men younger than 40 were less likely to present with localized disease than were those older than 40.—J.C. Thompson, M.D.

Reference

1. Griffin PM, et al: *Gastroenterology* 100:1033, 1991.

Prognostic Significance of Carcinoembryonic Antigen in Colorectal Carcinoma—Serum Levels Before and After Resection and Before Recurrence
Chu DZJ, Erickson CA, Russell MP, Thompson C, Lang NP, Broadwater RJ, Westbrook KC (Univ of Arkansas)
Arch Surg 126:314–316, 1991   22–9

Introduction.—Carcinoembryonic antigen (CEA) is used as a tumor marker, but it is not sufficiently specific or cost effective for the diagnosis of a particular tumor. The CEA level at the time of diagnosis of recurrence (RCEA) has in some instances been of prognostic value. The prognostic value of CEA determination preoperatively and postoperatively was assessed in 425 patients with colorectal carcinoma. The mean follow-up was 48 months.

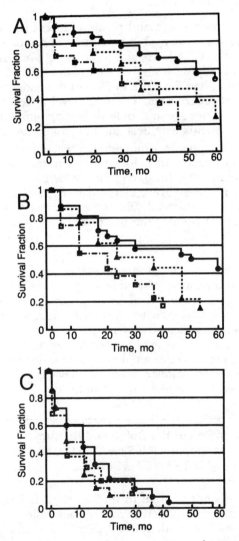

Fig 22–1.—Survival plots of patients according to tumor stage and preoperative carcinoembryonic antigen levels in 3 groups: less than 5 ng/mL (*solid line*), 5–10 ng/mL (*dotted line*), and greater than 10 ng/mL (*dashed line*). Survival plots for patients with stage 1 disease are not shown. **A,** patients with stage 2 tumors, $P = .03$ by log-rank test. **B,** stage 3 tumors, $P = .04$. **C,** stage 4 tumors, $P = .17$. (Courtesy of Chu DZJ, Erickson CA, Russell MP, et al: *Arch Surg* 126:314–316, 1991.)

Methods.—Preoperative CEA measurements were carried out within 1 month before resection of colorectal carcinoma; postoperative CEA measurements were made between 1 and 3 months after surgery; and RCEA measurements were made within 1 month of diagnosis of the recurrence. The patients were divided into 3 groups according to CEA levels of less than 5 ng/mL, between 5 and 10 ng/mL, and more than 10 ng/mL.

Findings.—The preoperative and postoperative CEA levels were predictive of recurrence and survival independent of tumor stage. Preoperative and postoperative CEA levels and tumor stage were significant prognostic variables of adjusted survival (Fig 22–1). The RCEA level at recurrence was more than 5 ng/mL in 79% of the patients and in 89% of the intra-abdominal recurrences. The CEA level at recurrence was predictive of postrecurrence survival only in a subgroup with locoregional disease and not in patients with liver and lung metastases.

Conclusions.—Carcinoembryonic antigen was effective in diagnosing intra-abdominal recurrences of colorectal carcinoma and projecting survival after development of local/regional recurrence of tumor. In the present series, RCEA levels were elevated in 89% of patients who had abdominal relapses of colorectal carcinoma. Because this recurrence site has the best treatment option, the use of periodic postoperative serum CEA tests may be justified.

▶ Why is a study like this still of interest? Well, for one thing, it confirms once again that postoperative elevations of previously normal CEA levels suggest recurrence, especially in patients who had high levels preoperatively that returned to normal after colectomy. A major interest arises from reports of higher resection rates when recurrences are detected by CEA before clinical deterioration (1), as well as improvement in tumor response rates to regional infusion when recurrences are detected by elevations of CEA (2). We still do not know whether elevation of the CEA level is proportional to either the size or the aggressiveness of the recurrent tumor.—J.C. Thompson, M.D.

Synchronous Carcinoma of the Colon and Rectum
Slater G, Aufses AH Jr, Szporn A (Mt Sinai Med Ctr, New York)
Surg Gynecol Obstet 171: 283–287, 1990   22–10

Background.—It is not unusual to find more than 1 site of colorectal carcinoma at the time of surgery; synchronous lesions are reported at rates of 2% to 11%. The incidence and distribution of synchronous carcinoma were reviewed.

Methods.—The records of 1,000 patients seen from 1976 to 1981 with newly diagnosed adenocarcinoma of the colon and rectum were examined. Synchronous carcinomas were defined as adenocarcinomas separated by normal bowel wall that clearly were not metastatic.

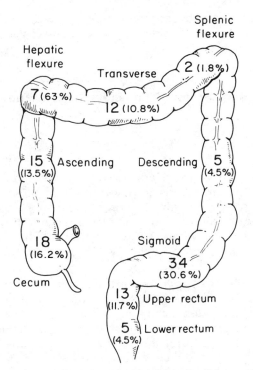

Fig 22–2.—Location of 111 synchronous carcinomas of the colon and rectum in 54 patients. (Courtesy of Slater G, Aufses AH Jr, Szporn A: *Surg Gynecol Obstet* 171:283–287, 1990.)

Findings.—Fifty-four patients (5%) had synchronous carcinoma, and 3 of them had 3 sites of disease. These patients had a mean age of 72 years, compared with a mean of 69 years for all patients. Stage of disease was comparable in the patients with and those without synchronous carcinoma. Benign polyps were seen in 70% of patients with synchronous carcinoma and in 30% of the others. Fifteen patients with single carcinomas and 3 with synchronous carcinomas had polyps that were noted to have carcinoma in situ. The distribution of synchronous carcinomas is shown in Figure 22–2.

Conclusions.—A significant number of patients with adenocarcinoma of the colon or rectum have synchronous lesions. They tend to be older than those without synchronous lesions and to have an increased incidence of associated polyps. It is important to identify synchronous lesions preoperatively, preferably by colonoscopy.

▶ When you find that a patient has a colorectal cancer, you must determine whether or not another colorectal cancer is present. The best way to do this is by colonoscopy, but if we were to apply this nationwide, the extra cost for colonoscopic examination versus barium enema study might be difficult to justify. Not surprisingly, the other major metaplastic lesion, adenomatous polyp, was also found more commonly in patients with synchronous tumors, providing yet another bit of evidence that these polyps act as signposts of cancer.—J.C. Thompson, M.D.

Second-Look Surgery for Colorectal Cancer: The Second Time Around
Martin EW Jr, Carey LC (Univ of South Florida)
Ann Surg 214:321–327, 1991   22–11

Background.—To proceed effectively with cytoreductive surgery in patients with recurrent colorectal cancer, it is believed that all cancerous tissue must be removed. Only this criterion qualifies a patient as potentially curable. Also, the carcinoembryonic antigen (CEA) level must return to baseline values within 1 postoperative month. Patients enrolled in the Radioimmunoguided Surgery (RIGS) protocol were assessed several years after second-look surgery.

Methods.—Eighty-six patients with colorectal cancer were treated and assessed for 2-, 3-, 4-, and 5-year survival after second-look procedures. Patients with extra-abdominal tumor involvement were eliminated according to preoperative evaluation criteria. Patients received a saturated potassium iodide preparation before B72.3 monoclonal antibody radiolabeled with 2 mCi of iodine-125 by the IODOGEN technique was administered. Precordial monitoring of biological clearance was done

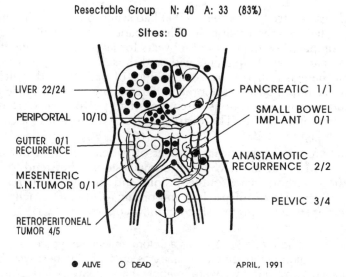

Resectable Group   N: 40   A: 33   (83%)

Sites: 50

LIVER 22/24

PERIPORTAL   10/10

GUTTER   0/1
RECURRENCE

MESENTERIC
L.N.TUMOR 0/1

RETROPERITONEAL
TUMOR 4/5

PANCREATIC 1/1

SMALL BOWEL
IMPLANT 0/1

ANASTAMOTIC
RECURRENCE   2/2

PELVIC 3/4

● ALIVE   ○ DEAD   APRIL, 1991

Fig 22–3.—Two-, 3-, 4-, and 5-year survival rates in resectable RIGS-positive second-look patients (1986–1989). (Courtesy of Martin EW Jr, Carey LC: *Ann Surg* 214:321–327, 1991.)

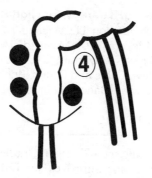

Fig 22–4.—Pelvic recurrence in the resectable group. (Courtesy of Martin EW Jr, Carey LC: *Ann Surg* 214:321–327, 1991.)

weekly with a handheld gamma-detecting probe. Surgery was performed once the drug was cleared from the blood.

Results.—The mean interval between injection and surgery was 24 days. Overall, 62% of the patients were judged resectable by the traditional methods of palpation and inspection, but only 47% were considered resectable after reexploration with the gamma-detecting probe. Survival data were determined for those considered resectable according to the RIGS method (Figs 22–3 and 22–4), those nonresectable by traditional methods, and those nonresectable by the new method. Two-year survival rates were 95%, 36%, and 53%, respectively. Three-year survival rates were 83%, 7%, and 30%, respectively. Also, 74% of the resectable patients survived after 4 years, and 60% survived after 5 years. There were no survivors in either nonresectable group after 4 years.

Conclusions.—As the extrahepatic RIGS-positive tissue is assessed successively, a more accurate curative resection can be done. The use of the new method improved the selection of resectable patients having second-look surgery for recurrent colorectal cancer.

▶ This sort of Star Wars approach to detecting recurrences has been a major goal of tumor immunologists for the past 2 decades. What you would really like to know is how often the surgeons found it impossible to eradicate the site of an intraoperative signal indicating a metastasis. Also of interest would be the duration of the operation. One can envision that a patient might have multiple signals, requiring multiple attempts at excision, each monitored by multiple frozen-section biopsies. Nonetheless, the ability to get 22 of 24 patients with hepatic metastases out alive and 10 of 10 patients with periportal metastases out alive is remarkable. As with any new bright idea, a fair amount of healthy skepticism is warranted, but we all look forward to future reports on the efficacy of this innovation.—J.C. Thompson, M.D.

Effective Surgical Adjuvant Therapy for High-Risk Rectal Carcinoma

Krook JE, Moertel CG, Gunderson LL, Wieand HS, Collins RT, Beart RW, Kubista TP, Poon MA, Meyers WC, Mailliard JA, Twito DI, Morton RF, Veeder MH, Witzig TE, Cha S, Vidyarthi SC (Duluth Community Clinical Oncology Program, Minn; Mayo Clinic and Found, Rochester, Minn; Mayo Clinic Scottsdale, Ariz; Saskatchewan Cancer Found, Regina, Canada; Duke Univ; et al)

N Engl J Med 324:709–715, 1991 22–12

Background.—As an adjunct to surgery, radiation treatment reduces local recurrence but does not improves survival in patients with rectal cancer. A previous report suggested that combined radiation and chemotherapy improves survival compared to surgery alone but not compared to adjuvant radiation, which is often regarded as standard therapy. A combination regimen was designed to optimize the effects of chemotherapy, decrease recurrence, and improve survival in comparison with adjuvant radiation alone.

Methods.—Included were 204 patients with rectal carcinoma that was either deeply invasive or metastatic to regional lymph nodes. All of the patients had undergone potentially curative resection. Patients were assigned randomly to a group receiving postoperative radiation alone or a group receiving sequential postoperative chemotherapy and radiation treatments. Postoperative radiation consisted of 4,500–5,040 cGy in a 5-week period. The combined treatment group received radiation plus fluorouracil, which was both preceded and followed by a cycle of systemic treatment with fluorouracil plus semustine. The median follow-up was longer than 7 years.

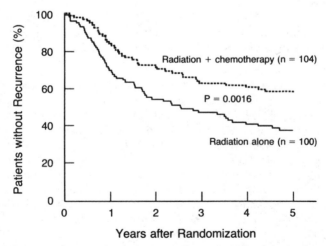

Fig 22–5.—Recurrence-free interval according to treatment group. The P value has been adjusted for imbalances in prognostic variables. (Courtesy of Krook JE, Moertel CG, Gunderson LL, et al: N Engl J Med 324:709–715, 1991.)

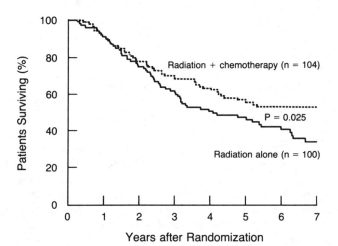

Fig 22–6.—Survival according to treatment group. The *P* value has been adjusted for imbalances in prognostic variables. (Courtesy of Krook JE, Moertel CG, Gunderson LL, et al: *N Engl J Med* 324:709–715, 1991.)

Results.—Combined treatment reduced the recurrence of rectal cancer by 34% (Fig 22–5), initial local recurrence by 46%, and distant metastasis by 37%. The combined treatment group had a 36% reduction in the rate of cancer-related deaths and a 29% reduction in the overall death rate (Fig 22–6). Nausea, vomiting, diarrhea, leukopenia, and thrombocytopenia were seen as acute toxic effects of the combined regimen, but they were seldom severe. Of all patients receiving radiation, 6.7% experienced severe, delayed treatment-related reactions, usually small bowel obstruction requiring surgery. The 2 treatment groups had comparable frequencies of these complications.

Conclusions.—In patients who have rectal carcinoma with a poor prognosis, combined postoperative local treatment with radiation plus fluorouracil and systemic therapy with a fluorouracil-based regimen improves results compared with postoperative radiation alone. Improvements are seen in both recurrence rate and survival. The addition of fluorouracil appears to be crucial in reducing the rate of local recurrence.

▶ For years, common knowledge among surgeons held that radiation and chemotherapy were without effect in patients with colorectal cancer. Radiation treatment as a surgical adjunct has been shown to diminish local recurrence, but has not improved survival. This report and reports from the National Colon Cancer Group in Pittsburgh suggest that all is not lost. The demonstration in this study of an absolutely clear-cut improvement in local recurrence, distal metastases, and, most importantly, death rate after combined fluorouracil and radiation therapy should mobilize attention all over the world. We have been particularly interested in the intraoperative administration of radiation therapy in patients with rectal cancer.—J.C. Thompson, M.D.

Loop Colostomies Are Totally Diverting in Adults

Morris DM, Rayburn D (Louisiana State Univ, Shreveport)
Am J Surg 161:668–671, 1991   22–13

Background.—The loop colostomy, with a rod placed beneath the loop to facilitate exteriorization, is formed more easily and quickly than an end colostomy. Some physicians have argued that the loop colostomy is not totally diverting and have relied on an end colostomy and mucous fistula or Hartmann's pouch. Patients with loop colostomies were studied to discover whether loop colostomies are totally diverting.

Patients.—Twenty-three patients with loop colostomy were given barium by mouth when they were seen for closure of the colostomy. Serial abdominal x-ray films were obtained during 24 hours.

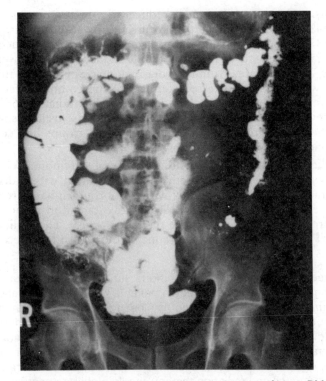

Fig 22–7.—Barium test result—loop colostomy of left colon. (Courtesy of Morris DM, Rayburn D: *Am J Surg* 161:668–671, 1991.)

Findings.—Scout films revealed that even vigorous bowel preparation did not cause passage of barium into the distal colon. Even in long-established loop colostomies, there was no passage of barium into the distal limb of the colon in any patient (Fig 22–7).

Conclusion.—Data on these patients indicate that a loop colostomy in any segment of the colon, constructed over a rod and matured immediately, totally diverts the fecal stream. Barium studies revealed no passage of barium into the distal colon even after vigorous bowel preparation. Because a loop colostomy is easily created and closed and is totally diverting, it should be used instead of a divided colostomy whenever possible.

▶ One of the favorite ploys of wise old men at morbidity and mortality conferences in the past, when discussing the resident's grief at finding that the emergency loop colostomy did not solve the problems of the patient with the perforated sigmoid diverticulitis, was to point out, sanctimoniously, that you could not expect a loop colostomy totally to divert the fecal stream; and, further, that the patient was in trouble because of continued spillage from the perforation caused by feces that somehow jumped over the rod that was supporting the right upper quadrant loop colostomy into the distal orifice of the colostomy, then traveled downward and escaped from the leaking perforation. The fallacy, I believe, is that the *bête noire* here is leaving a leaking perforation in the belly. The perforation just continues to suppurate and fester, and the patient will not be well until it is removed. It is nearly impossible to drain adequately the site of a perforated sigmoid. The current authors from Shreveport have studied the problem and have shown by barium that there is no passage into the distal colon in a loop colostomy.

The message here is that the proper treatment is to take out the perforated segment of the sigmoid in the first place if at all possible. You can then create a proximal sigmoid or descending colon colostomy and the patient will get well.—J.C. Thompson, M.D.

Reversal of Hartmann's Procedure: Timing and Operative Technique
Roe AM, Prabhu S, Ali A, Brown C, Brodribb AJM (Derriford Hosp, Plymouth, England)
Br J Surg 78:1167–1170, 1991   22–14

Background.—Hartmann's operation is often still carried out for cancer when the patient's condition demands a simpler procedure, or when the surgeon is relatively inexperienced in primary reconstruction. No objective guidelines exist for timing or performing the reversal operation.

Patients.—Data were reviewed on 69 patients who underwent reversal procedures between 1984 and 1990. Forty-eight patients initially had diverticular disease and 21 had cancer. One third of the patients had reversal within 4 months of Hartmann's operation. During the same period, 107 patients had a Hartmann procedure without reversal.

Results.—Operative mortality was 3%, and 4% of reversal operations were followed by anastomotic leakage. Nearly one third of the patients had significant morbidity. Delayed closure had no apparent advantage over earlier operation. Complication rates also were similar in patients having hand-sewn and stapled anastomoses.

Conclusions.—Reanastomosis after a Hartmann operation is safe in terms of operative mortality and anastomotic leakage, but significant morbidity does occur in nearly a third of the patients. An experienced operator is essential. It may be best to carry out primary resection and anastomosis initially in carefully selected patients. In severely ill patients with peritonitis, the Hartmann procedure can be lifesaving.

▶ In an ideal world, I would go around doing Hartmann's resections and leaving it up to somebody else to do the later reanastomosis. The problem is, of course, that the rectal end is usually shortened by scarring and, because it was not long enough to begin with, the stump is difficult to mobilize, the hole is deep, and the pelvis is narrow. We find that use of the EEA stapling device facilitates dissection when it is stuck into the rectal stump and used as a mobilizing lever. The presence of the stapler in the rectum allows for early identification and greatly facilitates dissection, especially posteriorly.

It is interesting that nearly half again as many patients had a Hartmann's procedure without closure than had closure. The similarity of leakage in stapled and hand-sewn anastomosis again tells us that the stapler is a facilitator, not a magic wand.—J.C. Thompson, M.D.

23 The Liver and the Spleen

Warning: Fatal Reaction to the Use of Fibrin Glue in Deep Hepatic Wounds: Case Reports
Berguer R, Staerkel RL, Moore EE, Moore FA, Galloway WB, Mockus MB
(Denver Gen Hosp; Univ of Colorado)
J Trauma 31:408–411, 1991   23–1

Introduction.—An adverse reaction occurred in a patient undergoing bronchopleural fistula closure with fibrin glue.

Case Report.—Man, 36, was brought to the emergency room with a gunshot wound. The bullet track entered the medial segment of the left lobe of the liver and went through the hepatic parenchyma to the right. Fibrin glue and balloon tamponade of the bullet track were used. The patient's blood pressure was 105/85 mm Hg and his heart rate, 85 beats per minute. He received 6 units of packed red blood cells and 5 units of platelets. Within 15 seconds of application of fibrin glue and inflation of a Foley balloon in the bullet track, the severe hypotension developed and diffuse bleeding was observed from all cut surfaces. The patient sustained intraoperative cardiac arrest and died.

Methods.—Bovine thrombin was administered intravenously to an adult male mongrel dog. Within 20 seconds there was a profound decrease in systemic arterial pressure, sinus tachycardia, and a sharp increase in pulmonary arterial pressure. After 15 minutes, hemodynamic parameters gradually returned to baseline values with fluid resuscitation.

Conclusion.—The sudden hypotension is attributed to the use of fibrin glue because of the immediacy of cardiovascular collapse after injection in 2 similar patients. In both patients, clinical findings could be explained by an anaphylactic reaction of a component of the fibrin glue. Cryoprecipitate and bovine thrombin are antigenic and could cause this reaction. An alternate hypothesis is that thrombin caused direct activation of the coagulation cascade with resultant intravascular coagulation and vasomotor shock. Trauma surgeons should be alerted to the possibility of a severe reaction to injection of fibrin glue into deep hepatic injuries. Fibrin glue should be reserved for unique solid organ injuries not amenable to conventional surgery.

▶ It is obviously important for surgeons to be cognizant of this potential complication. A marked inflammatory response and aneurysmal dilatation have been associated with vascular anastomoses performed using the glue. The authors' finding that, in another patient, hypertension was not associated with any evidence of coagulopathy suggests that glue can continue to be used provided that fluid resuscitation and vasopressins are available if needed. The glue does have advantages affecting hemostasis in given situations. The first line of defense for diffuse ooze should be packing, cautery, or the use of an argon coagulator.—S.I. Schwartz, M.D.

Management of Haemangioma of the Liver: Comparison of Results Between Surgery and Observation

Yamagata M, Kanematsu T, Matsumata T, Utsunomiya Y, Ikeda Y, Sugimachi K (Kyushu Univ, Fukuoka, Japan)
Br J Surg 78:1223–1225, 1991

23–2

Background.—Although cavernous hemangioma is the most common benign liver tumor, its incidence, natural history, and surgical indications have not been clearly defined. Thirty-three patients with hepatic hemangioma were treated during a 10-year period.

Patients.—There were 17 men and 16 women; the mean age was 51 years. The diagnosis was made by hepatic angiography. Symptoms of ep-

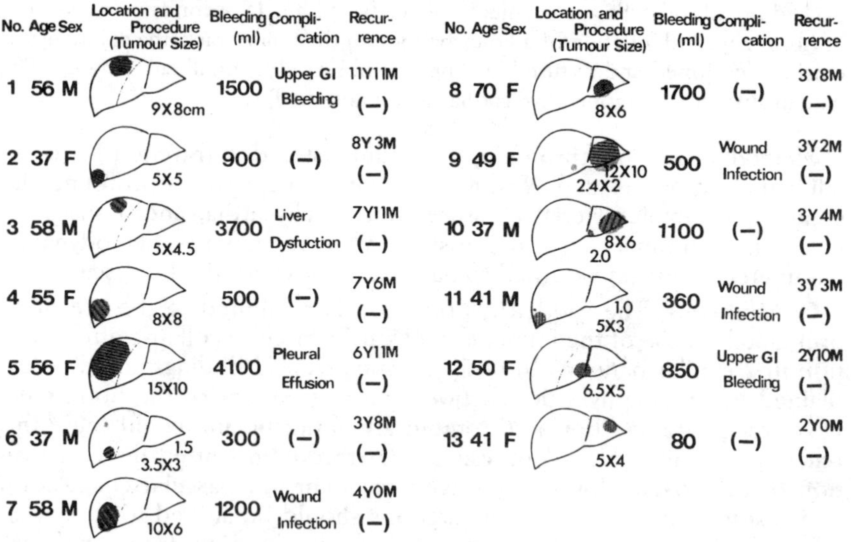

No.	Age	Sex	Location and Procedure (Tumour Size)	Bleeding (ml)	Complication	Recurrence
1	56	M	9X8cm	1500	Upper GI Bleeding	11Y11M (−)
2	37	F	5X5	900	(−)	8Y3M (−)
3	58	M	5X4.5	3700	Liver Dysfuction	7Y11M (−)
4	55	F	8X8	500	(−)	7Y6M (−)
5	56	F	15X10	4100	Pleural Effusion	6Y11M (−)
6	37	M	3.5X3 / 1.5	300	(−)	3Y8M (−)
7	58	M	10X6	1200	Wound Infection	4Y0M (−)
8	70	F	8X6	1700	(−)	3Y8M (−)
9	49	F	2.4X2 / 2X10	500	Wound Infection	3Y2M (−)
10	37	M	8X6 2.0	1100	(−)	3Y4M (−)
11	41	M	5X3 / 1.0	360	Wound Infection	3Y3M (−)
12	50	F	6.5X5	850	Upper GI Bleeding	2Y10M (−)
13	41	F	5X4	80	(−)	2Y0M (−)

Fig 23–1.—Results for the surgically treated patients. *Filled circle,* location of tumor; *open area,* region excised. Three patients had symptoms: case 2, right back pain; case 3, right hypochondrial pain; case 6, epigastric pain. *Abbreviations: GI,* gastrointestinal; Y, years; M, months. (Courtesy of Yamagata M, Kanematsu T, Matsumata T, et al: *Br J Surg* 78:1223–1225, 1991.)

igastric or back pain were present in 6 patients; none had Kasabach-Merritt syndrome. Multiple tumors were present in 10 patients, and only 1 patient had bilateral hemangiomas. Most of the lesions were in the right lobe. Operation was done in 13 patients, with the criteria of tumor larger than 5 cm, symptoms, rapid growth or rupture, and Kasabach-Merritt syndrome used as indications.

Outcomes.—There were no operative deaths. Two patients had upper gastrointestinal bleeding and 1 had liver dysfunction (Fig 23–1). The mean tumor size was 7.7 cm in the surgically treated group. Three patients had right lobectomy, 1 had left lobectomy, 3 had left lateral segmentectomy, and the rest had a subsegment or less resected. There were no recurrences up to 143 months postoperatively. In 2 patients residual tumor was left in the liver for anatomical reasons; the tumors had not increased in size at more than 3 years postoperatively. In the nonoperative group, no specific treatment was given. During a mean follow-up of 3 years, 11 months, none of the tumors ruptured or enlarged and 2 decreased in size.

Conclusions.—Most liver hemangiomas measuring less than 5 cm in diameter can be managed conservatively unless they are growing in size or the patient is symptomatic. Operative morbidity and mortality are low, however, so patients with potential exposure to trauma, rapid tumor growth, or severe symptoms may be considered for surgical treatment. The reported predominance of women among patients with hemangioma was not reflected in the present series.

▶ Our own experience has now extended to more than 40 resected cases. We agree whole-heartedly with the authors that lesions smaller than 5 cm can be observed. We have had the opportunity of observing several patients through pregnancy with sequential ultrasound and have noted essentially no growth. On the other hand, we have had 1 patient who has had a significant increase in the size of the hemangioma with intratumoral bleeding during the first trimester of her pregnancy. Interestingly, there was no growth of the hemangioma during her first pregnancy. We believe that operation is indicated for lesions that are exposed, those that have grown rapidly, and those to which pain can be attributed. We have had 1 patient with a large hemangioma complicated by thrombocytopenia related to platelet trapping. The recent modification that we have applied to our technical approach is the use of enucleation after inflow occlusion. This has minimized the amount of liver tissue removed (1).—S.I. Schwartz M.D.

Reference

1. Schwartz SI, Husser WC: *Ann Surg* 205:456 1987.

Intraabdominal Abscess Formation After Major Liver Resection
Andersson R, Saarela A, Tranberg K-G, Bengmark S (Lund Univ, Sweden)
Acta Chir Scand 156:707–710, 1990   23–3

Introduction.—Intra-abdominal sepsis complicates 10% to 30% of major liver resections. Data were reviewed on 138 patients who underwent major resection from 1970 to 1987. Right hepatectomy was the most common procedure. Ninety-nine patients received a single dose of antibiotic within 1 hour of the start of surgery.

Results.—Intra-abdominal abscesses developed in 11 patients (8%), forming in 8 after right hepatectomy (which was done in 63 patients). The risk was greater when a large amount of liver tissue was removed, when surgery lasted longer, and when there was more intraoperative bleeding. All but 1 of the patients with abscess has received antibiotic, but antibiotic treatment did not correlate significantly with abscess formation.

Outcome.—Nine patients who had an abscess underwent operative drainage, and 2 had percutaneous drainage under ultrasound guidance. A drain had been used in all 11 patients. Two patients who had abdominal abscesses died of multiple organ failure.

Implications.—Limiting leakage of blood and bile is the single best way of preventing intra-abdominal sepsis after major liver resection. Whether antibiotic prophylaxis can be helpful remains to be learned.

▶ The development of intra-abdominal abscess after major liver resection constitutes the most frequently encountered complication. Pace et al. (1) reported an incidence of 28.6%; in our own experience the incidence has been 18%. We have attempted to correlate this with length of operation and antibiotic coverage, and have noted no relationship with these factors. We have also followed the lead of Franco et al. (2) who had a series of liver resections that were carried out without abdominal drainage but in which abscesses also developed. From our experience, the abscesses have almost always been manageable by catheter drainage with insertion of the catheter under radiographic control; rarely is operative drainage required.—S.I. Schwartz, M.D.

References

1. Pace RR, et al: *Ann Surg* 209:302, 1989.
2. Franco D, et al: *Ann Surg* 210:748, 1989.

Results of Surgical Treatment of Hepatic Hydatidosis: Current Therapeutic Modifications
Moreno González E, Rico Selas P, Martínez B, García García I, Palma Carazo

F, Hidalgo Pascual M ("October 12" Univ Hosp, Madrid)
World J Surg 15:254–263, 1991

23–4

Patients.—The management of hydatid disease of the liver was contrasted in 322 patients who had a total of 443 cysts treated between 1974 and 1984, and 88 patients who had 118 cysts treated between 1985 and 1989. Both hepatomegaly and a palpable tumor were significantly less frequent in the group treated later. More than two thirds of both groups had a single cyst. Most children had univesicular cysts, but most of those in adults were multivesicular.

Management.—Total cystopericystectomy is aimed at removing all of the cyst by separating its fibrous surface from the adjacent liver parenchyma without opening the cavity. It was the most common procedure in both review periods. About one fourth of each group underwent partial cystopericystectomy. The liver was resected in 6.5% of the earlier patients and in 15% of the later group. Cholecystectomy was done in 33% and 43% of cases, respectively. Twenty percent of the earlier patients and 9% of the later group had exploration of the common duct.

Outcome.—Operative mortality was 2.4% in the earlier period and 1.1% in the second. Formation of biliary fistulas was more frequent after partial than after total cystopericystectomy. No relapses of hydatid disease occurred in the liver or any other abdominal site.

Conclusion.—It now is feasible to remove hydatid cysts from the liver with little risk. Liver resection should be considered only in exceptional circumstances.

▶ A 15-year North American experience was reported by Langer et al. (1) in which 40 patients were managed, 35 surgically. The best treatment for uncomplicated hydatid liver cysts was evacuation, scolecocidal, irrigation, and primary closure. The most commonly used method is capitonnage in which the cystic contents are removed, the cyst itself sterilized, and the residual cavity drained. The approach described in the present article, which reports that total cystopericystectomy is the preferred method, is relatively unique, and it is somewhat surprising that there is apparently little risk. It would seem that the simplicity of evacuation, irrigation, and closure would have some advantage.—S.I. Schwartz, M.D.

Reference

1. Langer JC, et al: *Ann Surg* 199:412, 1984.

Limited Hepatic Resection for Selected Cirrhotic Patients With Hepatocellular or Cholangiocellular Carcinoma: A Prospective Study

Paquet K-J, Koussouris P, Mercado MA, Kalk J-Fr, Müting D, Rambach W (Heinz-Kalk Hosp, Bad Kissingen, Germany)
Br J Surg 78:459–462, 1991

23–5

Background.—Views on the treatment of hepatocellular carcinomas (HCCs) have changed radically in recent years. With careful patient selection, the results of liver resection in cirrhosis are improved. Several authors have found that the operative risk is acceptable, and that resection can raise the survival rates of patients with HCC, especially those with small solitary tumors and no portal vein invasion or extrahepatic dissemination.

Methods.—Between 1983 and 1989, 123 cirrhotic patients with HCC or cholangiocarcinoma were seen at 1 center. Twenty-three patients were selected for surgical resection. These patients had tumors smaller than 5 cm that were not centrally located and were at least 1 cm away from main structures. Selection criteria also included no evidence of multicentricity or metastatic disease and a Child-Pugh classification of A or B with a urea-nitrogen synthesis rate of at least 6 g/day. Upper gastrointestinal endoscopy was used routinely to identify esophageal varices, found in 17 patients. Ten patients with a history of variceal hemmorrhage had preoperative endoscopic sclerotherapy. Controlled hypotension and hepatoduodenal ligament clamping were used during tumor resection.

Results.—The procedures included 12 bisegmentectomies, 10 segmentectomies, and 1 atypical resection. Operative mortality was 13%. Liver failure and sepsis were the causes of death. Overall, the recurrence rate was 26% and the late mortality, 30%. Thirteen patients were still alive as of the beginning of 1990. The 1-year survival was 77% and the 5-year survival, 49%.

Conclusions.—Carefully selected patients with small HCCs, liver cirrhosis, and portal hypertension may benefit from surgical resection of the tumor. When surgeons adhere to the methods outlined for perioperative care and operative management, resection is the treatment of choice for such tumors.

▶ The authors are to be complimented on the low operative mortality of 13% in cirrhotic patients undergoing an extensive operation. The fact that they have not had significant bleeding, particularly in the 12 bisegmentectomies, is unusual. This may represent the first Western experience analogous to that previously reported from the Orient. Fujio et at. (1) quoted a 5-year survival equivalent to that achieved in many series of noncirrhotic patients with hepatocellular carcinoma. The experience of most Western surgeons with hepatocellular carcinoma superimposed on cirrhosis is that rarely do the patients present with lesions smaller that 5 cm; resection is associated with high mortality, and the cure rate is extremely low. A prospective multicenter study evaluated the prediction of the first variceal hemorrhage in patients with cirrhosis of the liver and varices and indicated that bleeding was not predictable (2).—S.I. Schwartz, M.D.

References

1. Fujio N, et al: *World J Surg* 13:211, 1989.
2. The North Italian Endoscopic Club for the Study and Treatment of Esophageal Varices (University of Milan, Italy): *N Engl J Med* 319:983, 1988.

Hepatic Resection Versus Transplantation for Hepatocellular Carcinoma

Iwatsuki S, Starzl TE, Sheahan DG, Yokoyama I, Demetris AJ, Todo S, Tzakis AG, Van Thiel DH, Carr B, Selby R, Madariaga J (Univ of Pittsburgh)
Ann Surg 214:221–229, 1991   23–6

Introduction.—The role of orthotopic liver transplantation in the treatment of primary hepatobiliary malignancy has not yet been defined. The results after transplantation and after subtotal hepatic resection were compared in patients with hepatocellular carcinoma (HCC).

Patients.—During the past 10 years, 181 patients were treated for preoperatively identified HCC, 76 of whom were treated by hepatic resection and 105 by transplantation with associated cyclosporine-steroid therapy. Transplantation was used if hepatic resection was not anatomically feasible. Associated liver cirrhosis was present in 88 patients. All tumors were staged according to clinical, pathologic, and residual findings (pTNM classification).

Results.—The overall 5-year survival rates were 32.9% after hepatic resections and 35.6% after transplantation. Thus there was no difference in overall survival between the 2 treatments. Among hepatic resection-treated patients, those with fibrolamellar HCC survived significantly longer than those with non–fibrolamellar HCC, and those without liver cirrhosis survived significantly longer than those with HCC in a cirrhotic liver. However, in the transplantation-treated group, patients with fibrolamellar HCC or non–fibrolamellar HCC and patients with or without cirrhosis had similar survival rates. There was no 4-year survivor after hepatic resection among patients with HCC in the cirrhotic liver, but the 5-year survival rate after transplantation was 40.7%. During follow-up, 50% of the resection-treated patients and 42.9% of the transplantation-treated patients had a confirmed recurrence of HCC. Three-year survival was 50% after resection and 61% after transplantation. However, when comparing survival without recurrence, 3-year survival was 24% after resection but 54% after transplantation. This clear advantage for transplantation was considerably reduced for patients with multiple HCC or HCCs larger than 3 cm. Twelve hepatic resection-treated patients and 13 transplantation-treated patients lived for more than 5 years. For HCC associated with cirrhosis, survival after transplantation was significantly better at each pTNM stage. However, none of the patients with non-fibrolamellar HCC stage IV-A disease who received transplants survived for 5 years.

Recommendations.—Hepatocellular carcinoma confined to the liver should be treated by hepatic resection when it is anatomically and functionally feasible. Hepatocellular carcinoma confined to the liver should be treated by transplantation when liver function is poor, when the HCC cannot be removed by resection, or when both conditions are present.

▶ The figures are truly extraordinary and not in keeping with other results. It is of interest that after subtotal resection the results are significantly better with fibrolamellar carcinoma when compared to the total group, but the same does not pertain to the patients given transplants. The results are somewhat inexplicable in that no cirrhotic patients survived for 4 years after resection, but the 5-year survival after transplantation was about 41%. The 75% survival rate at 5 years in TNM stage I patients and, more particularly, the 50% rate in TNM stage III patients, subjected to transplantation is extraordinary.

In another series, many of the long-term survivors subsequent to transplantation for cirrhosis were patients in whom the tumor was found incidentally. I wonder how many of the patients in Iwatsuki et al's study fall into that category. As pointed out by Dr. Adson (1), any long-term results from Pittsburgh are significantly better than those reported in any other article. My own results substantiate those reported by Adson and Bismuth: that major resection for hepatocellular carcinoma in the cirrhotic patient has an extremely low yield. According to Bismuth (personal communication), the same pertains to transplantation.—S.I. Schwartz, M.D.

Reference

1. Adson MA, in Blumgardt L (ed): *Surgery of the Liver and Biliary Tract.* London, Churchill-Livingstone, 1988, pp 1153–1165.

Hepatocellular Carcinoma in Childhood: Clinical Manifestations and Prognosis
Ni Y-H, Chang M-H, Hsu H-Y, Hsu H-C, Chen C-C, Chen W-J, Lee C-Y (Natl Taiwan Univ, Taipei)
Cancer 68:1737–1741, 1991   23–7

Background.—In areas that are endemic for hepatitis B infection, hepatocellular carcinoma (HCC) is more common among childhood primary liver tumors than hepatoblastoma. In Taiwan, HCC is the fifth most common malignancy of children. The signs and symptoms of childhood HCC were examined along with factors affecting outcome.

Patients.—In a 25-year period, HCC was diagnosed in 71 children. There were 54 boys and 17 girls; the mean age was 9.7 years. Forty-three patients had a definitive histologic diagnosis and in 28 the diagnosis was made on a clinical basis. The diagnosis usually occurred in a late, advanced stage of the disease. The primary physical signs were hepatosplenomegaly, superficial venous engorgement, and ascites. The outcome was documented in 49 patients.

Outcome.—Prognosis was extremely poor. From the time of the first symptoms, only 10% of the patients survived for longer than 1 year, and only 2 patients survived for longer than 5 years. One of the long-term survivors had a small tumor with internal bleeding, and the other had a large tumor with abdominal distention. The tumor was resected in both patients, and reoperation for recurrence was done in the patient with the large tumor. Only 9.8% of the tumors were resectable. Factors that improved prognosis appeared to be resectability and nonicterus.

Conclusions.—The initial manifestations of HCC in children are similar to those in adults and have no prognostic significance. There is an overt association between HCC and hepatitis B surface antigen. In both age groups, males predominate. Improvement of prognosis requires earlier diagnosis to increase resectability.

▶ The article demonstrates the distinct difference in the biology of HCC and hepatoblastoma in children. The prognosis for HCC remains poor, and there is little influence of chemotherapy, unlike hepatoblastoma. Lin et al. (1) reported a 5-year survival of 18% after major hepatic resection in patients of all ages with HCC. It remains difficult to reconcile the figures from Japan. Fujio et al. (2) reports a 5-year survival of approximately 35% after resection for HCC and, if transarterial embolization and portal venue embolization are added, the 3-year survival approaches 70%. I would suspect that this represents a tumor that is biologically distinct from that which we see in Western civilization.—S.I. Schwartz, M.D.

References

1. Lin TY, et al: *Br J Surg* 74:839, 1987.
2. Fujio N, et al: *World J Surg* 13:211, 1989.

The Surgical Management of Children With Incompletely Resected Hepatic Cancer Is Facilitated by Intensive Chemotherapy
King DR, Ortega J, Campbell J, Haas J, Ablin A, Lloyd D, Newman K, Quinn J, Krailo M, Feusner J, Hammond D (Children's Cancer Study Group, Pasadena, Calif)
J Pediatr Surg 26:1074–1081, 1991   23–8

Background.—Historically, complete surgical resection of hepatic malignancy in children has provided the best chance for cure. However, total extirpation of the primary tumor at the time of diagnosis has been possible in less that 50% of children with this type of cancer. The efficacy of continuous-infusion doxorubicin and cisplatin (CI-DOX/CPPD) in the treatment of children with incompletely resected hepatic cancer was assessed.

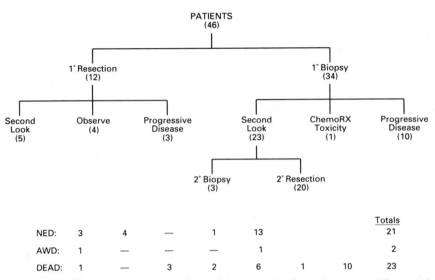

	NED:	3	4	—	1	13			Totals 21
	AWD:	1	—	—	—	1			2
	DEAD:	1	—	3	2	6	1	10	23

Fig 23–2.—*Abbreviations:* NED, no evidence of disease; AWD, alive with recurrence. The surgical management and outcome of the 46 evaluable patients. (Courtesy of King DR, Ortega J, Campbell J, et al: *J Pediatr Surg* 26: 1074–1081, 1991.)

Patients.—Forty-six evaluable children were included in the analysis. Of these, 32 had hepatoblastoma and 14 had hepatocellular carcinoma. Ten children had microscopic residual (stage II) tumors, 25 had gross residual (stage III) tumors, and 11 had distant metastasis (stage IV). Twelve children had initial incomplete resections. Tumor biopsy specimens were obtained from the remaining 34.

Outcomes.—A total of 70% of the children had an excellent clinical response to chemotherapy, with a reduction in both α-fetoprotein levels and measured tumor dimensions. Combined CI-DOX/CPDD clearly facilitated surgical management, permitting delayed hepatic resections in 20 of the 34 children whose tumors were biopsied initially and judged to be unresectable. The overall survival in this series was significantly better than that achieved historically. Of the children, 46% remained in complete clinical remission a mean of 30 months after diagnosis. The outcomes for those with hepatoblastoma were much better than the outcomes for those with hepatocellular carcinoma, with survivals of 63% and 17%, respectively. The 20 children who had delayed hepatic resections had survival rates comparable to those of the 12 children whose hepatic tumors were removed at initial laparotomy. However, children who underwent surgery after chemotherapy had a higher risk of postoperative complications that those who underwent initial hepatic resection (Fig 23–2).

Conclusions.—Complete resection of the hepatic tumor at initial laparotomy should continue to be the primary surgical goal in children with hepatic cancer. However, there might be a role for initial subtotal resection. If complete or subtotal resection is not possible, a biopsy should be done and chemotherapy should be begun. Preoperative diagnostic imaging studies seem to be a reasonably good way to assess resectability.

▶ The improved results with hepatoblastoma compared with hepatocellular carcinoma provide added evidence of the biological difference between these 2 lesions. In his discussion, Filler indicated that since 1986 at the Toronto Sick Childrens Hospital 14 patients were treated with preoperative chemotherapy and underwent resection, with a cure rate of 90%.—S.I. Schwartz, M.D.

One Hundred Patients With Hepatic Metastases From Colorectal Cancer Treated by Resection: Analysis of Prognostic Determinants
Doci R, Gennari L, Bignami P, Montalto F, Morabito A, Bozzetti F (Istituto Nazionale Tumori, Milan, Italy)
Br J Surg 78:797–801, 1991

23–9

Patients.—One hundred patients underwent "radical" liver resection of metastases from colorectal cancer from 1980 to 1989. Only 42% had a single metastasis involving less than one fourth of the liver parenchyma. In all cases at least 1 cm of normal tissue surrounded the tumor, and there was no microscopic invasion of the resection margins. Fifty patients had lobectomy and the others had nonanatomical resections.

Results.—There were no operative deaths, but 5 patients died after operation of hepatorenal failure, 4 of them after major resection. The estimated median operative blood loss was 900 mL. The median postoperative hospital time was 15 days. The actuarial survival rate at 5 years was 30%, but only 11% of patients were living without disease. Patients with Duke stage B tumors did significantly better than those with more advanced disease. Patients with single and multiple metastases had similar outcomes, but those with bilobar metastases did better than those with multiple metastases in 1 hepatic lobe.

Conclusions.—Resection is an effective approach to selected patients who have liver metastases of colorectal cancer. The stage of disease and the extent of liver involvement may be significant predictors of the outcome.

▶ This article affirms the data presented by the multi-institutional study in the United States (1) that reported a 5-year actuarial survival for 859 patients (33%) and a 5-year actuarial disease-free survival of 21%. It's of interest that in the present article there was no difference in outcome between patients with single and multiple metastases, and that the survival rate of patients with bilobar metastases was higher than that of patients with multiple unilobar metastases. As far as I know, this is the first series in which a significant number of patients underwent lobectomy and wedge resection of lesions of the residual lobe. The 5-year actuarial survival of 53% in 11 patients in this category is quite extraordinary. It would be important to assess other series.—S.I. Schwartz, M.D.

Reference

1. Registry of Hepatic Metastases: Surgery 103:278, 1988.

Cytoreductive Hepatic Surgery for Neuroendocrine Tumors

McEntee GP, Nagorney DM, Kvols LK, Moertel CG, Grant CS (Mayo Clinic and Found, Rochester, Minn)
Surgery 108:1091–1096, 1990   23–10

Objective.—Cytoreductive surgery, alone or in combination with other procedures, may give effective palliation for some patients with diffuse hepatic neuroendocrine tumors. Experience with palliative or curative hepatic resection of metastases in conjunction with treatment of primary lesions was reviewed to further define the role of cytoreductive surgery for such tumors.

Patients.—Subjects were 37 patients who had hepatic resection for metastatic neuroendocrine tumors during a 19-year period. The primary tumors were carcinoid in 24 cases and pancreatic islet cell tumors in 13.

Outcome.—Resections were considered to be potentially curative, i.e., left no gross residual tumor, in 17 patients (table). Of these, 9 patients had symptomatic endocrinopathies, 8 of whom obtained complete relief of symptoms. By a mean of 26 months later, 5 were alive with no evidence of disease. Of 7 patients with symptoms caused by the primary tumor, 6 obtained complete relief. By a mean of 14 months later, 5 were alive with no evidence of disease. Curative hepatic resection was done in 1 symptom-free patient who had abdominoperineal resection for a rectal carcinoid 5 years earlier. Overall, 11 of 17 patients were free of recurrence within a mean of 19 months.

Palliative resections were done in 20 patients. Of the 16 who had symptomatic endocrinopathies, 8 obtained complete relief and 5 were alive a mean of 11 months later. Complete relief lasted for a mean of 6 months. All 4 patients who had symptoms related to the primary tumor had complete relief, and 2 were alive and free of symptoms at 10 months and 101 months.

Conclusions.—Curative surgery should be considered for all patients who have completely resectable metastatic neuroendocrine malignancies. Even though the relief obtained is short lived, palliative surgery should be considered for some patients because it delays and may reduce the need for subsequent medical therapy.

▶ I have cared for 5 patients with carcinoid syndrome related to hepatic metastases from primary ileal lesions. The cytoreductive surgery in each of

| Primary | Duration of preoperative symptoms (mo) | Curative Resections | | | | | | |
		Preoperative tumor marker	Postoperative tumor marker	Largest metastasis excised (cm)	Clinical outcome	Duration of complete response (mo)	Current status	Postoperative survival (mo)
Endocrine-related symptoms								
Carcinoid	24	118	5	—	CR	6	ANED	6
Carcinoid	60	30	3.0	5	CR	34	ANED	34
Carcinoid	60	75	7.1	10	CR	3	AWD	52
Carcinoid	2	19	25.2	3	IR	—	AWD	59
Carcinoid	8	26	5.4	8	CR	50	AWD	92
Carcinoid	3	14	6.5	6	CR	6	DOD	49
Gastrinoma	6	1200	120	19	CR	8	ANED	8
Glucagonoma	4	2340	52	15	CR	4	ANED	4
Glucagonoma	4	481	—	20	CR	82	ANED	82
Local tumor symptoms								
Carcinoid	60	—	—	—	CR	8	ANED	8
Carcinoid	5	—	3.9	—	CR	16	ANED	16
Carcinoid	6	—	—	2	CR	28	ANED	28
Carcinoid	3	—	—	1	CR	18	DOD	60
Gastrinoma	48	2000	—	8	CR	5	ANED	5
Glucagonoma	5	1317	43	—	CR	13	ANED	13
Nonfunctional	5	—	—	—	IR	—	DOD	13
Symptom-free patient								
Carcinoid	—	—	—	3	—	1	ANED	1

Abbreviations: CR, complete relief; ANED, alive, no evidence of disease; AWD, alive, with disease; IR, incomplete relief; DOD, died of disease.
(Courtesy of McEntee GP, Nagorney DM, Kvols LK, et al: *Surgery* 108:1091–1096, 1990.)

these patients resulted in marked symptomatic improvement and return of the 5-HIAA to normal or near-normal levels within days. Three of the 5 patients survived without evidence of recurrent carcinoid syndrome for more than 5 years. In addition, we have seen a primary VIPoma of the liver with a watery diarrhea syndrome. Resection corrected the patient's symptom complex immediately but, unfortunately, she died of recurrence 3 years later.—S.I. Schwartz, M.D.

Prophylactic Sclerotherapy for Esophageal Varices: Long-term Results of a Single-Center Trial

Triger DR, Smart HL, Hosking SW, Johnson AG (Royal Hallamshire Hosp, Sheffield, England)
Hepatology 13:117–123, 1991   23–11

Background.—An alternative approach to prevention of variceal hemorrhage is endoscopic variceal sclerotherapy. A long-term, single-center study was carried out based on wedged hepatic vein pressure gradient (WHVPG) measurement in 99 patients, most of them not alcoholics.

Methods.—Patients were assessed during an 8-year period. Measurement of WHVPG determined the degree of risk for variceal hemorrhage; those whose pressure was 12 mm Hg or more were randomized to receive either sclerotherapy or no treatment. The other patients were not randomized but were merely followed regularly as dictated by their disease. All patients who had episodes of bleeding were treated by emergency endoscopy and sclerotherapy. Patients were stratified according to the presence of ascites. Patients were followed for a median of 61 months.

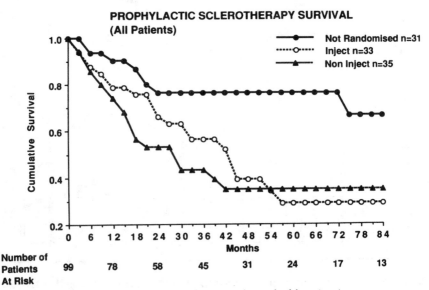

Fig 23–3.—Cumulative survival curves in all patients after wedged hepatic vein pressure measurement. (Courtesy of Triger DR, Smart HL, Hosking SW, et al: *Hepatology* 13:117–123, 1991.)

Results.—Survival was significantly longer among nonrandomized than randomized patients; however, the difference between those treated by sclerotherapy and controls was not significantly different (Fig 23–3). The 2-year survival rate was 80% in alcoholic cirrhotic patients compared to 43% in controls, but this difference was not sustained over 5 years. Among nonalcoholic patient groups, survival was identical; of 50 deaths, only 10 resulted from variceal bleeding. Bleeding occurred in 48% of patients with large varices compared to 20% of those with small varices. Alcoholic patients at low risk of variceal bleeding were accurately identified by a WHVPG of less than 12 mm Hg, but not nonalcoholic patients. Elective sclerotherapy seemed to cause only 4 episodes of variceal bleeding.

Conclusions.—On its own, prophylactic sclerotherapy does not improve survival in cirrhotic patients with esophageal varices. Factors other than variceal hemorrhage may be responsible for the difference in survival between alcoholic and nonalcoholic patients.

▶ A prognostic index was developed, and the authors plan to address patients with a predictably high incidence of bleeding and subject them to a variety of prophylactic regimens. Santangelo et al. (1) reported that in their experience, prophylactic sclerotherapy of large esophageal varices in patients with chronic alcoholic cirrhosis did not provide any clinical benefit. It has long been recognized that prophylactic portacaval anastomosis should not be performed in cirrhotic patients with varices (2).—S.I. Schwartz, M.D.

References

1. Santangelo WC, et al: N *Engl J Med* 318:814, 1988.
2. Resnick RH, et al: *Ann Intern Med* 70:675, 1969.

Injection Sclerotherapy for Bleeding Varices: Risk Factors and Complications
McKee RF, Garden OJ, Carter DC (Royal Infirmary, Glasgow)
Br J Surg 78:1098–1101, 1991   23–12

Background.—Injection sclerotherapy appears to reduce the number of bleeding episodes and improve survival in esophageal varices, but there is controversy as to the technique and timing of this treatment. An 8-year experience with injection sclerotherapy, focusing on identifying the risk factors for complications, was reviewed.

Patients.—Of 209 patients referred for management of esophageal varices, 163 underwent a total of 667 injection sclerotherapy treatments. Per treatment session, the overall mortality rate was 7%, with a 16% rate per acute session and a 2.4% rate per elective session. Of the 219 acute sessions, 160 were done within 72 hours of acute bleeding. Twenty of these patients had further variceal bleeding during their admission. Most of the sessions (84%) were uncomplicated.

Risk Factors.—There was a higher incidence of chest infection in patients with modified Child's grade C, in those who had rigid esophagoscopy, and after acute variceal bleeding. High-risk patients with recent bleeding were more likely to have postinjection bleeding. There were 8 esophageal perforations, all occurring after rigid esophagoscopy, 7 within 7 days of the first episode of bleeding. Six patients with perforation died. There were 15 cases of esophageal ulceration, all in patients who received 15 mL or more of sclerosant at 1 session. This complication developed after acute therapy in 13 patients and in 11 patients with recurrent bleeding. Strictures requiring dilatation developed in 8 patients, all but 1 of whom had had at least 5 previous treatments.

Conclusions.—Risk factors for complications from injection sclerotherapy include poor modified Child's grading, first episodes of bleeding, acute therapy, and use of the rigid esophagoscope. There appears to be no advantage to use of the rigid rather than the fiberoptic endoscope.

▶ Now that sclerotherapy generally represents the first line in the algorithm of treatment of bleeding varices, it is important that the complications are appreciated. The results of long-term injection sclerotherapy were evaluated by Terblanche et al. (1) in 245 patients; 140 survived little more than 3 months, but the varices were eradicated in 88% of these. In the group whose varices were eradicated, 30% had recurrence and one third of those bled. Garrett et al. (2) evaluated 177 patients who underwent sclerotherapy. They demonstrated that the influence of therapy on long-term survival is limited, with only 20% of class C patients surviving for more than 36 months.—S.I. Schwartz, M.D.

References

1. Terblanche J, et al: *Ann Surg* 210:725, 1989.
2. Garret KO, et al: *Surgery* 104:813, 1988.

Portocaval Shunt Versus Endoscopic Sclerotherapy in the Elective Treatment of Variceal Hemorrhage
Planas R, Boix J, Broggi M, Cabré E, Gomes-Vieira MC, Morillas R, Armegol M, De León R, Humbert P, Salvá JA, Gassull MA (Hosp Universitari "Germans Trias i Pujol," Barcelona)
Gastroenterology 100:1078–1086, 1991   23–13

Introduction.—In variceal bleeding, distal splenorenal shunt and portacaval anastomosis (PCA) do not appear to result in differences in survival or incidence of postoperative hepatic encephalopathy. Variceal rebleeding is more common after distal splenovenal shunting, which is technically more difficult. The effectiveness and safety of endoscopic sclerotherapy and PCA were compared in 82 consecutive cirrhotic patients who survived hemorrhage resulting from rupture of gastroesophageal varices.

Methods.—The patients were randomized to receive either PCA or endoscopic sclerotherapy; all were in either Child-Campbell class A or B. After exclusion of dropouts, there were 34 patients in the PCA group and 35 in the sclerotherapy group. There were no significant differences in the characteristics of the groups. The mean follow-up was 20.6 months.

Results.—The incidence of variceal rebleeding was 40% in the sclerotherapy group compared with 2.9% in the PCA group, with 8 of 14 episodes of bleeding occurring before completion of sclerotherapy. The incidence of rebleeding in the patients who completed sclerotherapy was 25%. The probability of at least 1 episode of hepatic encephalopathy by 2 years was 40% in the group having PCA compared with 12% in the group having sclerotherapy. Only 8.8% of patients who underwent surgery had disabling encephalopathy. The 2-year survival rates were 83% in the PCA-treated group and 79% in the group having sclerotherapy; the difference was not significant.

Conclusion.—In the prevention of variceal rebleeding, PCA appears to be a more effective therapy than endoscopic sclerotherapy and was preferred despite its greater incidence of hepatic encephalopathy. The role of this treatment in management of bleeding from gastroesophageal varices warrants reassessment.

▶ Rikkers et al. (1) addressed the issue of shunt surgery versus endoscopic sclerotherapy in the long-term treatment of variceal bleeding. He concluded that endoscopic therapy is an acceptable alternative to shunt surgery, but it is not a superior treatment. Patients with limited liver function might do better with sclerotherapy. Cello et al. (2) concluded that, although endoscopic sclerotherapy is as good as surgical shunting in the acute management of variceal hemorrhaging in poor-risk patients with massive bleeding, sclerotherapy-treated patients in whom varices are not obliterated and in whom bleeding continues should be considered for elective shunt therapy. Burroughs et al. (3) reported that staple transection of the esophagus as emergency treatment for variceal bleeding in patients with cirrhosis of the liver is as safe as sclerotherapy and more effective than a single sclerotherapy procedure.—S.I. Schwartz, M.D.

References

1. Rikkers LF, et al: *Ann Surg* 206:261, 1987.
2. Cello JP, et al: *N Engl J Med* 316:11, 1987.
3. Burroughs AK, et al: *N Engl J Med* 321:857, 1989.

Emergency Portosystemic Shunt in Patients with Variceal Bleeding

Spina GP, Santambrogio R, Opocher E, Gagliano G, Cucchiaro G, Pisani A, Macri M (Univ of Milan, Italy)

Surg Gynecol Obstet 171:456–464, 1990   23–14

Background.—Available methods of treating variceal bleeding may be complicated by early repetitive or persistent episodes of hemorrhage. Bleeding may lead to death in such patients, and aggressive therapy is needed. A prospective study of the use of emergency portosystemic shuts was performed in 35 cirrhotic patients who did not respond to nonsurgical treatment of variceal bleeding.

Patients.—All patients had undergone emergency sclerotherapy or had conservative treatment, or both. The male-to-female ratio was 26:9, and the mean age was 51.6 years. Four patients were in Child's category A, 20 were in category B, and 11 were in category C. The mean time between the start of bleeding and the shunt procedure was 96.7 hours, and the mean interval between hospitalization and the procedure was 31.6 hours.

Results.—Variceal bleeding was controlled permanently in all patients but 1. Varices disappeared in 18 patients and were reduced in 14. Three patients died, 2 of hepatic failure and 1 of bleeding ulcerations of the gastric fundus; 1 of these patients was in Child's category B and 2 were in category C. Twelve of the 32 patients who were discharged died within an average of 11.2 months after operation. Four died of hepatic failure, 3 of hemorrhaging duodenal ulcers, 2 of hepatomas, 2 of other neoplasia, and 1 of renal failure. The 5-year survival was 43%. Long-term survival was 21% for patients in Child's category C, compared to 55% for those in categories A and B. There were 6 cases of chronic encephalopathy —3 mild, 1 moderate, and 2 severe.

Conclusions.—To gain control of hemorrhage and prolong survival in patients in whom conservative treatment of variceal bleeding has failed, emergency portosystemic shunts should be used. In patients with severe hepatic disease, such shunts have only limited use, because these patients have poor results no matter what treatment is given.

▶ The authors in essence agree with the conclusion of Cello et al. (1). Villeneuve et al. (2) also reported that an emergency portacaval shunt produces acceptable long-term survival rates in patients with mild or moderate liver disease whose bleeding has not been controlled by other methods. In their experience, the operative mortality rate was 19% and 1- and 2- year survival rates were 78% and 71% respectively.—S.I. Schwartz, M.D.

References

1. Cello JP, et al: N Engl J Med 316:11, 1987.
2. Villeneuve JP, et al: Ann Surg 206:48, 1987.

Improved Survival After Prophylactic Portal Nondecompression Surgery for Esophageal Varices: A Randomized Clinical Trial
Inokuchi K and the Cooperative Study Group of Portal Hypertension of Japan (Saga Kohseikan Hosp, Fukuoka, Japan)
Hepatology 12:1–6, 1990   23–15

Introduction.—Prophylactic surgery for esophageal varices was assessed in a randomized trial in patients younger than age 70 years who were at high risk of variceal bleeding but had not bled previously. All were acceptable surgical risks.

Management.—Sixty patients were operated on, half undergoing esophageal transection. Ten patients received selective shunts, 8 had gastric transection, 7 underwent cardiectomy, and 5 had the Hassab procedure. The 52 patients not operated on did not undergo sclerotherapy or embolization.

Outcome.—Mortality rates during a median follow-up of about 4 years were 22% for the surgical group, including 2 operative deaths, and 44% for the group not operated on. Cumulative survival rates at 5 years were 72% and 45%, respectively, and were significantly different. Seven percent of the patients treated surgically and 46% of the nonsurgical group had variceal bleeding within 5 years.

Conclusion.—Portal nondecompression surgery apparently can prevent variceal bleeding in patients at risk and improve their survival.

▶ Conventional thinking has been that there is little case for prophylactic portal decompressive surgery because of the lack of predictability of bleeding and the concern for encephalopathy. The Japanese group has suggested that they can more precisely define the risk of bleeding and address the patients at risk with an operation that does not have a high incidence of associated encephalopathy. Nagasue et al. (1) reported 5-, 10-, 15-year survival rates of 85.5% in patients undergoing prophylactic distal spleen or renal shunt. It is difficult to reconcile these results with the recent report that endoscopic sclerotherapy provided no improvement in patients who had not bled. Santangelo et al. (2) reported that prophylactic sclerotherapy of large esophageal varices in patients with chronic alcoholic cirrhosis did not provide any clinical benefit.—S.I. Schwartz, M.D.

References

1. Nagasue N, et al: *World J Surg* 13:92, 1989.
2. Santangelo WC, et al: *N Engl J Med* 318:814, 1988.

Percutaneous Transjugular Portosystemic Shunt

Zemel G, Katzen BT, Becker GJ, Benenati JF, Sallee S (Baptist Hosp, Miami)
JAMA 266:390–393, 1991
23–16

Introduction.—Surgical portosystemic shunts effectively prevent re-bleeding in variceal hemorrhage secondary to portal hypertension, but surgical shunts are associated with a high rate of morbidity and mortality.

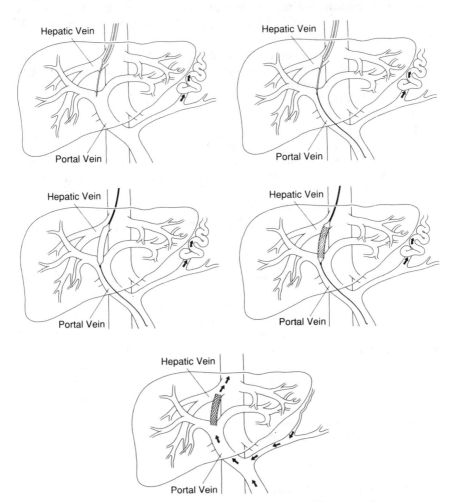

Fig 23–4.—*Top left*, modified Ross needle is advanced from a hepatic to a portal vein via a transjugular approach (*arrows* indicate hepatofugal flow in an enlarged coronary vein); *top right*, guidewire is advanced through the needle into the superior mesenteric vein; *middle left*, an 8-mm angioplasty balloon is advanced over the guidewire and expanded across hepatic parenchymal tract; *middle right*, Palmaz stent, mounted on an 8-mm angioplasty balloon, is expanded to bridge hepatic and portal veins; and *bottom*, final appearance of stent resulting in an intrahepatic shunt from portal to hepatic vein. Coronary vein is smaller and demonstrates return to hepatopetal flow. (Courtesy of Zemel G, Katzen BT, Becker GJ, et al: JAMA 266:390–393, 1991.)

A new technique—the Palmaz balloon expandable stent for creation of a transjugular intrahepatic portosystemic shunt (TIPS)—was evaluated.

Patients.—During a 9-month period, 8 patients with cirrhosis received a TIPS (Fig 23-4) for control of hemorrhage. Bleeding from esophageal varices occurred in 7 patients and from hemorrhoids in the eighth patient. Shunt patency and recurrent variceal hemorrhage were assessed during a mean follow-up period of 5 months.

Results.—The procedures were performed without technical failure and resulted in a brisk flow in the shunt and complete decompression of the gastroesophageal varices. Immediately after placement, the average pressure gradient was lowered from a mean of 36 mm Hg to 11 mm Hg. Liver function did not deteriorate during the first 4 months. All shunts remained patent throughout the follow-up period, although the patient with hemorrhoidal bleeding required shunt enlargment by balloon angioplasty.

Conclusion.—This early experience with TIPS suggests that the procedure is an effective means of portal decompression for the treatment of variceal hemorrhage. In patients with end-state liver disease, use of a TIPS may allow time for a suitable donor to be found.

▶ The technique offers exciting possibilities if patency is sustained. In 1982, Colapinto et al. (1) carried out balloon angioplasty within the liver parenchyma and created a track between the hepatic and portal-venous branches, but early shunt occlusion occurred. Richter et al. (2) reported an encouraging experience with the Palmaz balloon expandable stent. It would be interesting to determine whether shunt patency can be maintained; even if it can't, this may serve as a temporizing procedure in a patient who is bleeding acutely.—S.I. Schwartz, M.D.

References

1. Colapinto RF, et al: *Can Med Assoc J* 126:267, 1982.
2. Richter GM, et al: *Radiology* 174:1027, 1990.

The Sugiura Procedure for Patients With Hemorrhagic Portal Hypertension Secondary to Extrahepatic Portal Vein Thrombosis
Orozco H, Takahashi T, Mercado MA, Garcia-Tsao G, Hernandez-Ortiz J (Instituto Nacional de la Nutricion Salvador Zubiran, Mexico City)
Surg Gynecol Obstet 173:45–48, 1991   23–17

Introduction.—About 7% of patients with portal hypertension have extrahepatic portal vein thrombosis (EPVT) without associated hepatic disease. Selective shunts give good results in such cases but cannot be performed in all patients with EPVT. The Sugiura procedure offers comparable results and is a good alternative for selective shunts (Fig 23-5).

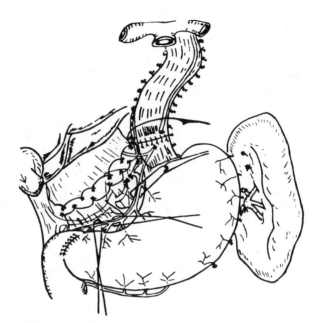

Fig 23–5.—Modification of the Sugiura procedure in accordance with Orozco and others. (Courtesy of Orozco H, Takahashi T, Mercado MA, et al: *Surg Gynecol Obstet* 173:45–48, 1991.)

Patients.—The Sugiura procedure was studied from 1979 through 1989 in a group of 27 patients (14 females, 13 males) whose mean age was 28 years. The cause of EPVT was unknown in 21 patients, 2 had protein C deficiency, 2 a history of omphalitis, 1 a history of pancreatitis, and 1, antithrombin III deficiency.

Results.—The Sugiura procedure was completed in 2 surgical stages in 14 patients and in 1 stage in 9. The single operative death resulted from sepsis and multiple organ failure. One patient died 6 months postoperatively. Two patients were treated for rebleeding at 3 years and 5 years postoperatively; the patient who rebled at 5 years died. Actuarial survival at 5 years and 10 years was 82%. One patient had mild postoperative encephalopathy.

Conclusion.—Some physicians recommend only supportive measures for the management of variceal bleeding secondary to EPVT, at least in young patients with good hepatic function. Results in the series recommend the Sugiura procedure as an effective alternative to other treatments that may result in higher rates of rebleeding, postoperative mortality, and encephalopathy.

▶ We have reported (1) that the majority of patients with EPVT who bleed stop bleeding spontaneously and have a normal life expectancy. There is no life expectancy without surgical intervention. Kahn et al. (2) reported that injection sclerotherapy markedly reduced the incidence of bleeding. Warren et al. (3) reported 70 patients with varices secondary to EPVT; selected distal spleen and renal shunts were carried out in 24 patients, resulting in a patency rate of more than 90% and late rebleeding in only 1%.—S.I. Schwartz, M.D.

References

1. Grauer SE, Schwartz SI: *Ann Surg* 1989:566, 1979.
2. Kahn D, et al: *Br J Surg* 74:600, 1987.
3. Warren WD, et al: *Ann Surg* 207:623, 1988.

Splenectomy for the Massively Enlarged Spleen
Danforth DN Jr, Fraker DL (Natl Cancer Inst, Bethesda, Md)
Am Surg 57:108–113, 1991   23–18

Background.—Enlargement of the spleen to a size of 1,500 g or more may require splenectomy. Because of underlying disease, the risk of postoperative morbidity and mortality are increased. A 33-year experience with 46 patients was reviewed to define the characteristics and postoperative course of these patients. These cases were identified in a review of 802 splenectomies. The median age of the group was 51 years, and the male:female ratio was 31:15.

Management.—The most common indication for surgery was hypersplenism (69.6% of cases), which was usually assocciated with anemia and thrombocytopenia (32.6% of cases). Thirty-one operations were done for malignancies, including chronic lymphocytic leukemia (11), chronic myelogenous leukemia (10), lymphoma (9), and hairy cell leukemia (1); 11 procedures were done for myeloid metaplasia and 4 were done for other nonmalignant conditions. Thirty patients had a midline incision and 4 had a thoracoabdominal incision.

Results.—The median blood loss (1,300 mL) in the 16 patients who did not have ligation of the splenic artery initially was not significantly different from the loss in those who did, 1,200 mL. The median weight of the spleen was 2,030 g. The postoperative complication rate was 39.1%, including infection in 11 patients and bleeding in 6. Reoperation was needed in 6 cases, 4 because of bleeding, 1 because of abscess, and 1 because of small bowel obstruction. The 30-day operative mortality was 19.6%. There was improvement in the parameters for which splenectomy was done in 29 patients and no change in 6.

Conclusions.—Splenectomy may be beneficial in many patients with massive splenomegaly, but the risk of postoperative morbidity and mortality is high. Patients should be selected carefully. The operation may be done earlier in the course of the disease to improve the benefits of the procedure.

▶ In general, the massively enlarged spleen is not difficult to remove, and we strongly advise against a thoracoabdominal approach because of the increased complications. Our own preference for incision is a long, and at times extended, left subcostal incision, frequently crossing to the right upper quadrant in a chevron fashion. We agree that little is to be gained by initial ligation of the splenic artery. The greatest number of complications in our experience relate to patients with myeloproliferative disorders. The complication that occurs relatively uniquely in these patients is thrombosis of the stump of the splenic vein extending into the portal and superior mesenteric veins causing ascites, renal failure, and death. We've seen this on at least 4 occasions and, as a consequence, have modified our preoperative preparation of patients with myeloid metaplasia to include antiplatelet-aggregating drugs and low-dose heparin. About 90% of our patients demonstrate a response in their platelet count returning to levels of more than $100,000/mm^3$ subsequent to splenectomy. Johnson and Deterling (1) identified 36 patients who underwent splenectomy for spleens that weighed more than 1,000g. Of 21 patients with drainage tubes, 8 had complications, as did 8 of 21 with preliminary early splenic arterial ligation.—S.I. Schwartz, M.D.

Reference

1. Johnson HA, Deterling RA: *Surg Gynecol Obstet* 168:131, 1989.

Immune Thrombocytopenia: Surgical Therapy and Predictors of Response

Davis PW, Williams DA, Shamberger RC (Children's Hosp, Boston)
J Pediatr Surg 26:407–413, 1991   23–19

Background.—Most children with immune thrombocytopenia purpura (ITP) experience early and spontaneous remission, with or without medical therapy. Those with complications or failure to have remission often undergo splenectomy, with a significant number of patients failing surgical therapy. Current methods of preparation for surgery and perioperative complications and responses to splenectomy were evaluated.

Methods.—During a 10-year period (1979–1989), 40 patients underwent splenectomy for ITP. Twenty-one had failed to respond to medical management and 19 had severe acute ITP. The most common symptoms were purpura (90%), epistaxis (32.5%), and petechial rash (20%); the median platelet count was $8,000/mm^3$.

Results.—There were few complications to splenectomy and no episodes of postsplenectomy sepsis. Within a mean follow-up of 15 months, 32 patients (80%) responded to splenectomy. The 8 patients in whom surgical therapy failed all had significant thrombocytopenia requiring further medical treatment. One of these patients was found to have an accessory spleen and responded after its removal (Fig 23–6). Patients with chronic ITP responded better to splenectomy (90%) than those with severe thrombocytopenia (68%). Splenectomy also failed in

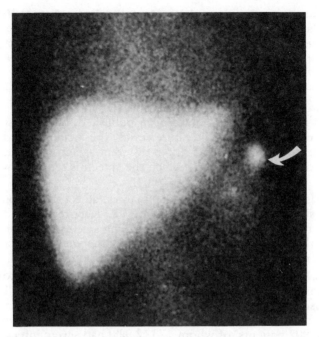

Fig 23–6.—Radionuclide scan of patient with recurrent thrombocytopenia 8 months after splenectomy. Scan demonstrates area of uptake in the left upper quadrant (*arrow*) consistent with accessory spleen. (Courtesy of Davis PW, Williams DA, Shamberger RC: *J Pediatr Surg* 26:407–413, 1991.)

the 1 patient not responsive to intravenous IgG therapy. Of 17 patients who received steroids immediately before surgery, 16 responded to splenectomy.

Conclusion.—Steroids and IgG were equally effective in pretreatment and allowed less frequent use of platelet transfusion. A response to steroids, IgG, or both was highly predictive (97%) of response to splenectomy, whereas a failure to respond to medical management predicted a 70% rate of surgical failure.

▶ The authors found that all patients with chronic ITP responding to steroids at one time also responded to splenectomy, although they indicate that 4 of 7 patients who failed to respond to steroid therapy did not respond to splenectomy. The data, looked at another way, indicate that 3 patients did respond and splenectomy therefore should not be withheld from steroid nonresponders. Use of preoperative treatment with steroids or IgG to elevate platelet counts is questionable. It has been our approach to operate on these patients in the severely thrombocytopenic state if necessary; we have seen no untoward effects. If there is any diffuse ooze related to the low platelet count, as soon as the spleen is removed improvement is noted. We rarely administer platelets intraoperatively to these patients.—S.I. Schwartz, M.D.

Postsplenectomy Sepsis and Its Mortality Rate: Actual Versus Perceived Risks

Holdsworth RJ, Irving AD, Cuschieri A (Ninewells Hosp and Med School, Dundee; Stracathro Hosp, Angus, Scotland)
Br J Surg 78:1031–1038, 1991   23–20

Introduction.—Numerous studies on whether the risk of infection is increased after splenectomy have been published, but the issue remains unresolved. In a collective literature review the incidence and nature of postsplenectomy infection, its risk in different age groups, and the effect of the underlying disorders for which the spleen is removed were examined.

Methods.—In the first part of the analysis, all 59 studies on postsplenectomy sepsis published from 1952 to 1987 were reviewed. This review yielded a total of 12,514 patients undergoing splenectomy for all indications. In the second part of the study, only the well-documented infections that developed after splenectomy were analyzed in detail.

Results.—Among the 12,514 patients undergoing splenectomy for all indications, 447 had severe infections (3.6%) and 221 died (1.8%). However, those incidence rates are likely to be inaccurate as many reports gave few details of the infections. The well-documented series yielded a total of 5,902 patients, of whom 173 (2.9%) had severe infection and 91 (1.5%) died. In children younger than 16 years, the incidence of postsplenectomy infection was 4.4% and the mortality rate was 2.2%. In adults, the incidences were .9% for infection and .8% for mortality. The differences were statistically significant. A particularly high incidence of infection was seen after splenectomy for thalassemia and Hodgkin's disease. The incidence of severe postsplenectomy infection in infants was 15.7%, and the mortality rate from infection was 6.7%. In children younger than 5 years, the rates were 10.4% for infection and 4.5% for mortality. *Streptococcus pneumoniae* was the single most important organism responsible for postsplenectomy sepsis, accounting for 57% of infections and 59% of deaths. *Hemophilus influenzae* was the second most common causative organism. Infection was most common in the first and second years after splenectomy. Children undergoing splenectomy for benign disease have been reported to be at increased risk for pneumococcal infection. However, this analysis of only well-documented cases found that children are no more susceptible to pneumococcal infection than to infection with any other organism.

Conclusions.—Severe infection after splenectomy for benign disease is uncommon except in infants and children less than 5 years of age. However, the presence of a coexistent disorder can increase the risk substantially.

▶ The issue of overwhelming postsplenectomy infection is real, but it is probably blown out of proportion. The present article puts the situation in appropriate perspective. Green et al. (1) provide data indicating that the risk of major infections is significantly higher in adults undergoing splenectomy. In patients underoing splenectomy for trauma, the mortality rate caused by overwhelming sepsis is not appreciably higher. Schwartz et al. (2) reported that the incidence of fulminant sepsis after splenectomy was 0.1 case/100 years of follow-up. Infections were significantly more frequent in patients who had malignancy or were treated with immunosuppression. Malangoni et al. (3) reported their personal experience and added the reports of 4 other groups, totaling 3,315 patient years of observation, and indicated that the rate of serious infection was 1/331 patient-years of observation. There were no sepsis-related deaths and only 1 fulminant infection.—S. I. Schwartz, MD

References

1. Green JB, et al: *J Trauma* 26:999, 1986.
2. Schwartz PE, et al: *JAMA* 248:2279, 1982.
3. Malangoni MA, et al: *Surgery* 96:775, 1984

Severe Late Postsplenectomy Infection

Cullingford GL, Watkins DN, Watts ADJ, Mallon DF (Univ of Western Australia, Nedlands, Western Australia)
Br J Surg 78:716–721, 1991   23–21

Background.—The occurrence of severe, often fatal, septic episodes after splenectomy has been recognized for several decades, but the incidence and mortality of these episodes have not been defined. The records of 1,490 patients who underwent splenectomy between 1971 and 1983 were reviewed to establish the risk of severe late postsplenectomy infection in Western Australia.

Methods.—The period chosen was one in which prophylactic antibiotic therapy was rarely prescribed and pneumococcal vaccination was not available or yet in routine use. The relative risk of contracting infection after splenectomy was compared with the rate of infection in the Western Australian population. Patients were categorized according to the indication for splenectomy.

Results.—Severe late postsplenectomy infection developed in 33 (2.2%) of the 1,490 splenectomized patients. None had received antibiotic prophylaxis or pneumococcal vaccine. Three had meningitis, 8 had pneumococcal pneumonia, and 22 had septicemia. The incidence was lower among patients undergoing splenectomy for trauma than for in other categories (surgery for malignant or nonmalignant conditions and hematologic or lymphoproliferative disorders). Compared with the general population, patients undergoing splenectomy have a 12.6-fold increased risk of late septicemia developing. No significant increase was found in the incidence of pneumococcal pneumonia or meningitis.

Summary of Studies on Late Postsplenectomy Infection Rates per 100 Person Years Exposure

First author*	All splenectomy indications				Splenectomy for trauma *			
	PYE	Incidence sepsis/100 PYE	Mortality sepsis/100 PYE	Incidence OPSI /100 PYE	PYE	Incidence sepsis/100 PYE	Mortality sepsis/100 PYE	Incidence OPSI /100 PYE
O'Neal	944	ns	0·74	ns	303	3·30	0	0
Schwartz	1090	4·77	0·09	0·09				
Standage	879	ns	2·28	ns				
Pedersen	2381	0·88	0·25	ns				
Malangoni	1203	0·25	0	0	1203	0·25	0	0
Chaikof	4837	ns	0·70	0·08	1406	0·57	0	0
Sekikawa	1406	0·57	0	0	734	1·91	0·14	0·14
Green	734	1·91	0·14	0·14	105	1·90	0	0·95
Green	105	1·90	0	0·95	3855	0·21	0·03	0·03
Present study (P)	7825	0·42	0·08	0·04	7246	0·59	0·03	0·04
Combined	21 404	0·89 †	0·35	0·06 †				

Abbreviations: P, population study; OPSI, overwhelming postsplenectomy infection; PYE, person years exposure; ns, not stated.
* Trauma excludes iatrogenic trauma or incidental splenectomy unless indicated.
† Corrected to exclude studies where sepsis type not stated.
(Courtesy of Cullingford GL, Watkins DN, Watts ADJ, et al: *Br J Surg* 78:716–721, 1991.)

Nearly half (42%) of the severe late postsplenectomy infections occur-rect more than 5 years after splenectomy.

Conclusion.—Because of low incidence of severe late postsplenec-tomy infection (table), statistical evaluation of preventive measures is dif-ficult. Modifications of surgical practice and recognition of the risks in splenectomized patients may reduce the incidence and severity of infec-tion.

▶ Although there is a real increase in postsplenectomy infection, the inci-dence is very low. The data demonstrate that splenectomy for trauma is as-sociated with the lowest incidence of late postsplenectomy infection. The 3 patients who had overwhelming sepsis did have a prodromal period. Dun-combe et al. (1) showed that early recognition and treatment of infection re-duce the severity of infection and halt progression to overwhelming sep-sis.—S.I. Schwartz, M.D.

Reference

1. Duncombe AS, et al: *Lancet* 1:570, 1987.

24 The Biliary Tract

A Valved Hepatic Portoduodenal Intestinal Conduit for Biliary Atresia

Tanaka K, Shirahase I, Utsunomiya H, Katayama T, Uemoto S, Asonuma K, Inomata Y, Ozawa K (Kyoto Univ, Japan)

Ann Surg 213:230–235, 1991

24–1

Introduction.—Ascending cholangitis is a serious complication after many types of biliointestinal reconstruction. The only procedure to regularly avoid this complication, hepatic portocholecystostomy, cannot be performed in many cases. A newly developed intestinal valve designed to reduce the incidence of cholangitis and improve survival was evaluated.

Patients.—Forty-six consecutive infants with biliary atresia underwent surgery between May 1978 and August 1989. The mean age at operation was 59 days. At follow-up, ranging from 5 months to 11 years, the patients were assessed for bile drainage, presence of cholangitis, and valvular competence.

Technique.—The porta hepatis structures are dissected by means of the Kasai operation. A biliointestinal anastomosis is then constructed with a valved hepatic portoduodenal intestinal conduit. The intestinal valve is an intussuscepted muscular valve, fixed with 8–10 interrupted sutures (Fig 24–1).

Results.—Bile drainage was achieved in 39 patients (85%) after the initial operation. Ten patients died; 6 survived with jaundice and 30 without jaundice. Nine patients with apparent bile drainage had cholangitis, a condition that was tractable in 5 and refractory in 4. Eight patients without cholangitis required reoperation after bile drainage ceased abruptly. Bile flow was restored in 2 of these patients.

Conclusion.—Use of a valved hepatic portoduodenal intestinal conduit improved the survival rate in these infants with biliary atresia. The antireflux valve is effective in preventing ascending cholangitis and bile flow into the duodenum. The 5-year jaundice-free survival rate was 64%.

▶ The rate of 85% bile drainage after the initial operation is quite similar to the rate reported by Lilly et al. (1) of 82%. In Lilly's experience, biliary obstruction remained relieved for more than a year in 57% of the 72 patients, but 21 of these patients had clinical signs of portal hypertension and 17 had antibiotic-resistant cholangitis. If the latter complication can truly be pre-

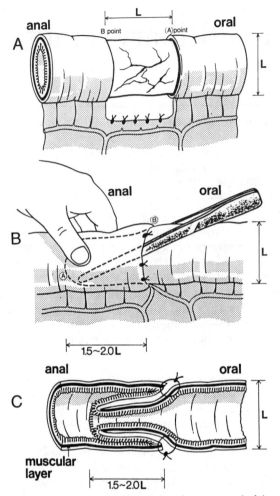

Fig 24–1.—Construction of an intussusceptal muscular valve. **A,** removal of the seromuscular layer; **B,** intussusception and valvular fixation; and **C,** cross-section of the valve. (Courtesy of Tanaka K, Shirahase I, Utsunomiya H, et al: *Ann Surg* 213:230–235, 1991.)

vented by the use of this valve, it represents a significant contribution.—S.I. Schwartz, M.D.

Reference

1. Lilly JR, et al: *Ann Surg* 210:289, 1989.

Surgical Techniques and Long-Term Results in the Treatment of Choledochal Cyst

Joseph VT (Singapore Gen Hosp)
J Pediatr Surg 25:782–787, 1990   24–2

Background.—Data on 52 patients who were treated for choledochal cyst from 1961 to 1988 were reviewed.

Methods.—Ultrasonography was the most useful diagnostic procedure. There were 45 type I cysts. Surgical treatment of choledochal cysts from 1961 to 1973 most often used internal drainage procedures. Cyst excision became almost exclusively the procedure of choice after 1973. Complete cyst excision was performed on 34 patients. The excision was successful if dissection of the distal part of the cyst was performed in a clear, bloodless field working directly on the cyst wall beneath the overlying loose areolar tissue. A Roux-en-Y retrocolic hepaticojejunostomy completes the procedure.

Results.—There were no operative deaths, and there was no anastomotic leakage. One patient who had undergone cyst excision of a type I cyst later died of cholangiocarcinoma. Of the 5 patients with associated cirrhosis of the liver, 1 eventually underwent successful liver transplantation because of ascites and bleeding esophageal varices. Cholangitis developed in 3 of the 10 patients who had internal drainage procedures; reoperations were performed 10, 11, and 20 years after the initial surgery despite the fact that the original stoma was judged to be adequate.

Conclusion.—The surgical excision of choledochal cyst and hepaticojunostomy, using the same surgical procedure for types I–IV cysts was successful. Operative cholangiograms are not helpful in most patients. Anastomosis of the cyst wall at the gastrointestinal tract ultimately results in stricture and cholangitis.

▶ This lesion is generally managed by pediatric surgeons, and cyst excision with anastomosis of the proximal duct to the intestine is the treatment of choice. Occasionally, the symptoms are delayed until adulthood and associated hepatobiliary pathology may complicate the presentation. Hopkins et al. (1) reported 7 cases with complications, including cholangitis, hepatic abscess, pancreatitis, and malignancy within the cyst. Two of their patients presented during pregnancy, and treatment was delayed until after delivery.—S.I. Schwartz, M.D.

Reference

1. Hopkins NF, et al: *Ann R Coll Surg Engl* 72:229, 1990.

Gallstone Dissolution With Methyl *tert*-Butyl Ether in 120 Patients: Efficacy and Safety

Leuschner U, Hellstern A, Schmidt K, Fischer H, Güldütuna S, Hübner K, Leuschner M (Johann Wolfgang Goethe Univ, Frankfurt/Main, Germany)
Dig Dis Sci 36:193–199, 1991   24–3

Introduction.—In 1985, Thistle et al. introduced the use of methyl *tert*-butyl ether (MTBE) to dissolve cholesterol gallstones. The agent is instilled into the gallbladder after percutaneous transphepatic puncture and is immediately reaspirated.

Methods.—Percutaneous transhepatic litholysis with MTBE was attempted in 120 of 612 patients seen since 1986 with cholesterol gallbladder stones. The gallbladder was punctured under fluoroscopic control with a pigtail catheter. Enough MTBE was used to just cover the stones.

Results.—Attempted gallbladder puncture succeeded in all but 3 patients and, in 113 of these 117 cases, the stones dissolved. Treatment lasted for 4 hours on average for solitary stones and 10 hours when multiple stones were present. The mean hospital stay was 3½ days. Bile leakage developed in 3 patients. One third of the patients had some residue present at the end of treatment, and 2 had recurrent stones. None of the 6 patients who had cholecystectomy had gross evidence of erosion or ulceration of the gallbladder wall. Histologic findings were unrelated to treatment time.

Conclusions.—Contact litholysis with MTBE is an improvement in gallstone treatment. The changes in the gallbladder after treatment are probably a result of the presence of stones, not the treatment.

▶ With the advent of laparoscopic cholecystectomy, the indications for gallstone dissolution have been reduced. It certainly represents an expensive modality, amplified by the fact that all patients are given ursodeoxycholic acid each day for the next 3 months. The statement that should appear in bold relief, related to the appropriateness of removing stones as contrasted with removing the gallbladder, is that made by Langenbuch when he reported his first elective cholecystectomy and indicated that the gallbladder was removed not because it contained stones but, rather, because it formed stones.—S.I. Schwartz, M.D.

Laparoscopic Cholecystectomy: Experience With 375 Consecutive Patients

Bailey RW, Zucker KA, Flowers JL, Scovill WA, Graham SM, Imbembo AL (Univ of Maryland)
Ann Surg 214:531–541, 1991   24–4

Introduction.—Early reports of laparoscopic general surgery indicated considerable reductions in hospital and recovery times, as well as less postoperative discomfort and improved cosmetic results. Concern over major complications persists, however. Experience with 375 patients undergoing laparoscopic cholecystectomy was reviewed. Thirty-four patients had acute cholecystitis, gallstone pancreatitis, or cholangitis; the remaining 341 underwent the procedure on an elective basis.

Technique.—A 4-puncture method is used. Pneumoperitoneum is established using CO_2 and either a "closed" or "open" approach. Operative visualization is with a miniaturized video camera attached to a 10-mm laparoscope. Intraoperative cholangiography is carried out after identification of the cystic duct. The gallbladder is dissected from the liver by monopolar electrocautery. The gallbladder is removed via the umbilical incision by applying an 11-mm penetrating forceps to its neck. The umbilical fascia is closed with an absorbable suture.

Results.—Twenty patients were converted to laparotomy and cholecystectomy, for an overall success rate of 95%. Ninety percent of patients were discharged within 24 hours of the procedure. Operative cholangiography showed choledocholithiasis in 5 of 141 patients. Two retained stones were found in the 214 patients not having cholangiography. Three patients required reoperation for perioperative complications. The overall rate of morbidity was 3.5%. The 1 postoperative death was caused by myocardial infarction.

Conclusions.—Laparoscopic cholecystectomy can be done with the efficacy, morbidity, and mortality expected from open operation while enhancing patient recovery. Such improvements as a 3-dimensional video system may make this approach even more useful.

▶ The procedure is certainly here to stay, but there is some concern that the overall complication rate of .8% reported by the authors will not be matched by the experience of many. There is also an increasing literature on ambulatory cholecystectomy (1). It is feasible that similar hospitalization periods can be achieved for open cholecystectomy. But it has been the experience at our institution that at 1 week subsequent to the operation, the patients undergoing laparoscopic cholecystectomy can perform at a higher level of activity compared to those undergoing open cholecystectomy.—S.I. Schwartz, M.D.

Reference

1. Ledet WP: *Arch Surg* 125:1434, 1990.

Appraisal of Laparoscopic Cholecystectomy

Graves HA Jr, Ballinger JF, Anderson WJ (Vanderbilt Univ; Centennial Med Ctr, Nashville)
Ann Surg 213:655–664, 1991   24–5

Objective.—Three general surgeons performed a total of 304 laparoscopic cholecystectomies at separate private hospitals between 1989 and 1990. Indications were the same as for open surgery.

Patients.—More than 80% of the patients were women and the average age was 50 years. All but 10% of the patients were evaluated ultrasonically. Ten patients had acute cholecystitis.

Outcome.—Almost all (93%) of the procedures were successful. Twenty-one patients required an open operation, usually because of problems in defining the anatomy secondary to inflammatory changes. There were no conversions for uncontrolled bleeding, and no patient required later laparotomy. Four of the 10 patients with acute cholecystitis had successful laparoscopic surgery. The average operating time was 99 minutes. Cautery was used in 59% of patients and laser dissection in the remainder. Complications occurred in 2% of patients; prolonged ileus being the most frequent. Eighty-six percent of patients were admitted on the day of surgery, and 75% were discharged within 24 hours.

Discussion.—Laparoscopic cholecystectomy can be done with little morbidity. Although patients recover rapidly and are satisfied with the procedure, it is recommended that symptomatic cholelithiasis remain the indication.

A Prospective Analysis of 1,518 Laparoscopic Cholecystectomies

Meyers WC, for The Southern Surgeons Club (Duke Univ)
N Engl J Med 324:1073–1078, 1991   24–6

Background.—Laparoscopic cholecystectomy has gained widespread popularity. To assess the procedure's results, 1,518 operations performed by 59 surgeons were studied prospectively.

Methods.—Twenty surgical groups participated. Data on all patients were submitted on standard forms, after which, surgeons were questioned about their definitions of complications. The average age was 47 years, and 75% were women. Symptoms suggestive of gallbladder disease were present in 99% of the patients, 96% had cholelithiasis, and 90% had gross anatomical or histologic evidence of gallbladder inflammation.

Results.—Ultrasonography was done preoperatively to document gallbladder abnormalities in 96.5% of patients. Of all operations, about 5% were converted to open cholecystectomy, usually when the surgeon was unable to identify gallbladder anatomy because of inflammation. Sixty-five patients had unexpected operative findings of disease, including acutely inflamed organs in 14, common bile duct disease in 21, gallbladder cancers in 4, benign gallbladder adenomas in 2, cholesterolosis in 8, duodenal diverticulum in 1, and other cancers in 2. The procedure lasted for an average of 90 minutes. The complication rate was 5%, the most common complication being wound infection. Intra-abdominal abscesses and hepatic duct injuries also were seen. One patient died of a ruptured abdominal aortic aneurysm 3 days after the procedure. The mean hospital stay was 1.2 days.

Conclusions.—Laparoscopic cholecystectomy compares favorably to conventional cholecystectomy. The overall rate of bile duct injury was .5%, but this is probably outweighed by the low rates of death, hemorrhage, and pulmonary problems. The incidence of undetected common duct stones was about 2%, probably because of selection of low-risk patients, the preoperative use of endoscopic retrograde cholangiopancreatography, and selective use of cholangiography. When coincidental duct stones are found, the surgeon must choose between conversion to conventional surgery, postoperative endoscopic retrograde cholangiopancreatography, and expectant therapy.

▶ The number of articles extolling the advantage of laparoscopic cholecystectomy suggests that the verdict is in and approval is declared. Schrimer and associates (1) reported a conversion rate of 8.5% and a complication rate of 4%. Overall, 87% of the patients were discharged on the first postoperative day and returned to normal activities within a week after discharge. Frazee et al. (2) demonstrated that laparoscopic cholecystectomy also offers improved pulmonary function compared to the open technique and lessens the pulmonary risk.—S.I. Schwartz, M.D.

References

1. Schirmer BD, et al: *Ann Surg* 213:665, 1991.
2. Frazee RC, et al: *Ann Surg* 213:651, 1991.

The Importance of Intraoperative Cholangiography During Laparoscopic Cholecystectomy
Phillips EH, Berci G, Carroll B, Daykhovsky L, Sackier J, Paz-Partlow M (Cedars-Sinai Med Ctr, Los Angeles)
Am Surg 56:792–795, 1990   24–7

Background.—Stones often reform after nonsurgical treatment of gallstone disease. With laparoscopic cholecystectomy (LC), however, the lithogenic organ is removed. The procedure also has the advantage of shortening the hospitalization, disability, pain, and visible scarring associated with standard cholecystectomy. Cystic duct cholangiography should be performed before structures are transected, and a clip should be placed on the dissected cystic artery before cholangiography is performed. Cholangiography is useful for assessing the length of the cystic duct and determining its proximity to the extrahepatic ductal system, an important feature when performing LC because the surgeon is likely to dissect close to the common duct.

Technique.—After the cystic duct and artery are identified, a clip is placed at the base of the cystic artery and another at the junction of the cystic duct and gallbladder. With a microscissors a transverse incision is made in the cystic duct. During fluoroscopic cholangiography 25% hypaque solution serves as a contrast material. Multiple films should be exposed. After a review of the cholangiogram, the catheter is removed and the cystic duct and artery are clipped and then divided. The gallbladder is dissected by a retrograde technique.

Results.—Fifty-eight patients were treated with LC, and the procedure was successful in 56. Five patients required opening. The gallbladder was removed intact in 40 patients. Fifty-three patients had successful cholangiography, but in 5 it was impossible to cannulate the small cystic duct lumen. Twenty-seven patients who were unopened left the hospital the first postoperative day, and 42 patients were able to return to full activity within 7 days.

Conclusions.—Laparoscopic cholecystectomy may become the standard procedure for elective gallbladder removal, but the safety of the technique must be established. Preoperative cholangiography can prevent the most serious complication, common duct injury. Cholangiography should be attempted on all patients scheduled for LC.

▶ The authors' suggestion that cholangiography be performed on a routine basis during LC is not endorsed by most. In the major series carried out to date, fewer than 25% of patients had cholangiography. We must await cumulative data regarding the 2 subsets of patients—1 having cholangiography and 1 not having it who undergo LC. For those who use cholangiography selectively, the criteria should certainly be the same as those used for patients undergoing standard cholecystectomy.—S.I. Schwartz, M.D.

Outpatient Cholecystectomy Simulated in an Inpatient Population
Treen DC Jr, Downes TW III, Hayes DH, McKinnon WMP (Ochsner Clinic and Alton Ochsner Med Found, New Orleans)
Am Surg 57:39–45, 1991   24–8

Background.—Surgeons have been gradually reducing the duration of in-hospital convalescence of patients after uncomplicated elective cholecystectomy. In many cases the hospital stays have been reduced to 24–48 hours or less. The feasibility, safety, and efficacy of elective cholecystectomy on an outpatient basis were evaluated.

Methods.—Forty patients were enrolled in an inpatient protocol simulating the outpatient experience. Their results were compared with those of 19 patients managed by conventional postoperative techniques. Oral liquids were begun in the recovery room, and intravenous fluids were discontinued 4 hours after surgery. Enteral analgesics and antiemetics were given on the ward. The patients in the protocol group were then randomized in a double-blind manner to receive metoclopramide or placebo postoperatively to evaluate its effect on the early tolerance of oral intake.

Results.—Twenty-three percent of the protocol group had nausea without emesis, and another 28% had nausea with emesis. These percentages were not significantly different from those in the control group. The patients treated with metoclopramide did not have a lower incidence of nausea or emesis; however, they did tolerate oral liquids sooner after surgery than the group given placebo. After being released from the recovery room, 20% of the protocol group requested parenteral narcotics for pain relief. Postoperative urinary catheterization was needed in 23% of the protocol patients and in 26% of the controls. There were no major complications.

Conclusions.—Outpatient cholecystectomy can be done without jeopardizing the patient's safety or comfort. Such an approach results in substantial financial savings. Metoclopramide may also permit earlier tolerance of enteral fluids after surgery.

▶ This is yet another article demonstrating that cholecystectomy can be performed on an outpatient basis. Ledet (1) reported 200 consecutive outpatient cholecystectomies. The morbidity was thought to be comparable to that of laparoscopic cholecystectomy. Patients were able to return to work within 4–5 days if they had sedentary jobs.—S.I. Schwartz, M.D.

Reference

1. Ledet WP: *Arch Surg* 125:1434, 1990.

Choledocholithiasis: Endoscopic Sphincterotomy or Common Bile Duct Exploration

Stain SC, Cohen H, Tsuishoysha M, Donovan AJ (Los Angeles County–Univ of Southern California Med Ctr)
Ann Surg 213:627–634, 1991   24–9

Objective.—A prospective, randomized trial was carried out in 52 patients with biliary stone disease to compare surgery alone with surgery after endoscopic sphincterotomy. The 26 patients in each group were comparable demographically and with respect to indications for treatment.

Results.—Stones were absent in 88% of patients after surgery alone and in 65% after both sphincterotomy and surgery. Five patients had more than 20 residual common bile duct stones. One patient in each group had major bleeding, but there were no deaths. Professional costs were similar for successful procedures in the 2 groups. Patients were hospitalized somewhat longer if common duct exploration was necessary.

Discussion.—The findings do not support the use of endoscopic sphincterotomy to clear the common bile duct of stones before surgery.

▶ Miller et al. (1) reported that complication rates, success rates, and death rates were comparable in patients undergoing surgical versus endoscopic management of common bile ducts. Patients treated with endoscopic papillotomy have a significantly shorter hospital stay. If the endoscopist can achieve equivalent results, it seems that this would be preferable procedure. As success rate of endoscopic retrograde cholangiopancreatography and endoscopic extraction for stones improve, the need for common duct exploration will be reduced. The anticipated scenario of the future is endoscopic removal of stones from the duct, followed by laparoscopic cholecystectomy.—S.I. Schwartz, M.D.

Reference

1. Miller BM, et al: *Ann Surg* 207: 135, 1988.

Combined Endoscopic Sphincterotomy and Laparoscopic Cholecystectomy in Patients With Choledocholithiasis and Cholecystolithiasis
Aliperti G, Edmundowicz SA, Soper NJ, Ashley SW (Washington Univ)
Ann Intern Med 115:783–785, 1991   24–10

Introduction.—Laparoscopic cholecystectomy is becoming the preferred surgical treatment for patients with symptomatic cholelithiasis alone who do not require stone removal from the common bile duct. Symptomatic patients with both gallbladder and common bile duct calculi are still treated with open cholecystectomy.

Methods.—A combined endoscopic-laparoscopic procedure was used to treat 326 symptomatic patients with simultaneous cholecystolithiasis and choledocholithiasis. Preoperative endoscopic retrograde cholangiography was performed in 31 patients because of liver enzyme abnormalities in the absence of acute cholecystitis. If calculi were confirmed during the preoperative examination, sphincterotomy was performed and the ducts were cleared.

Results.—Stones in the common bile duct were suspected in 31 of the 326 patients (9.5%) and were confirmed in 18 (5.5%), who then underwent sphincterotomy. Of the 18 patients treated for common bile duct stones, 5 had gallstone pancreatitis, 1 had cholangitis, and 5 had abnormal liver enzyme levels, 5 had ultrasonographic confirmation of common bile duct stones, and 2 had a dilated common bile duct. Of the 13 patients who did not have common bile duct stones, 5 had gallstone pancreatitis, 6 had abnormal liver enzyme levels, and 2 had a dilated common bile duct. The length of hospital stay varied, depending on the patient's diagnosis. The procedure failed in 1 patient in whom acute cholecystitis developed with empyema and a right upper-quadrant phlegmon 7 days after sphincterotomy and who had to have conventional cholecystectomy. In 10 patients, endoscopic retrograde cholangiography with sphincterectomy was performed at admission and laparoscopic cholecystectomy was performed on the next day; 4 patients remained hospitalized between the 2 procedures, with hospital stays of 6–12 days. Total and postoperative hospital stays and postoperative disability for patients treated with the combined procedure were significantly shorter than they were for 12 age-matched controls who had conventional cholecystectomy with common bile duct exploration.

Conclusion.—The early results of combined preoperative endoscopic sphincterotomy and laparoscopic cholecystectomy in the treatment of patients with simultaneous cholecystolithiasis and choledocholithiasis suggest that it is safe and effective.

▶ Duodenoscopic sphincterotomy has been associated with excellent results in patients who have retained or have recurrent duct stones after previous cholecystectomy (1). The long-term outlook was comparable to that in patients who were operated on. Heinerman et al. (2) advocated preoperative endoscopic retrograde cholangiopancreatography (ERCP) and stone removal before cholecystectomy. This approach reduced the incidence of surgical complications significantly and also reduced the time of recovery. I predict that the combination of ERCP, sphincterotomy, and laparoscopic cholecystectomy for choledocholithiasis and cholecystolithiasis will become the standard in the future.—S.I Schwartz, M.D.

References

1. Hawes RH, et al: *Gastroenterology* 98:1008, 1990.
2. Heinerman PM, et al: *Ann Surg* 209:267, 1989.

Decision for Surgical Management of Perforation Following Endoscopic Sphincterotomy
Bell RCW, Van Stiegmann G, Goff J, Reveille M, Norton L, Pearlman NW
(Univ of Colorado; Denver Veterans Hosp)
Am Surg 57:237–240, 1991   24–11

Introduction.—The most serious complication of endoscopic sphincterotomy (ES) is perforation; the associated mortality is 25%. Timely diagnosis of this complication may be difficult, and appropriate treatment is controversial.

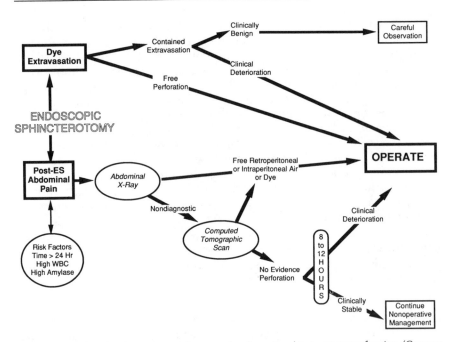

Fig 24–2.—Algorithm for treatment of suspected endoscopic sphincterotomy perforation. (Courtesy of Bell RCW, Van Stiegmann G, Goff J, et al: *Am Surg* 57:237–240, 1991.)

Methods.—The diagnosis and management of duodenal perforation resulting from ES were evaluated in 441 ES procedures done by a single endoscopist in an 8-year period. Most patients had common bile duct stones (56%) or sphincter of Oddi dysfunction (40%). In 8 patients (1.8%) there were proven perforations.

Results.—There were common duct stones in 4 patients, sphincter of Oddi dysfunction in 3, and recurrent sepsis in 1. Clinical evidence of perforation consisted of fever, tachycardia, or abdominal tenderness. In 1 patient, radiologic evidence consisted of extraluminal dye extravasation at the time of ES. The 5 patients in whom free retroperitoneal or free intraperitoneal air was seen on plain abdominal film underwent laparotomy and were treated with wide drainage of the retroduodenal area or drainage of a discrete abscess. Both patients who were operated on within 8 hours survived. The remaining 6 patients were operated on within a mean of 43 hours after ES; 2 eventually died as a result of multiple organ failure.

Conclusions.—Radiographic evidence of free retroperitoneal or intraperitoneal air was the most important determinant of perforation. Physical and laboratory findings were of little diagnostic value. Both medical and operative treatment are more likely to be successful when initiated within 24 hours of ES perforation. An algorithm was developed for treatment of suspected ES perforation (Fig 24–2).

▶ It is important to stress that endoscopic procedures are not totally benign. Miller et al. (1) reported comparable complications, success rates, and death rates for endoscopic papillotomy and common bile duct exploration. In the group of 156 patients undergoing endoscopic papillotomy, gastrointestinal hemorrhage occurred in 6, duodenal perforation in 5, biliary spesis in 4, and pancreatitis in 1.—S.I. Schwartz, M.D.

Reference

1. Miller BM, et al: *Ann Surg* 207:135, 1988.

Bleeding After Endoscopic Sphincterotomy as an Underestimated Entity
Mellinger JD, Ponsky JL (Mt Sinai Med Ctr, Cleveland; Case Western Reserve Univ)
Surg Gynecol Obstet 172:465–469, 1991   24–12

Introduction.—Hemorrhage is reported in 2% to 9% of patients who undergo endoscopic sphincterotomy (ES), but the frequency of occult bleeding after this procedure is unknown.

Methods.—Data were reviewed concerning 75 patients who underwent ES between 1986 and 1989. The most frequent indications were choledocholithiasis and papillary stenosis.

Findings.—Nine patients had clinical bleeding after sphincterotomy, and 27 had hematologic evidence of bleeding without clinical signs or symptoms. The average fall in hematocrit was 5% (equivalent to 1.6 g of hemoglobin per dL). The recognition of bleeding at the time of sphincterotomy was 85% specific but only 47% sensitive in predicting postprocedural bleeding. Three patients had significant delayed hemorrhage. Endoscopic intervention was required for bleeding in 7 patients.

Implications.—Bleeding is apparently much more frequent after ES than previously thought. Significant delayed bleeding is a possibility. Early detection of bleeding and its aggressive management will limit mortality and morbidity.

▶ The article is selected to emphasize that endoscopic procedures are not without complications. The reported total postsphincterotomy bleeding rate of 48% indicates that bleeding should be anticipated, evaluated, and addressed in an appropriate fashion to reduce the morbidity and mortality of major bleeding, which fortunately is quite rare.—S.I. Schwartz, M.D.

Transduodenal Exploration of the Common Bile Duct in Patients With Nondilated Ducts

Rataych RE, Sitzmann JV, Lillemoe KD, Yeo CJ, Cameron JL (Francis Scott Key Med Ctr, Balitmore; Johns Hopkins Med Inst)
Surg Gynecol Obstet 173:49–53, 1991   24–13

Introduction.—It may be technically difficult to explore the small common bile duct, and there is a significant risk of duct injury or late stricture. An alternative means of examining the duct without choledochotomy is transduodenal common duct exploration after sphincteroplasty (TCDE/S).

Technique.—The duodenum is mobilized after cholecystectomy, and a biliary Fogarty catheter is inserted via the cystic duct into the duodenum. The balloom is then inflated and withdrawn snugly against the ampulla. A duodenotomy and standard sphincteroplasty follow. The sphincteroplasy is at least 1 cm in length. After the duct is irrigated, it is ligated and the duodenotomy is closed in 2 layers.

Experience.—Twenty-eight patients with nondilated bile ducts underwent TCDE/S. Common duct stones or sludge were recovered from 17 of them. Possible reasons for failure to retrieve stones in 11 patients include false positive cholangiographic findings, stone passage into the bowel during catheter insertion, and falsely negative findings on duct exploration. There were no perioperative deaths, but 2 patients had asymptomatic hyperamylasemia, and pancreatitis developed in 1. In all, 29% of patients had complications. Twenty patients were asymptomatic after a mean follow-up of 38 months.

Conclusion.—Apparently, TCDE/S is an effective and safe means of exploring the nondilated common bile duct.

▶ This technique, which was proposed by Peel et al. (1), merits a place among the procedures used by biliary tract surgeons. The article demonstrates that deliberate transduodenal exploration should not be associated with significant morbidity, and the development of a fistula should represent a rarity.—S.I. Schwartz, M.D.

Reference

1. Peel A, et al: *Ann R Coll Surg Engl* 55:236, 1974.

Combined Surgical and Interventional Radiological Approach for Complex Benign Biliary Tract Obstruction

Schweizer WP, Matthews JB, Nudelmann LI, Triller J, Halter F, Gertsch P, Blumgart LH (Univ of Berne, Switzerland)
Br J Surg 78:559–563, 1991   24–14

Introduction.—The most complex benign biliary tract obstructions are difficult to manage by surgery alone. Interventional radiologic or endoscopic techniques have also been unsuccessful as primary therapy in these cases. A multidisciplinary approach combining the advantages of surgery and interventional radiology appears to minimize the need for repeated surgery.

Patients.—During a 30-month period, 17 of 58 patients with benign biliary strictures were selected for the combined approach. Most (15) of these patients had undergone previous hepatobiliary operations. All had right upper abdominal pain, as well as jaundice and fever. Ten of 17 patients had complex postcholecystectomy strictures and 7 had strictures resulting from inflammatory disease, hepatic resection, or congenital problems. A Roux-en-Y hepaticojejunostomy was performed and an extended limb of the jejunum brought to the abdominal wall to create access for a later radiologic approach (Fig 24–3).

Results.—There were no deaths in the first month, but 1 patient died 4 months after surgery because of infected ascites. The only serious intraoperative complication, an injury to the portal vein, was repaired immediately. Overall, at a mean follow-up of 16 months, 7 results were judged excellent, 6 good, 2 fair, and 2 poor. The outcome in these patients suggests a modification of the Bismuth method of classification.

Conclusion.—In patients unlikely to achieve long-term clinical success by surgical, radiologic, or endoscopic techniques alone, the combined approach described here may avoid major surgical reinterventions. Permanent radiologic access is established because of the risk of recurrent stricture or intrahepatic stone formation.

▶ The management of the high benign biliary fistula constitutes one of the

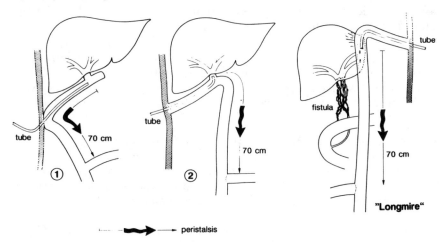

Fig 24–3.—Variations of the Roux-en-Y reconstruction allowing access for radiological intervention. (Courtesy of Schweizer WP, Matthews JB, Nudelmann LI, et al: *Br J Surg* 78:559–563, 1991.)

most demanding surgical exercises, and this large series reports a laudatory incidence of excellence and good results. Planning a surgical procedure that will facilitate subsequent radiologic dilatation is most appropriate. I've had personal success with dilatation of biliary strictures through a stomatized jejunal limb as described by Russel et al. (1).—S.I. Schwartz, M.D.

Reference

1. Russel E, et al: *Acta Radiol Diag* 26:283, 1985.

Long-Term Results of Choledochoduodenostomy in the Treatment of Choledocholithiasis: Assessment of 225 Cases

Parrilla P, Ramirez P, Sanchez Bueno F, Perez JM, Candel MF, Muelas MS, Robles R (Univ of Murcia, Spain)
Br J Surg 78:470–472, 1991   24–15

Patients.—Among 2,610 patients operated on for biliary stone disease from 1979 through 1988, 225 (8.6%) underwent choledochoduodenostomy. More than 60% of these patients had a preoperative diagnosis of choledocholithiasis. Thirty had previously undergone cholecystectomy.

Outcome.—Four percent of the patients had intra-abdominal complications after choledochoduodenostomy. Six had an intra-abdominal abscess and 3 had an external biliary fistula. One biliary fistula was fatal, and 3 patients died of pulmonary complications. The overall morbidity rate was 21%. Six of 8 patients with cholangitis and anastomotic stenosis were reoperated on. Other complications included bile gastritis and bile duct bezoar. About one fourth of the patients with colic had either asymptomatic stenosis or sump syndrome. More than two thirds of the patients were asymptomatic after a mean follow-up of 4½ years.

Discussion.—The basic indication for choledochoduodenostomy is a bile duct more than 12 mm in diameter. If marked stenosis is present postoperatively with consequent stone formation, surgery should be done to reconstruct the anastomosis. Endoscopic papillotomy is not very useful because bile stasis is related to the supra-anastomotic bile duct.

▶ Choledochoduodenostomy has stood the test of time as a procedure to deal with common duct stones within in a dilated common duct. The sump syndrome is actually an extreme rarity. Escudero-Fabre et al. (1) followed 71 patients subsequent to choledochoduodenostomy for 5–15 years. Cholangitis was observed in only 3 of them. The sump syndrome did not develop in any. Most authors have emphasized that choledochoduodenostomy should not be performed in a nondilated duct, and that the stoma itself should be at least 14 mm.—S.I. Schwartz, M.D.

Reference

1. Escudero-Fabre A, et al: *Ann Surg* 213:635. 1991.

Combined Portal Vein and Liver Resection for Carcinoma of the Biliary Tract

Nimura Y, Hayakawa N, Kamiya J, Maeda S, Kondo S, Yasui A, Shionoya S
(Nagoya Univ, Japan)
Br J Surg 78:727–731, 1991   24–16

Patients.—Surgical resection was possible in 170 of 216 patients seen from 1975 through 1989 with biliary tract carcinoma. Of 107 patients undergoing hepatectomy, 29 had combined portal vein and liver resection for advanced biliary tract carcinoma. Sixteen of these patients had cancer of the bile duct.

Management.—The superior mesenteric artery was clamped temporarily during segmental excision and end-to-end anastomosis of the portal vein. The anastomosis employed a continuous extraluminal over-and-over suture of 5-0 polypropylene with 2 guy stitches. Sixteen patients had segmental excision of the portal vein, and 13 underwent wedge resection of the vessel wall.

Results.—Operative mortality was 17%. Patients had an actuarial survival rate of 48% at 1 year, 29% at 3 years, and 6% at 5 years. Forty-six patients with unresectable cancer had a median survival of 3 months and a 1-year actuarial survival of 13%. None of these patients survived for 3 years. The difference in survival between the resected and comparison groups was significant. Ten patients with gallbladder carcinoma who survived the combined operative procedure had a median survival of 19 months.

Conclusion.—Combined portal vein and liver resection seems to be a reasonable operative approach to selected patients with advanced cancer of the biliary tract.

▶ The operations carried out represented technical feats and the reported operative mortality rate of 17% is reasonable. It is somewhat disappointing that the actuarial 5-year survival rate was only 6%. We appreciate that an occasional patient with carcinoma of the bile duct will survive for a long period of time. The Japanese have had a major role in extending surgery for carcinoma of the biliary tract and pancreas. Tashiro et al. (1) reported on tumor and vascular resection in 27 patients with biliary and pancreatic cancer. Portal vein resection was carried out in 23 patients; the mortality rate was 8%. Nine of 14 patients were alive after 2 years. This approach is recommended for patients with vascular involvement without lymph node metastases.—S.I. Schwartz, M.D.

Reference

1. Tashiro S, et al: *Surgery* 109:481, 1991

Role of Radiation After Operative Palliation in Cancer of the Proximal Bile Ducts

Grove MK, Hermann RE, Vogt DP, Broughan TA (Cleveland Clinic Found)
Am J Surg 161:454–458, 1991   24–17

Patients.—Surgery was done in 51 patients with histologically confirmed proximal blue duct cancers from 1977 through 1985. Thirty patients had lesions confined to the hilar region, and 21 had extensive infiltration of the liver or distant metastasis.

Management.—One patient had resection, and 6 had biopsy alone. The remaining 44 patients underwent transtumoral dilation and intubation. Thirty patients received adjunctive radiotherapy. Twenty-seven received external beam irradiation in a mean dose of 3,766 cGy, and 3 received less than 1,000 cGy.

Results.—Patients with metastatic disease had a mean survival of 6 months, which was not influenced by postoperative irradiation. In patients lacking metastatic or advanced local disease, radiotherapy significantly lengthened the mean survival from 4.5 months to 12 months. The median survival improved from 2 months to 12 months. The operative mortality was 14%.

Conclusion.—External beam radiotherapy appears to improve the survival time of patients given palliative surgical treatment for tumors of the proximal bile duct. More aggressive resection followed by external or intracavity irradiation might further improve the outlook.

▶ The pendulum continues to swing back and forth about the efficacy of radiation in patients undergoing palliative treatment of hilar tumors. Iwasaki et al. (1) indicated that the noncurative resection plus intraoperative radiation therapy, combined with postoperative external radiation therapy, appeared to improve the prognosis. By contrast, Molt et al. (2) demonstrated no change in long-term survival associated with radiation therapy. The advent of brachytherapy, which could be administered through the catheters, may provide a more effective method of managing these patients.—S.I. Schwartz, M.D.

References

1. Iwasaki Y, et al: *World J Surg* 12:91, 1988.
2. Molt P, et al: *Cancer* 57:536, 1986.

Cholangiocarcinoma Complicating Primary Sclerosing Cholangitis

Rosen CB, Nagorney DM, Wiesner RH, Coffey RJ Jr, LaRusso NF (Mayo Clinic and Found, Rochester, Minn)
Ann Surg 213:21–25, 1991   24–18

Introduction.—Cholangiocarcinoma may occur in association with primary sclerosing cholangitis (PSC). Data were reviewed on 30 patients seen during an 8-year period. Primary sclerosing cholangitis was diagnosed on the basis of its classic radiographic feature on cholangiography, elevation of the serum level of alkaline phosphatase to at least twice the upper limit of normal before the development of cholangiosarcoma, and findings on liver biopsy. The 19 men and 11 women had a mean age of 43 years and included 5 who were part of a trial of therapy with D-penicillamine. In addition, 70 patients with PSC were followed prospectively for an average of 30 months.

Results.—In the review series the mean time between the diagnoses of PSC and cholangiocarcinoma was 52 months; the interval was at least 2 years in 12 patients, and the diagnoses were synchronous in 9. Classic cholangiographic features were present in 26 patients, and 25 had inflammatory bowel disease. At the time of diagnosis of cholangiosarcoma, 23 of the 30 patients were alive. Jaundice, weight loss, and abdominal discomfort were the most common symptoms. Liver biopsy was done in 21 patients; 1 had stage I disease, 8 had stage II disease, 6 had stage III disease, and 6 had stage IV disease. These findings often precluded effective therapy; the overall median survival was 5 months (Fig 24-4). There were 6 intrahepatic and 18 extrahepatic cholangiocarcinomas, and 6 were of indeterminate origin. Among the 70 patients in the follow-up study, 12 died and 5 were found to have cholangiocarcinoma at autopsy.

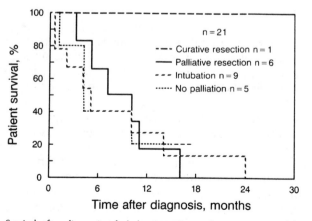

Fig 24–4.—Survival after diagnosis of cholangiocarcinoma by treatment modality. (Courtesy of Rosen CE, Nagorney DM, Wiesner RH, et al: *Ann Surg* 213:21–25, 1991.)

Conclusions.—Because cholangiocarcinoma may develop in PSC, liver transplantation may be considered earlier in the course of the disease. For patients with both conditions, however, the disease may recur after liver transplantation. More study is needed to determine whether PSC is a premalignant condition.

▶ It is accepted that orthotopic liver transplantation is the most effective treatment for patients with end-stage liver disease caused by sclerosing cholangitis (1). The present article suggests that the indications have to be extended, however, because of the potential for carcinoma. The differential diagnosis between sclerosing cholangitis per se and cholangiocarcinoma is essentially impossible short of histologic evaluation. The question can be asked whether the benign process evolves into a malignant one, whether the 2 coexist, or whether the initial diagnosis of sclerosing cholangitis was erroneous. Currently, the data suggest that primary sclerosing cholangitis rarely transforms into a malignant lesion. I am in agreement with the authors that this issue needs to be studied further. The cure rate for cholangiocarcinoma is so poor, and the survival rate is so short, that an alteration in therapeutic consideration is called for.—S.I. Schwartz, M.D.

Reference

1. Marsh JW Jr, et al: *Ann Surg* 207:21, 1988.

Surgical Management of 552 Carcinomas of the Extrahepatic Bile Ducts (Gallbladder and Periampullary Tumors Excluded): Results of the French Surgical Association Survey
Reding R, Buart J-L, Lebeau G, Launois B (Hôsp Pontchaillou; Ctr Hosp–Univ, Rennes, France)
Ann Surg 213:236–241, 1991   24–19

Introduction.—Data were reviewed on 552 patients with primary carcinoma of the extrahepatic bile duct to compare long-term survival rates of patients treated with palliative surgery with those undergoing resection. There were upper-third lesions in 307 patients, middle-third in 7, and lower-third bile duct carcinomas in 101; the remaining patients had diffuse lesions.

Methods.—Of the patients, 41 were operated on after failure of percutaneous or biliary drainage, whereas 511 had surgery as the initial therapeutic procedure. The resectability rates were 32% for upper-third, 47% for middle-third, 51% for lower third, and 6% for diffuse carcinomas. Hepatic resection was combined with tumor excision in 49 patients.

Results.—Resected patients were significantly younger than nonresected patients and had a lower incidence of chronic respiratory disease, cardiac insufficiency, and cirrhosis. The operative mortality rate of 26% increased significantly after exploratory or decompressive surgery

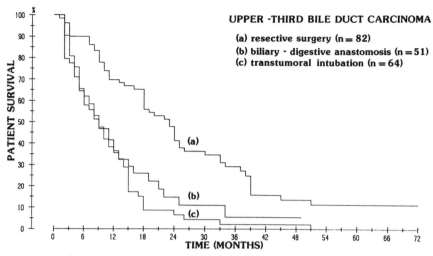

UPPER -THIRD BILE DUCT CARCINOMA

(a) resective surgery (n = 82)
(b) biliary - digestive anastomosis (n = 51)
(c) transtumoral intubation (n = 64)

Fig 24–5.—Survival curves (operative death excluded) in patients operated on for upper-third bile duct carcinoma according to the type of surgical management: *a*, resective surgery (n = 82); *b*, biliary-digestive anastomosis without resection (n = 51); *c*, transtumoral intubation (n = 64). Statistical significance: *a* vs. *b*: P < .001; *a* vs. *c*: P < .001; *b* vs. *c*: NS. (Courtesy of Reding R, Buard J-L, Lebeau G, et al: *Ann Surg* 213:236–241, 1991.)

than after tumor resection in upper-third tumors. In patients with diffuse carcinomas, operative mortality rates were 45% after exploratory surgery, 36% after transtumoral intubation, 25% after biliary digestive anastomosis, and 33% after resective surgery. The resectability rate for upper-third tumors was 51% from 1974 to 1987 compared with 10% before 1974. The operative mortality rate for proximal carcinomas was 16% with resection and 31% with palliative surgery. The overall 1-year survival after exclusion of operative deaths was 68% after tumor resection compared with 31% after palliative surgery (Fig 24–5). The long-term results correlated with local and regional extension of the disease.

Conclusion.—Resection of extrahepatic bile duct carcinomas is often associated with worthwhile long-term survival, particularly in an upper-third localization.

▶ The survival rates for patients with carcinoma of the biliary tract remain low, and long-term survival of 10% has been reported by most authors. Ouchi et al. (1) analyzed prognostic factors in 146 resections in patients with carcinoma of the biliary tract. They reported a 5-year survival of about 45% that is not in keeping with most series. They pointed out that papillary lesions should be considered separately because they have different biology. It would have been interesting for the French study to have indicated the percentage of papillary lesions in the group that survived beyond 5 years. The role of intraoperative or postoperative radiation in the treatment of bile duct cancer has not been defined, and both improvement and lack of improvement in the survival of those statistics has been reported.—S.I. Schwartz, M.D.

Reference

1. Ouchi K, et al: *Arch Surg* 124;248, 1989.

Radical Resection for Carcinoma of the Ampulla of Vater
Monson JRT, Donohue JH, McEntee GP, McIlrath DC, van Heerden JA, Shorter RG, Nagorney DM, Ilstrup DM (Mayo Clinic and Found, Rochester, Minn)
Arch Surg 126:353–357, 1991   24–20

Introduction.—Because of recent attention to the improved outcome of patients undergoing radical resection for pancreatic carcinoma, data were reviewed on 104 consecutive patients who underwent radical resection for ampullary cancer from 1965 to 1989.

Results.—Frequent clinical findings included jaundice in 67% of the patients, significant weight loss in 42%, and anemia in 27%. Radical subtotal pancreatectomy was performed in 87 patients (84%). The remaining 17 underwent total pancreatectomy. The postoperative mortality was 5.7%. There was intra-abdominal hemorrhage in 3 patients, infarction in 1, leaking pancreatojejunal anastomosis in 1, and pulmonary embolus in 1. Follow-up for the 98 surviving patients ranged from 8 months to 21.5 years. The median survival was 2.8 years, with a 1-year survival of 81%, a 3-year survival of 48%, a 5-year survival of 34%, and a 10-year survival of 25%. Twenty patients were alive more than 5 years after surgery and 13 were alive more than 10 years after surgery; 8 patients died of tumor re-

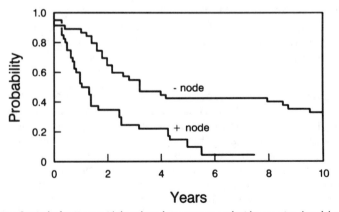

Fig 24–6.—Survival of patients with lymph node metastases and without regional nodal spread after radical resection for ampullary carcinoma. (Courtesy of Monson JRT, Donohue JH, McEntee GP, et al: *Arch Surg* 126:353–357, 1991.)

currence more than 5 years after resection. Patient gender, presence of jaundice, and weight loss had no significant influence on survival. Survival was significantly impaired by microscopic lymphatic invasion, regional nodal metastasis, tumor grade, and the epithelium of origin. Of 17 patients who had total pancreatectomy, 16 died, compared with 55 of the 87 who had radical subtotal pancreatectomy. The 5-year survival rate of those with documented lymph node metastases was 16%, compared with 43% for those without regional nodal metastases (Fig 24–6).

Conclusion.—Radical resection for ampullary cancer can be performed with low morbidity and mortality and should be the procedure of choice for ampullary carcinoma.

▶ This large series emphasizes that the lesion has the best prognosis among malignant tumors of the extrahepatic bile duct and pancreas. Doubtless this relates to the biology of the tumor. Chiappetta et al. (1) reviewed the experience with ampullectomy for excision of adenocarcinoma of the ampulla. The overall 5-year survival was 23%. The operative death rate associated with ampullectomy for carcinoma was 3%, as contrasted with 14% for pancreatoduodenectomy. The 5-year survival rate after ampullectomy was 23%, whereas that for 187 patients without node metastases who underwent pancreatoduodenectomy was 39%. It was therefore concluded that ampullectomy is probably best reserved for localizing fungating lesions in patients regarded as poor risks for pancreatoduodenectomy.—S.I. Schwartz, M.D.

Reference

1. Chiappetta A, et al: *Am Surg* 52:603, 1986.

25 The Pancreas

Differences of Pancreatic Stone Morphology and Content in Patients With Pancreatic Lithiasis

Mariani A, Bernard JP, Provansal-Cheylan M, Nitsche S, Sarles H (U 315 IN-SERM; CRMC 2 CNRS Campus de Luminy, Marseille, France)

Dig Dis Sci 36:1509–1516, 1991

25-1

Objective.—Differences between pancreatic stones were sought in 25 patients, 20 of whom had calcified stones, and 5, radiolucent stones. Most of the former patients were alcoholics, and 4 of the 5 with lucent stones were nonalcoholic women.

Findings.—The calcified stones ranged from compact, resistant structures to coralliform and brittle calculi. All stones in the same patient were identical. In coralliform stones, organic fibrils of varying size were

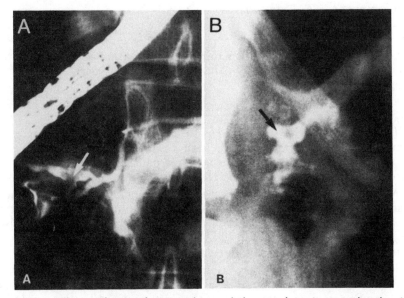

Fig 25–1.—Follow-up of a case of x-ray-translucent calculus. **A,** endoscopic retrograde catheterism of the pancreatic ducts in a nonalcoholic woman. A radiolucent pancreatic calculus is present in a dilated duct of Santorini (*arrow*). **B,** an x-ray film of the abdomen of the same patient after 7 years. Pancreatic calculi are visible. The biggest calculus corresponds to the radiolucent stone previously observed. It is now covered by a calcified shell (*arrow*). (Courtesy of Mariani A, Bernard JP, Provansal-Cheylan M, Nitsche S, et al: *Dig Dis Sci* 36:1509–1516, 1991.)

strongly attached to mineral crystals. A larger mass of stone correlated with a lower content of lithostathine (pancreatic stone protein). The lucent stones consisted of amorphous material solubilized at acidic pH, which corresponded to degraded forms of lithostathine. In 1 patient followed for 7 years, a radiolucent core developed that became wrapped secondarily in a calcified shell (Fig 25-1).

Interpretation.—Two distinct processes, which are not always associated in the same patient, lead to pancreatic stone formation. One is precipitation of calcium carbonate, an important feature of chronic alcoholic pancreatitis, and the other is precipitation of insoluble, degraded forms of lithostathine. The link between these processes remains to be established.

▶ One of the gurus of gallstone composition refers to himself as a biliary geologist. Perhaps Professor Sarles can establish that claim for the pancreas. I was not familiar with radiolucent ("transparent") pancreatic stones, but they made up 20% of this series and differed from calcified stones in that 4 of 5 patients with radiolucent stones were nonalcoholic. The translucent stones apparently are associated with some specific protein. We do not know anything about the differential prognosis of these 2 kinds of rocks. Is it a French phenomenon?—J.C. Thompson, M.D.

Acute Edematous Pancreatitis Impairs Pancreatic Secretion in Rats
Murayama KM, Drew JB, Nahrwold DL, Joehl RJ (VA Lakeside Med Ctr, Chicago; Northwestern Univ)
Surgery 107:302–310, 1990   25–2

Introduction.—The cause and pathophysiology of acute pancreatitis remain poorly understood and, as a result, treatment has remained mostly supportive. Little is known about pancreatic secretory function after the induction of experimental pancreatitis.

Methods.—To determine whether acute pancreatitis impairs pancreatic exocrine function, cholecystokinin (CCK)-stimulated pancreatic secretion was measured in conscious rats bearing gastric, duodenal, bile, and pancreatic fistulas before and after supramaximal intravenous administration of caerulein to induce acute pancreatitis.

Results.—Marked hyperamylasemia developed immediately after caerulein administration. Both basal and stimulated flow of pancreatic juice and protein secretion decreased significantly 24 hours after induction of pancreatitis, despite a return of the plasma amylase levels to baseline.

Conclusion.—These results suggest that exocrine pancreatic function is impaired in acute pancreatitis. In this model of pancreatitis, there is evidence that digestive enzymes localize within vacuoles containing lysosomal hydrolases, which can activate trypsinogen. The vacuoles discharge active enzymes preferentially into the pancreatic tissue, producing acute inflammation and hyperamylasemia.

▶ Gomez, in our lab, has shown that suppression of CCK release by stimulating feedback inhibition (by instillation of bile salts) can ameliorate pancreatitis in mice (1). Another mechanism for feedback suppression of CCK release is via intraduodenal trypsin. Interference with pancreatic enzyme secretion in edematous pancreatitis would diminish trypsin delivery to the duodenum and increase CCK release, which might further enhance development of pancreatitis, a sort of endogenous loop to worsen the pancreatitis. The other model for experimental pancreatitis in rats (produced by a choline-deficient, ethionine-supplemented diet) results in much greater destruction and would presumably cause even greater interference with pancreatic secretion. In both instances, CCK release could be greatly diminished by intraduodenal instillation of bile salts to allow a check on the putative role of CCK in ongoing pancreatitis.—J.C. Thompson, M.D.

Reference

1. Gomez G, et al: *J Clin Invest* 86:323, 1990.

Acute Necrotizing Pancreatitis: Management by Planned, Staged Pancreatic Necrosectomy/Débridement and Delayed Primary Wound Closure Over Drains
Sarr MG, Nagorney DM, Mucha P Jr, Farnell MB, Johnson CD (Mayo Clinic and Found, Rochester, Minn)
Br J Surg 78:576–581, 1991   25–3

Introduction.—Pancreatic débridement, or necrosectomy, has markedly improved survival over drainage alone in the management of severe, necrotizing pancreatitis. Present management has evolved from use of controlled open lesser sac drainage for pancreatic abscess to staged necrosectomy with delayed primary closure over drains whenever possible.

Patients and Methods.—The medical records and intravenous contrast-enhanced CT scans of 23 patients with acute necrotizing pancreatitis with parenchymal or peripancreatic necrosis were studied. Patients were classified by the Ranson and Imrie criteria and APACHE II scoring. Clinical staging was correlated statistically with postoperative morbidity.

Findings.—Findings of extraluminal gas on CT or culture-positive CT-guided needle aspirations of peripancreatic fluid collections were indications for operative intervention (Figs 25-2—25-4). The remaining patients were treated surgically because of a deteriorating clinical course. After the initial necrosectomy, the peripancreatic area was further débrided for several days. In 14 patients, closure after final necrosectomy was done in a delayed primary fashion with multiple Penrose or soft, closed suction drains. The wound was partially closed in another 4 pa-

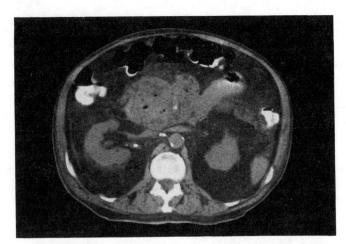

Fig 25–2.—Computed tomography showing extraluminal gas, diagnostic of pancreatic abscess. (Courtesy of Sarr MG, Nagorney DM, Mucha P Jr, et al: *Br J Surg* 78:576–581, 1991.)

tients and "marsupialized" in the remaining 5. Four of 23 patients died, and 12 of 23 patients had significant morbidity. However, only 1 patient experienced recurrent intra-abdominal abscess.

Conclusion.—Patients with acute necrotizing pancreatitis treated with staged necrosectomy and débridement with delayed primary closure over drains had significant long-term related morbidity and mortality of 17%. However, this closure method minimized the incidence of recurrent intra-abdominal abscess related to persistent necrosis and undrained fluid.

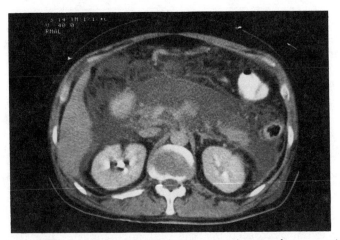

Fig 25–3.—Dynamic contrast-enhanced CT demonstrating patchy areas of no pancreatic enhancement in head and body of pancreas in a severely toxic patient with noninfected pancreatic necrosis. (Courtesy of Sarr MG, Nagorney DM, Mucha P Jr, et al: *Br J Surg* 78:576–581, 1991.)

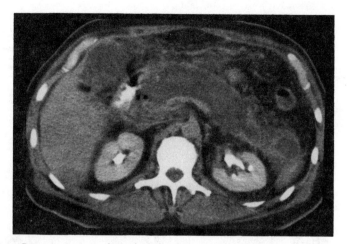

Fig 25–4.—Dynamic contrast-enhanced CT demonstrating lack of pancreatic parenchymal enhancement throughout entire gland. At operation, this patient had isolated necrosis of the entire pancreas. (Courtesy of Sarr MG, Nagorney DM, Mucha P Jr, et al: *Br J Surg* 78:576–581, 1991.)

▶ Patients with acute necrotizing pancreatitis die, usually with sepsis, and the focal point of the sepsis seems to be colonization of necrotic pancreatic and peripancreatic tissues by transmigratory colonic organisms. A careful staged program for open drainage and repeated removal of necrotic material should help, and the authors' overall mortality of 17% speaks well for this treatment in this group of highly threatened patients. In our experience, the morbidity rate in this group is nearly 100%. Once again, the central role of CT is clearly demonstrated in diagnosis, assessment of progress of the disease, and in planning for surgical intervention.—J.C. Thompson, M.D.

Total Pancreatectomy With Preservation of the Duodenum and Pylorus for Chronic Pancreatitis
Easter DW, Cuschieri A (Univ of Dundee, Scotland)
Ann Surg 214:575–580, 1991   25–4

Introduction.—Pancreatectomy can relieve the debilitating pain that often complicates severe chronic pancreatitis, but in turn it can lead to nutritional complications. Duodenum-preserving total pancreatectomy was performed in 8 patients who had severe, unrelenting pain requiring large opiate doses.

Technique.—The operation begins by detaching the greater omentum and exposing the pancreatic bed (Fig 25–5). Sharp dissection is used to create a plane between the duodenum and pancreas. A band of pancreatic tissue overlying the ampulla is fractured to enter the dissected plane on the lateral aspect of the bile duct. A similar technique is used for anterior separation. The pancreatic tail and

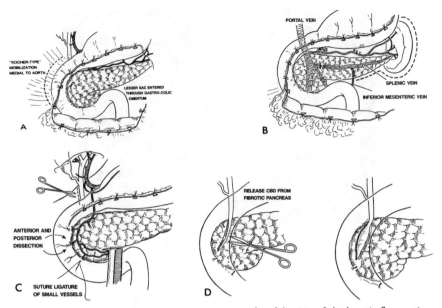

Fig 25–5.—A, detachment of the greater omentum and mobilization of the hepatic flexure gives access to the bed of the pancreas. The peritoneum well lateral to the duodenum is opened, and the duodenum, paraduodenal areolar tissue, and head of the pancreas are mobilized to the level of the aorta. **B,** the splenic artery is divided along the upper border of the pancreas distal to the origin of the common hepatic artery. The spleen and tail of the pancreas are lifted out of the retroperitoneum by dividing the leinorenal ligament. The inferior mesenteric vein is taken where encountered, and the splenic vein is taken at its junction with the portal vein. **C,** the branches of the right gastric artery to the duodenum are preserved, but the distal gastroduodenal artery (or pancreaticoduodenal) is divided at the surface of the pancreas. The intrapancreatic bile is liberated with scissors dissection. Small vessels at the pancreatic-duodenal interface are suture ligated when encountered. **D,** the distal common bile duct is freed from its intrapancreatic course anteriorly, meeting the prior dissection posterolaterally. Once liberated from the fibrotic pancreatic tissue, the common bile duct "balloons out". (Courtesy of Easter DW, Cuschieri A: *Ann Surg* 214:575–580, 1991.)

spleen are lifted from the retroperitoneum after dividing the splenic artery. The right gastric artery branches to the duodenum are preserved.

Results.—Six of the 8 patients had good relief of pain and an undoubted improvement in the quality of their lives. There were no problems with controlling diabetes, and no patient required treatment for hypoglycemic attacks. In 1 patient a colonic adenocarcinoma developed, and another had a bleeding duodenal ulcer after omitting H$_2$-blocker treatment.

Conclusions.—Total pancreatectomy can be done while preserving the duodenum and pylorus in patients with chronic pancreatitis. The risk of stenosis can be reduced by retaining a narrow rim of pancreas between the bile duct and duodenum. Antiulcer treatment is required indefinitely.

► This clearly is a technical tour de force. The problem, of course, is that the head of the pancreas and the descending duodenum share the same blood supply, and taking out the pancreas often injures that blood supply. The authors state that they totally removed the pancreas, but they do not tell us how they excise the small rim of tissue that lies to the right of the intrapancreatic portion of the distal common bile duct, shown in the last drawing in Fig 25–5. They had only 2 operative complications (1 bleeding, 1 duodenal perforation) in a patient, and the median operating time was between 3 and 3.5 hours.

We have been reluctant to subject patients with chronic pancreatitis to total pancreatectomy, because most of them are alcoholics and the combination of labile diabetes and alcoholism is a bad one. The authors state that they had no instances of postoperative hypoglycemia requiring attention. The late complications were duodenal stricture, 2 cases of bleeding, and 1 of cholangitis; 6 of the 8 patients reported good relief of pain, but 2 require constant medication. This looks like an interesting effort, and we look forward to a longer period of follow-up. The problem of how to deal with painful chronic pancreatitis in patients who do not have a dilated pancreatic duct remains unsolved.—J.C. Thompson, M.D.

Treatment of Pancreatic Pseudocysts With Octreotide
Gullo L, Barbara L (Univ of Bologna, Italy)
Lancet 338:540–541, 1991   25–5

Introduction.—Pancreatic pseudocysts complicating chronic pancreatitis often cause persistent pain. Because drainage procedures are invasive and not without risk, the effect of treatment with octreotide, a long-acting somatostatin analog that inhibits pancreatic secretion, was evaluated.

Study Design.—Seven consecutive patients with chronic pancreatitis and ultrasound evidence of pseudocyst received subcutaneous injections of octreotide, .1 mg 3 times daily for 2 weeks. One patient received a second course of treatment.

Results.—The mean diameter of the pseudocysts was 7.8 cm. Four patients had a rapid and marked reduction in pseudocyst size and complete reflief of pain. One of these patients had regrowth of the cyst and responded to a second course of octreotide therapy (Fig 25–6). There were no significant side effects.

Conclusions.—Octreotide-induced suppression of pancreatic secretion can aid the resolution of painful pseudocysts in some patients with chronic pancreatitis. The effect appears to last for some months at the least.

► We won't really be able to evaluate this proposed treatment until the patients have been followed for a year or more. Early resolution in 4 of 7 pa-

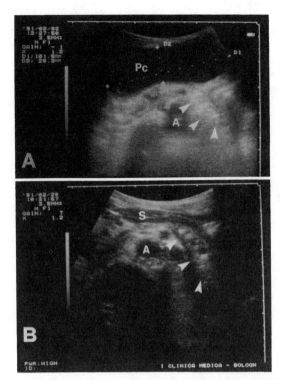

Fig 25–6.—*Abbreviations:* A, aorta; S, Stomach; Pc; pseudocyst. Abdominal ultrasonographs of a patient before and after a second course of treatment—transverse scans at the epigastrum. **A,** a large Pc is seen extending anteriorly from the pancreas (diameter, 10 cm). **B,** after 4 weeks of treatment with octreotide, the Pc is no longer seen. (Courtesy of Gullo L, Barbara L: *Lancet* 338:540–541, 1991.)

tients given the somatostatin analog is interesting, but we do not know what the recurrence rate is nor how long the involution of the pseudocyst will persist. It is of interest that the authors failed to mention the problem of pain at the site of injection, which led patients taking somatostatin for the dumping syndrome to cease taking the drug (see Abstract 20–7).—J.C. Thompson, M.D.

Invasive Treatment of Pancreatic Fluid Collections With Surgical and Nonsurgical Methods
Szentes MJ, Traverso LW, Kozarek RA, Freeny PC (Virginia Mason Med Ctr, Seattle)
Am J Surg 161:600–605, 1991   25–6

Introduction.—Pancreatic fluid collections such as pseudocysts, peripancreatic accumulations, and intrapancreatic collections develop in 2% to 18% of patients with pancreatitis.

Methods.—Data on 75 patients with a total of 107 pancreatic fluid collections were reviewed; those with phlegmon or necrosis at initial diagnosis were excluded. In 75 patients, 1 or more drainage procedures were performed.

Results.—Most of the 59 patients who were followed for a mean of 10 months after drainage were treated initially nonoperatively. Surgical drainage was performed in 34 patients. Morbidity rates were 20% to 25% for patients who had invasive nonsurgical drainage, those who had both invasive drainage and surgery, and those treated only by surgery. Rates of successful drainage exceeded 80% in all groups. Mortality was 8% in patients who had invasive nonsurgical drainage and 5% in those who had both forms of drainage. None of those who had surgery alone died.

Conclusion.—Nonoperative invasive methods represent an effective approach to treating pancreatic fluid collections, especially in patients whose fluid collections are unrelated to alcoholism or biliary tract disease and are symptomatic or persistent.

▶ The obvious problem here is patient selection. There is no question but that percutaneous drainage of pancreatic fluid collections may provide definitive solutions to difficult problems. Retrospective studies carry the obvious bias in that more difficult cases end up being treated by an operation. Even so, it was interesting that those patients who had surgery only had no deaths compared to 8% and 5% in the other series. The high rate of successful drainage in patients with percutaneous drainage alone means, in one sense at least, that the simplest problems were handled by this method. I do not know that it would be morally justified, but the only way to answer the question definitively is to do a prospective trial with randomization of the different means of treatment. I do not think that would be justified, because some patients are not truly candidates for one or the other modes of treatment. Simple problems, in general, can be handled simply, and more complex problems often require surgical intervention.—J.C. Thompson, M.D.

Pancreatic Regeneration After Partial Pancreatectomy
Parekh D, Townsend CM Jr, Rajaraman S, Ishizuka J, Thompson JC (Univ of Texas, Galveston)
Am J Surg 161:84–89, 1991   25–7

Introduction.—The pancreas has the capacity to grow and regenerate after acinar cell injury, but spontaneous regeneration of the remnant after partial pancreatectomy appears to be limited. The influence of trophic hormones on pancreatic regeneration is not well understood.

Methods.—Rats were used to study the effect of the trypsin inhibitor FOY-305, which stimulates endogenous cholecystokinin (CCK), on pancreatic regeneration after partial pancreatectomy. The animals received

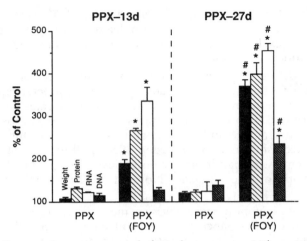

Fig 25–7.—Percentage increase over control of growth measurements in the pancreas after treatment with FOY-305 for 13 days or 27 days after pancreatectomy (n = 6 to 8). *Closed bars* indicate pancreatic weight; *cross-hatched bars*, protein content; *open bars*, RNA content; *stippled bars* DNA. (CON = duodenal and parabiliary segment in group 1 rats, control = 100%, * vs. pancreatectomy; # vs. pancreatectomy + FOY [13 days]) (Courtesy of Parekh D, Townsend CM Jr, Rajaraman S, et al: *Am J Surg 161:84–89, 1991.*)

FOY-305 or water only for 13 days or 27 days by gavage feeding after partial pancreatectomy or sham surgery.

Results.—Administration of FOY-305 significantly increased weight of the pancreatic remnant as well as its RNA and protein content. The DNA content was increased at 27 days. Augmentation of growth was greater at 27 days than in animals treated for 13 days (Fig 25–7). Only hypertrophy was evident at 13 days, whereas hyperplasia also was noted after prolonged treatment. Animals treated with FOY-305 had an increased number of secretory granules in the pancreatic acinar cells.

Conclusion.—Endogenous CCK stimulates pancreatic regeneration after partial removal of the organ. FOY-305 may prove useful in treating pancreatic insufficiency after either subtotal pancreatectomy or chronic pancreatitis.

▶ The ability of the liver to regenerate after partial hepatectomy is a wonder of the world; after unilateral nephrectomy, the opposite kidney enlarges by 50% to 60%. Little is known about pancreatic regeneration. This study indicates that endogenous CCK specifically stimulates the remaining pancreas to regenerate after partial resection. Actual hyperplasia takes some time to occur, as shown in Fig 25–7. At 13 days, the CCK releaser (FOY) has greatly stimulated cellular hypertrophy, as indicated by RNA, but has done little to increase the number of cells, as shown in the DNA level. Two weeks later, however, the striking increase in DNA indicates that new cells are forming. Stimulation of the endogenous release of CCK may be a practical clinical adjuvant either to resection or destruction by inflammation in patients with pancreatic insufficiency.—J.C. Thompson, M.D.

Glucose Metabolism After Pancreas Autotransplantation: The Effect of Open Duct Versus Urinary Bladder Drainage Technique

Barone GW, Flanagan TL, Cornett G, Pruett TL, Hanks JB (Univ of Virginia)
Ann Surg 213:159–165, 1991   25–8

Introduction.—Glucose metabolism and insulin secretion after pancreas transplantation may be influenced by the method used to drain the pancreatic duct. Altered glucose metabolism has been observed after pancreatic autotransplantation with intraperitoneal ductal drainage. An alternative technique, which is associated with reduced morbidity and mortality in clinical and animal models, is duct drainage into the urinary bladder.

Methods.—Glucose and insulin levels were estimated after oral glucose and stable hyperglycemic challenge in dogs undergoing pancreas autotransplantation with either intraperitoneal drainage (PAT), or with anastomosis of the urinary bladder to the pancreatic duct (PAT/B).

Results.—Animals in the PAT group had an increased integrated glucose response to oral glucose tolerance testing and a blunted insulin response to the hyperglycemic clamp. Those in the PAT/B group, in contrast, had a significantly reduced glucose response to oral glucose and an exaggerated insulin response to the hyperglycemic challenge, approximating normal control values. The amount of glucose metabolized during hyperglycemic challenge was depressed in both groups of animals.

Conclusions.—Draining the pancreatic duct into the urinary bladder at the time of pancreas autotransplantation "normalizes" peripheral insulin levels and improves the glucose response to an oral challenge. Nevertheless, graft recipients may remain insensitive to endogenous insulin.

▶ Hyperinsulinemia is common after pancreatic transplantation and is thought to be a result of drainage of the pancreatic vein into the systemic venous system. Why then does the intraperitoneally drained pancreas (the vein of which is anastomosed to the iliac) not show hyperinsulinemia? The study demonstrates clearly that in experimental pancreatic transplantation, as in clinical pancreatic transplantation, the use of the bladder for drainage of pancreatic juice appears to provide the best results. Even so, however, pancreatic transplantation in treatment for diabetes will not be highly efficacious until we solve the techniques that allow transplantation of isolated islet tissue alone. In whole organ or segmental organ grafts, 95% of the immunogenic transplanted pancreatic tissue is acinar; it is not only unnecessary, but it is highly dangerous. Pancreatitis with leakage of pancreatic juice is one of the great hazards of allotransplantation of the pancreas. Because pancreatic transplantation is designed to treat insulin insufficiency, we need to transplant beta cells, and the recent report of a few successful isolated islet transplantations in man are highly encouraging.—J.C. Thompson, M.D.

Glucagonoma Syndrome Is an Underdiagnosed Clinical Entity

Edney JA, Hofmann S, Thompson JS, Kessinger A (Univ of Nebraska)
Am J Surg 160:625–629, 1990   25–9

Introduction.—Glucagonomas are the rarest islet cell tumors. Despite a well-defined clinical syndrome characterized by necrolytic migratory erythema, diabetes mellitus, glossitis, anemia, and weight loss, the diagnosis of glucagonomas is often delayed. Data were reviewed on 7 patients treated for glucagonomas from 1974 to 1988.

Data Analysis.—All 7 patients had the classic cutaneous manifestation of glucagonoma syndrome consisting of a disseminated desquamating pruritic rash that had been present for 1–6 years before diagnosis (Fig

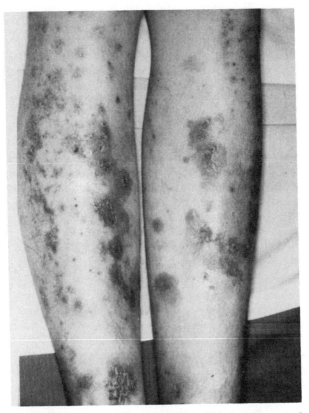

Fig 25–8.—The classic necrotic erythematous rash (NME) of the glucagonoma syndrome. (Courtesy of Edney JA, Hofmann S, Thompson JS, et al. *Am J Surg* 160:625–629, 1990.)

25–8). Stomatitis also was present in 5 patients and cheilitis in 3. Other symptoms included unexplained weight loss, intestinal ulceration, constipation, and amenorrhea. The mean serum glucagon level was 2,051 pg/mL (range, 435–5,000 pg/mL). There was no correlation between serum glucagon levels and the severity and duration of symptoms. All patients had abnormal glucose tolerance. There was extensive disease at the time of initial operation in 5 patients; 3 underwent aggressive cytoreductive surgery and the other 2 underwent biopsy only. Serum glucagon levels returned to normal after resection in 4 patients, but increased with recurrence of tumors in 2. The remaining 2 patients with small localized tumors underwent distal pancreatectomy and splenectomy and were free of disease at 2 years and 6 years postoperatively.

Conclusion.—Glucagonomas are not rare, as previously thought. Prompt recognition of this syndrome at a stage when surgical cure is feasible may increase survival. Partial pancreatectomy is recommended for patients with localized lesions, whereas aggressive cytoreductive surgery in patients with more extensive disease results in prolonged remission.

▶ There is undoubtedly a tendency to misdiagnose patients with rare diseases, and symptomatic pancreatic endocrinopathies are undeniably rare. Nonetheless, when you have only 7 patients, it is difficult to be sure that your own experience is typical, or atypical, because removal of only 4 patients would leave the authors presumably believing that they had seen their just share of a rare disease. Glucagonomas are rare. I once saw 4 patients with this syndrome in 1 day, but they represented, in all probability, nearly all of the glucagonoma patients in Holland. In 22 years, we have seen 2.

Only 2 of 7 patients were free of disease after operation. The authors suggest that patients with metastatic disease should undergo resection of as much tumor as possible, and I would certainly agree with that plan. So-called debulking operations are usually useless or meddlesome in patients with standard cancers, but patients with tumors that secrete active peptides often improve with reduction of the tumor mass. Our experience is that the necrolytic erythema migrans dermatitis is absolutely classic and is recognizable from photographs. The patients we have seen have been sent to us by dermatologists who recognize the disease from pictures. If you can find a patient with a localized tumor, you can take it out and the patient will be well. Otherwise, the patient will often live for an unusually long time with metastatic disease.—J.C. Thompson, M.D.

26 The Endocrine Glands

Natural History, Treatment, and Course of Papillary Thyroid Carcinoma
DeGroot LJ, Kaplan EL, McCormick M, Straus FH (Univ of Chicago)
J Clin Endocrinol Metab 71:414–424, 1990   26–1

Introduction.—A group of 269 patients with papillary thyroid carcinoma were followed for an average of 12 years after diagnosis. The basic treatment plan consisted of near-total thyroidectomy followed by low-dose radioiodine ablation of residual thyroid tissue that was performed 6–12 weeks postoperatively. If necessary, reablation was performed subsequently, and patients were monitored by whole body ^{131}I scanning.

Management.—Total or near-total thyroidectomy was performed in 66% of the patients; 12% underwent lobectomy or a more limited procedure. Neck dissection was performed at the time of thyroidectomy or within 6 months of diagnosis in 23% of the patients. Hypoparathyroidism developed in 6%.

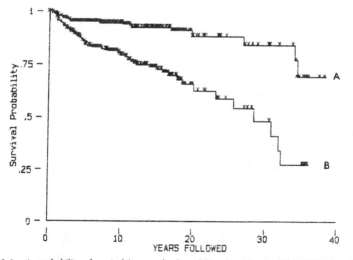

Fig 26–1.—**A**, probability of survival (cancer deaths only) analyzed by the Kaplan-Meier method, for the entire group of patients with papillary cancer. A small number of patients contribute to the observations beyond 30 years of follow-up. In all Kaplan-Meier plots, *the number or letter above the survival plot* indicates the last period of observation for each patient in the surviving group. **B**, probability of surviving without disease for the entire group of patients analyzed by the Kaplan-Meier method. (Courtesy of DeGroot LJ, Kaplan EL, McCormick M, et al: *J Clin Endocrinol Metab* 71:414–424, 1990.)

Course.—The overall mortality from cancer was 8% (Fig 26–1). The clinical class at diagnosis correlated closely with the outcome. Age at diagnosis also was an important variable. Less extensive surgery correlated significantly with an increased risk of recurrence, especially in patients whose tumors were larger than 1 cm. Mortality was especially high in patients older than 45 years who had class III or IV disease and a tumor larger than 2.5 cm.

Conclusion.—Patients with clinical class I or II disease (intrathyroidal disease and cervical node involvement) whose tumors are larger than 1 cm probably should undergo lobectomy with at least subtotal lobectomy contralaterally, followed by radioiodine ablation of residual thyroid disease. The best treatment for patients with smaller tumors remains uncertain.

▶ I am surprised that a major journal would publish another paper on the natural history of papillary cancer of the thyroid, but it does serve to remind us that this disease usually has a remarkably benign course, despite extrathyroidal spread when first seen in young people. The older the patient, the worse the prognosis. In fact, you can say that for thyroid cancer in general, regardless of the type. Young people do well, old people do badly. In tumors 1 cm or less in size, especially if they are located peripherally, we do a simple lobectomy. If they are greater than 1 cm or are located near the isthmus, we will do a total lobectomy on one side and a 95% dissection on the other. If the tumor is greater than 2 cm in size and near the isthmus, or if both sides are involved, we will do a total thyroidectomy. We do not routinely do a total thyroidectomy in all patients because the risk of the operation is greater than the risk of leaving behind an incidental tumor. A classic radical neck dissection is not indicated. If nodes are involved, these should be removed individually. Postoperative ablation of thyroid remnant tissue with ^{131}I seems indicated in patients with all but minimal disease.—J.C. Thompson, M.D.

Avoiding Reoperation for Indeterminate Thyroid Nodules Identified as Malignant After Surgery

Block MA, Dailey GE III, Muchmore D (Scripps Clinic Med Group Inc, La Jolla, Calif)
Arch Surg 126:598–602, 1991   26–2

Introduction.—Occasionally, a thyroid nodule that is indeterminate on needle biopsy and also on frozen section examination is found later to be malignant. If only lobectomy is performed, the question arises of whether to remove the remaining thyroid tissue to facilitate radioiodine therapy. One approach is to perform contralateral subtotal or near-total lobectomy when an indeterminate nodule is present. The remaining thyroid tissue can be ablated subsequently by radioiodine if desired.

Methods.—Data on 37 patients treated for indeterminate thyroid nodules from 1980 to 1989 were reviewed. All 37 had a cellular lesion that was indeterminate as carcinoma on fine-needle aspiration biopsy.

Results.—A malignant thyroid nodule was found in 11 patients; 2 others had an incidental occult papillary carcinoma in extranodular thyroid tissue. None of the patients required reoperation. Radioiodine therapy was administered to 3 patients postoperatively. In no patient did permanent hypoparathyroidism or recurrent laryngeal nerve damage develop.

Conclusion.—The occurrence of cancer in 30% of these patients with indeterminate thyroid nodules justifies more than unilateral lobectomy as the initial procedure. How much thyroid tissue can be ablated effectively by radioiodine is uncertain. It seems wise to administer thyroid hormone after subtotal thyroidectomy in these patients. Subtotal thyroidectomy, apart from avoiding reoperation, allows thorough evaluation and may preclude the later occurrence of nodules contralaterally.

▶ I am not sure that I agree with this admonition, but it does have justification. I would think that if the indeterminant nodule were located peripherally and less than 1 cm in size, a unilateral lobectomy would suffice. The problem is that these patients are told they have cancer, and the word so frightens them that they want to receive every possible treatment, including radioablation of the remaining thyroid tissue. The less thyroid tissue in the neck, the easier it is to accomplish radioablation. That is the basis for the authors' suggestion.—J.C. Thompson, M.D.

Combination Therapy for Anaplastic Giant Cell Thyroid Carcinoma

Schlumberger M, Parmentier C, Delisle M-J, Couette J-E, Droz J-P, Sarrazin D (Institut Gustave-Roussy, Villejuif; Institut Jean Godinot, Reims; Ctr François Baclesse, Caen, France)
Cancer 67:564–566, 1991   26–3

Introduction.—Anaplastic giant cell carcinoma of the thyroid gland is one of the most important malignant tumors that occurs in man. Most deaths have resulted from local tumor invasion. Only exceptional patients have lived longer than a year. Data were reviewed on 20 patients treated prospectively by both chemotherapy and external radiotherapy since 1981.

Methods.—Doxorubicin, 60 mg/m², and cisplatin, 90 mg/m², were administered to 12 patients aged 65 years or younger at 4-week intervals; also, 17.5 Gy of external photon-beam therapy was given. Mitoxanthone, 14 mg/m², was administered to 8 older patients every 4 weeks combined with the same radiotherapy.

Results.—There was a complete response of neck tumors in 5 patients, 4 of whom had previous surgery. Distant metastases did not respond and caused 14 deaths. Only 3 patients lived longer than 20 months. Severe treatment-related toxicity occurred in 12 patients; 3 had cardiotoxic effects.

Conclusion.—These combined treatment regimens have yielded results similar to those achieved with other protocols. Toxicity remains the chief factor limiting treatment of anaplastic giant cell thyroid carcinoma. Gross removal of tumor from the neck is indicated whenever possible, but it should not delay chemotherapy and radiotherapy. A trial combining chemotherapy with hyperfractionated external radiotherapy is in progress.

▶ I disagree almost completely with the recommendations for thyroidectomy in these patients. Recurrence is rapid, and you can almost watch the tumor grow. Early invasion of the trachea is common, and the wound often becomes a suppurating stinking mass with malignant tissue growing out of it. There is no good way to handle this lesion, and everyone should acknowledge that point. We tell our residents that someday they will be called to the Emergency Room to see a patient in advanced respiratory distress with a huge mass in the neck, and there will be someone there urging an emergent tracheostomy. Tracheostomy should be avoided as there are often 5–8 cm of highly vascular tumor tissue between the skin and the trachea, and many patients have exsanguinated in attempts at tracheotomy. The patient should undergo endotracheal intubation and radiotherapy should be instituted immediately in an attempt to shrink the tumor so the patient can breathe. Nothing seems to interfere with the progress of this disease, so that it appears correct to cause the patient as little trouble as possible. Operative interventions are frequently disastrous and never help, in my experience.—J.C. Thompson, M.D.

A Current Analysis of Primary Lymphoma of the Thyroid
Skarsgard ED, Connors JM, Robins RE (Univ of British Columbia)
Arch Surg 126:1199–1204, 1991   26–4

Introduction.—Primary thyroidal lymphoma comprises about 5% of all thyroid malignancies. Data were reviewed on 27 patients seen in a 9-year period with lymphoma confined to the thyroid or related nodes.

Clinical Features.—The 24 women and 3 men had a median age of 67 years; all but 4 patients were older than age 50. Nearly all patients had a nontender, rapidly enlarging thyroid mass. Symptoms were present for a median of 8 weeks before patients were seen. Half of the patients had dysphagia and 6 others had stridor. The median size of the presenting mass was 8 cm. In most cases the diagnosis was established by incisional or excisional biopsy of the thyroid or cervical nodes. Six patients had a high-grade lymphoma.

Treatment and Outcome.—Patients with smaller tumors received a brief course of multidrug chemotherapy, followed by involved-field radiotherapy. Those with larger tumors had more intense or prolonged chemotherapy and received irradiation only if disease persisted. Half of the patients had complications of treatment. The projected survival at 5 years was 70%, and disease-free survival was 70% after a median follow-up of 4 years. All patients with disease limited by the thyroid capsule survived. Favorable prognostic factors included the absence of dysphagia, a tumor mass less than 10 cm in diameter, and a lack of mediastinal node disease.

Recommendations.—Multidrug chemotherapy and irradiation now are the chief measures for thyroid lymphoma. Selected patients may undergo surgery if tumor can be resected without jeopardizing the recurrent nerves or parathyroid glands.

▶ There must be an epidemic of thyroid lymphoma in British Columbia! Twenty-seven patients in 9 years comes out to 3 patients per year in a plain old university hospital, not a world-famous center for thyroid treatment. The authors' recommended treatment of chemotherapy and irradiation instead of surgery led to a 5-year actuarial survival of 70%. I believe that thyroidectomy plus postoperative chemotherapy and irradiation would do better than that. The possibility of cure is so high in localized lymphomas that every effort should be made to maximize the chances of cure.—J.C. Thompson, M.D.

Total Parathyroidectomy Alone or With Autograft for Renal Hyperparathyroidism?
Higgins RM, Richardson AJ, Ratcliffe PJ, Woods CG, Oliver DO, Morris PJ (Univ of Oxford; Nuffield Orthopaedic Hosp, Oxford, England)
Q J Med 79:323–332, 1991   26–5

Introduction.—From 5% to 10% of patients with renal hyperparathyroidism and end-stage renal failure require removal of the parathyroid glands. The results of parathyroidectomy were reviewed in 76 patients who underwent neck exploration for renal hyperparathyroidism between 1977 and 1990. Thirteen patients had the surgery after renal transplantation. The patients had a total of 80 operations.

Outcome.—Ten patients had subtotal parathyroidectomy, whereas 49 had total removal and implantation of part of 1 gland as an autograft. Nine other patients had total parathyroidectomy without autografting; in 8 of these only 3 glands were found. Patients who remained on dialysis after total parathyroidectomy with autografting were at high risk of recurrent hyperparathyroidism. Nearly one third of the patients required partial removal of the autograft. Recurrences were rare in renal transplant recipients whose renal function was good, regardless of the type of surgery. Increased parathormone was infrequent when the creatinine clearance exceeded 40 mL/min (Fig 26–2). Bone disease improved after total parathyroidectomy without autografting in patients on dialysis. Cryopreserved parathyroid tissue functioned in 2 of 3 patients.

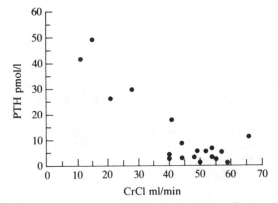

Fig 26–2.—The relationship between the PTH level and creatinine clearance in patients who received renal transplants. The minimum follow-up after transplantation is 1 year. Ten patients underwent parathyroidectomy after transplantation, 9 before. The operations performed were subtotal parathyroidectomy (5), total parathyroidectomy with an autograft (11), exploration in which only 3 glands were found and removed (3). (Courtesy of Higgins RM, Richardson AJ, Ratcliffe PJ, et al: *Q J Med* 79:323–332, 1991.)

Conclusion.—Total parathyroidectomy with autografting is appropriate after successful renal transplantation and in dialysis patients who are likely to receive a renal transplant. Those not likely to have transplantation may be best served by total parathyroidectomy without autografting.

▶ The message here is that unless the renal insufficiency is controlled, forearm grafting of the parathyroid is apt to be unnecessary and may even require later removal. The world experience with parathyroidectomy in patients with renal hyperparathyroidism is that there are no substantial differences in the short-term outcome of either total parathyroidectomy with a forearm implant as compared with ordinary subtotal parathyroidectomy (3 to 3.5 glands removed). Only if you could be sure of excellent renal function after a successful kidney transplantation would total parathyroidectomy with forearm implantation appear justified in these patients with secondary hyperparathyroidism.—J.C. Thompson, M.D.

The Role of Adrenalectomy in Cushing's Syndrome
Sarkar R, Thompson NW, McLeod MK (Univ of Michigan)
Surgery 108:1079–1084, 1990   26–6

Introduction.—Adrenalectomy continues to have an important role in the treatment of Cushing's syndrome. It is the preferred treatment for adrenal adenoma, adrenocortical carcinoma, and primary adrenocortical hyperplasia. In addition, bilateral adrenalectomy is used in selected patients with Cushing's disease or ectopic adrenocorticotropic hormone (ACTH) syndrome.

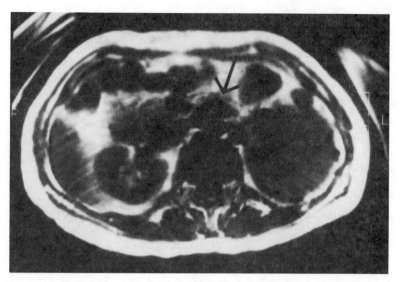

Fig 26–3.—An MRI scintiscan in a 72-year-old-woman with a 13-cm left adrenal tumor shows intra-vascular extension of the tumor into the adrenal gland and left renal vein. The *arrow* points to the in-travascular tumor thrombus in the left renal vein as it crosses the aorta. Magnetic resonance imaging is now the preferred study for demonstrating vascular involvement (intravascular extension) in adrenocor-tical carcinoma. (Courtesy of Sarkar R, Thompson NW, McLeod MK: *Surgery* 108:1079–1084, 1990.)

Methods.—From 1975 to 1989, 44 patients with clinical or biochemical evidence of Cushing's syndrome underwent adrenalectomy. In 20 patients there were adrenal adenomas, 13 in association with symptomatic Cushing's syndrome; 12 others had a diagnosis of Cushing's disease. There was adrenal hyperplasia in 6 patients, adrenocortical cancer in 4, and ectopic ACTH-producing neoplasms in 2. The patients with adrenocortical carcinomas (Fig 26–3) had florid Cushing's syndrome for less than a year.

Results.—All but 1 of the patients with adrenal adenoma underwent unilateral adrenalectomy; those with Cushing's disease had bilateral operations. There was 1 postoperative death; 3 patients had complications. There was complete remission of disease in 41 patients, and 39 were free of recurrent Cushing's disease on long-term follow-up.

▶ In a review by Brunicardi et al. (1) in this section in 1987, I commented on the multiple therapeutic approaches to Cushing's disease that those authors had suggested might be an institution-specific phenomenon. That is, some approaches appear to work well in some institutions, and other approaches in other institutions. It is clear that in Michigan, adrenalectomy is the treatment of choice, and the authors state that it provides prompt relief from the morbidity of the syndrome regardless of the cause. Despite many attempts to treat Cushing's syndrome with transsphenoidal hypophysectomy, adrenalectomy remains a common treatment. Adrenalectomy should be bilateral unless a truly functioning adrenal tumor can be localized to one side. The authors report complete remission in 41 of 44 patients. Of these, all but 2 were without recurrence on long-term follow-up.—J.C. Thompson, M.D.

Reference

1. Brunicardi FC, et al: *Surgery* 98:1127, 1985.

Efficient Management of Adrenal Tumors
Schwarz RJ, Schmidt N (Univ of British Columbia)
Am J Surg 161:576–579, 1991   26–7

Background.—Three hormonally mediated syndromes resulting from adrenal tumors are hypertensive virilizing, and Cushing's syndrome. Computed tomography, MRI, and scintigraphic techniques have improved the accuracy of preoperative diagnosis and localization of adrenal neoplasms.

Methods.—Data were reviewed on 121 patients with primary adrenal tumors operated on during a 20-year period. All aspects of the investigative process were examined to identify discriminating factors among the various diagnoses to minimize the time and cost of the process. Primary adrenal tumors included 57 cortical adenomas, 35 pheochromocytomas, 15 carcinomas, 8 cases of cortical hyperplasia, and 6 miscellaneous tumors. The mean time from onset of symtoms to diagnosis in patients seen with an identifiable syndrome was 48.3 months.

Findings.—Computed tomography was the most sensitive localizing technique with a sensitivity of 98%. The diagnostic sensitivity of other

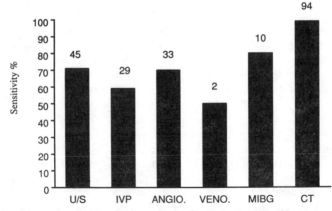

Fig 26–4.—Diagnostic sensitivity of radiographic localization techniques. *Abbreviations: U/S*, ultrasound; *IVP*, intravenous pyelogram; *ANGIO*, angiography; *VENO*, venography; *MIBG*, meta-iodobenzyl-guanidine; *CT*, computed tomography. (Courtesy of Schwarz RJ, Schmidt N: *Am J Surg* 161:576–579, 1991.)

techniques was 80% for metaiodobenzylguanidine, 71% for ultrasound, 70% for angiography, 59% for intravenous pyelography, and 50% for venography (Fig 26–4). A flank approach in surgery resulted in a shorter postoperative stay compared with an anterior approach.

Conclusion.—Computed tomography was the most sensitive localizing investigation for all categories of adrenal pathology. Supplementing CT with meta-iodobenzylguanidine scanning may be helpful in selected cases. Observation of asymptomatic nonfunctioning adrenal tumors less than 4 cm in diameter is recommended. Postoperative hospital stay and complication rates are not strongly influenced by the operative approach.

▶ It is probably not very helpful to lump all adrenal pathology together because the various conditions differ so much in their epidemiology, difficulty of diagnosis, severity of symptomatology, metabolic aberrations, difficulty of planning and executing therapy, and prognosis. Because the authors of this study operate on patients with adrenal tumors, they put them all together and wrote a paper about it. Their recommendations for simplified treatment appear worthwhile, namely, to observe (i.e., not operate on) adrenal tumors less than 4 cm in size found on incidental CT scanning; the diagnostic study of choice is enhanced CT (which they found to have a falsely negative rate of only 2%). They recommend an operative approach through the flank because it leads to a shorter postoperative stay.—J.C. Thompson, M.D.

Case Report: Unusual Appearance of a Giant Adrenal Pseudocyst
Lee SH, Goodacre BW, Scudamore CH (Univ of British Columbia)
Clin Radiol 43:349–351, 1991   26–8

Background.—Pseudocysts are uncommon and account for only 39% of adrenal cysts. Adrenal pseudocysts can grow to 20 cm in maximum diameter with a curvilinear calcification around the periphery. One patient's pseudocyst was observed for 4 years because of her reluctance to undergo surgery. The appearance of the giant adrenal pseudocyst on plain radiographic and CT images suggested the diagnosis of an hydatid cyst because of the distribution of calcification within the lesion.

Case Report.—Woman, 64, complained of right-sided abdominal pain and swelling. Radiography and CT revealed a large right upper quadrant mass with multiple areas of amorphous punctate calcification, irregular mural nodules, and a calcified daughter cyst. Hydatid disease of the liver was diagnosed. The patient was lost to follow-up until 4 years later when she was seen again with right-sided abdominal pain. The patient appeared healthy, but the mass had tripled its volume and free fluid was present beneath the right hemidiaphragm. The mass was excised because of concern over impending rupture. The mass weighed 3,496 g and measured 22 × 18 × 16 cm. The pseudocapsule had an organized fibrin wall with no epithelial or endothelial lining. There was no evidence of hydatid disease or malignancy.

Discussion.—On CT, the mass appeared to lie within the liver, and the multiple, amorphous irregular calcifications suggested a diagnosis of hydatid cyst or adrenal tumor. At surgical excision, the mass was found to arise from the right adrenal gland, and a diagnosis of hemorrhagic adrenal pseudocyst was made. This appears to be the first case report of an adrenal pseudocyst with this pattern of calicification observed on plain abdominal radiography and CT.

▶ This is presented as a gee-whiz case to be included in the general Clinical/ Pathologic Conference category of what is round, weighs 8 kilos, and hangs from the navel? In this instance, it was an adrenal cyst of unknown etiology. I just couldn't resist the CT (see the full-length article).—J.C. Thompson, M.D.

Surgical Pathology of Gastrinoma: Site, Size, Multicentricity, Association With Multiple Endocrine Nepolasia Type 1, and Malignancy
Donow C, Pipeleers-Marichal M, Schröder S, Stamm B, Heitz PU, Klöppel G (Free Univ of Brussels; Univ of Hamburg; Univ of Zurich)
Cancer 68:1329–1334, 1991   26–9

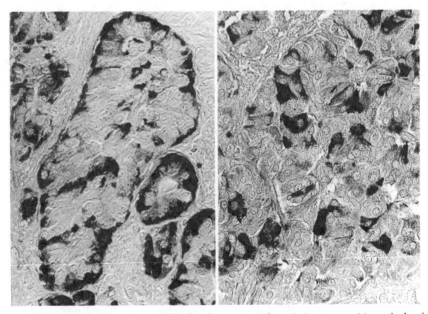

Fig 26–5.—Duodenal gastrinoma with trabecular pattern and gastrin immunoreactivity at the basal pole of the cells (magnification, ×600) **(left)**. Pancreatic gastrinoma with mixed solid-trabecular pattern and uneven gastrin immunoreactivity (magnification, ×600) **(right)**. (Courtesy of Donow C, Pipeleers-Marichal M, Schröder S, et al: *Cancer* 68:1329–1334, 1991.)

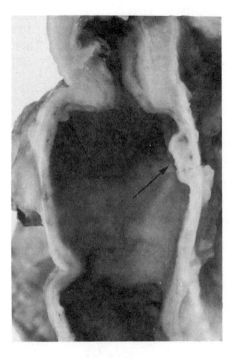

Fig 26–6.—Minute duodenal gastrinomas (*arrows*) in a patient with ZES and MEN-1. (Courtesy of Dorow C, Pipeleers-Marichal M, Schröder S, et al: *Cancer* 68:1329–1334, 1991.)

Introduction.—Pancreatic and duodenal specimens from 26 patients with sporadic Zollinger-Ellison syndrome (ZES) were examined for the presence of gastrinoma. Eighteen patients with multiple endocrine neoplasia type 1 (MEN-1), 17 of whom had ZES, also were studied immunocytochemically.

Findings.—Gastrin-positive tumors (Fig 26–5) were found in 38 patients. Nine of the 18 patients with MEN-1 had duodenal gastrinomas, 1 had a pancreatic tumor, and 2 had periduodenal lymph node lesions. Most duodenal gastrinomas were multiple (Fig 26–6). All patients with sporadic ZES had a solitary gastrinoma, 14 in the pancreas and 10 in the duodenum. Two of these patients had only periduodenal nodal lesions. Eighteen sporadic gastrinomas were malignant, as were 8 lesions in patients with ZES and MEN-1.

Conclusions.—Gastrinomas associated with the MEN-1 syndrome tend to occur in the duodenum and to be multicentric. Solitary gastrinomas are seen mainly in sporadic ZES, in either the pancreas or duodenum.

▶ Most recent studies have suggested that duodenal involvement is extremely common in patients who have ZES with both sporadic and MEN-1 disease. There is absolutely no question but that gastrinomas in the MEN-1 syndrome are multicentric. It seems impossible to render one of those patients eugastrinemic; however, they all so seem to live for years and years with their multicentric tumors. It does appear wise at operation always to study the duodenum carefully, either by endoscopy or by opening the duodenum, because the number of small intramural gastrinomas is high and they are often multiple, even in the sporadic form of the disease.—J.C. Thompson, M.D.

Subject Index

A

Abdomen
  abscess formation after liver resection, 376
  intra-abdominal (see Intra-abdominal)
  trauma
    aminoglycoside combinations vs. beta-lactams in, 64
    peritoneal lavage enzyme after, 160
Abscess
  intraabdominal, after liver resection, 376
Achalasia
  cardiomyotomy for, laparoscopic, 319
Acidosis
  lactic, bicarbonate in, 7
Acquired immunodeficiency syndrome (see AIDS)
Acute phase response
  in cancer and interleukin-6, 143
Adenocarcinoma
  colorectal under 40, 361
  esophagus, and Barrett's esophagus, 321
  gastroesophageal junction, and Barrett's esophagus, 321
Adenomatous
  colorectal polyps, cholecystectomy as risk for, 360
Adhesion
  molecule ELAM-1 and memory T cells, 110
Adrenal
  pseudocyst, giant, 449
  tumors, efficient management, 448
Adrenalectomy
  in Cushing's syndrome, 446
AIDS
  surgery in, indications and outcomes, 1
  surgical disease in, case review, 3
  (See also HIV)
Airway
  management in surgical critical care, early tracheostomy for, 197
Alcoholic
  beverage consumption in colorectal cancer and polyps, 360
Allografts
  burn, and donor-specific tolerance, 97
Alveolar
  macrophage chemotaxis in burns with smoke inhalation, 93
Aminoglycoside
  combinations in abdominal trauma, 64
Ampulla of Vater
  carcinoma, radical resection, 424
Amputation
  stump, below-knee, microvascular free flap to salvage, 312

Analgesia
patient-controlled
    in burns in children, 96
    in head and neck surgery, 193
Anaplastic
  thyroid carcinoma, combination therapy, 443
Anastomosis
  intestinal, in Crohn's disease, 348
Aneurysm
  aortic, abdominal
    natural history, 295
    repair, with myocardial revascularization, 251
    surgery, case review, 296
  Marfan, of aorta, graft for, 280
  popliteal artery, surgery results, 306
Angiogenesis
  fumagillin analogues inhibiting, 156
  induction in irradiated tissue, and oxygen dose, 68
  tumor, in breast carcinoma, 156
Angiogenic
  peptides in islet transplant in diabetes (in rat), 128
Angioplasty
  coronary, failed, coronary artery bypass in, 249
  in renal artery stenosis, atherosclerotic, 311
Annulus
  aortic, myth of, 216
Anti-B-cell monoclonal antibodies
  in marrow and organ transplant, 133
Anti-idiotypic antibodies
  immunomodulating kidney and heart transplants, 122
  monoclonal (see Monoclonal antibody, anti-idiotypic)
Anti-tumor necrosis factor
  monoclonal antibodies, Kupffer cell and MHC class II antigens, 17
Antibiotics
  artificial skin for sustained release, 163
  combination of topical and systemic, 85
  prophylactic , in Clostridium difficile disease, 87
Antibody(ies)
  anti-idiotypic, immunomodulating kidney and heart transplants, 122
  monoclonal (see Monoclonal antibody)
  yttrium-90 anti-tac, in xenograft transplant (in primate), 112
Anticoagulation
  in thromboembolic complications of advanced cancer, 314
Antigen
  blood-group, A, in lung cancer, 157

K

Kidney
cell subpopulations, lymphoproliferative
responses against (in dog), 121
hyperparathyroidism, total
parathyroidectomy in with
autograft, 445
transplant (*see* Transplantation, kidney)
trauma, preliminary vascular control for,
59
tubular epithelial cells, cytokine
regulation of ICAM-1 expression
on, 120
(*See also* Renal)
Kupffer cell
antigen, anti-TNF monoclonal
antibodies preventing hemorrhagic
suppression, 17

L

Laparoscopy
in cardiomyotomy for achalasia, 319
in cholecystectomy (*see*
Cholecystectomy, laparoscopic)
Larynx
preservation in glossectomy, 187
Lavage
peritoneal, enzyme after abdominal
trauma, 48
Leiomyosarcoma
of vena cava, inferior, 316
Leukocyte
adhesion molecule-1, endothelial, in
colon carcinoma, 158
endothelial adhesion molecules in heart
transplant, 125
scan with ^{111}In-oxyquinoline, 88
Leukocytosis
tumor necrosis factor in, 139
Leukotriene
receptor blockade reducing bile acid
gastric mucosal injury, 325
Limbs (*see* Extremities)
Lipid
peroxides and antioxidants in septic
shock, 20
Lithiasis
pancreatic, pancreatic stone in, 427
Liver, xxxv
cancer incompletely resected in
children, chemotherapy in, 381
carcinoma, hepatocellular (*see*
Hepatocellular carcinoma)
cell subpopulations, lymphoproliferative
responses against (in dog), 121

in conduit for biliary atresia, 403
hemangioma, management results, 374
hydatidosis, surgery results, 376
injury, parenchymal, total mesh
wrapping in, 57
metastases from colorectal cancer,
resection in, 383
protein synthesis in cancer and
interleukin-6, 143
resection
in biliary tract carcinoma with portal
vein resection, 419
intraabdominal abscess after, 376
limited, in cirrhosis with carcinoma,
377
in liver metastases from colorectal
cancer, 383
vs. transplant in hepatocellular
carcinoma, 379
steatosis, polymyxin B in, during
parenteral nutrition (in rat), 10
surgery, cytoreductive, from
neuroendocrine tumors, 384
wounds, fibrin glue in, fatal reaction to,
373
Lung
cancer
limited small-cell, surgery of, 207
non-small-cell, blood-group antigen A
in, 157
carcinoma, care pattern national survey,
203
compliance, static, and ibuprofen in
septic lung injury (in pig), 28
injury, septic, ibuprofen in (in pig), 28
permeability, microvascular, after smoke
inhalation, 54
(*See also* Pulmonary)
Lymphatics, xxxi
Lymphoblastoid
cell tumorigenicity and interleukin-6 (in
mice), 144
Lymphocyte
phytohemagglutinin-stimulated,
interleukin 1 receptor expression
and, 108
responses, antidonor cytotoxic, in
transfusions, 104
tumor-infiltrating, 142
T Lymphocyte
hyporesponsiveness, cytotoxic, after
kidney transplant, 116
Lymphoid
tissue, replacement in small bowel
transplant, 131
Lymphokine
release and OKT3 F(AB)$_2$ fragments,
109

Author Index